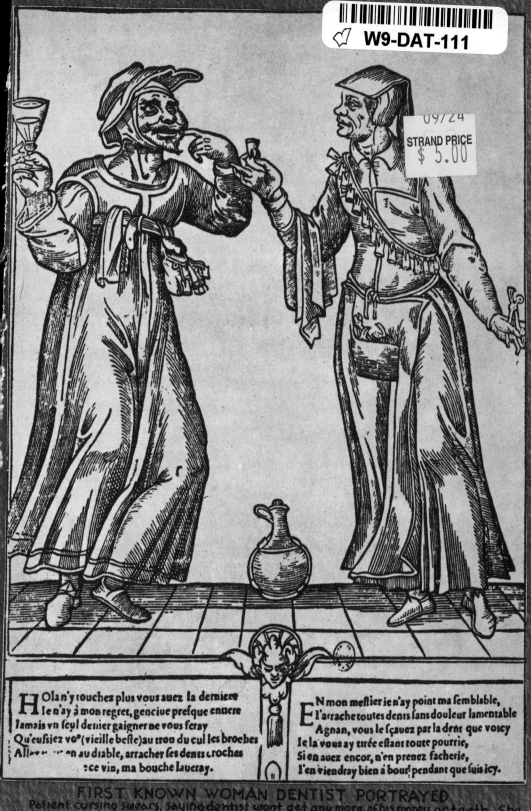

W9-DAT-111

09/24
STRAND PRICE
$ 5.00

HOla n'y touchez plus vous auez la derniere
Ie n'ay à mon regret, genciue presque entiere
Iamais vn seul denier gaigner ne vous seray
Qu'eussiez vo°(vieille beste)au trou du cul les broches
Alle... ...en au diable, arracher ses dents croches
:ce vin, ma bouche laueray.

EN mon mestier ie n'ay point ma semblable,
E l'arrache toutes dents sans douleur lamentable
Agnan, vous le sçauez par la dent que voicy
Ie la vous ay tirée estant toute pourrie,
Si en auez encor, n'en prenez facherie,
I'en viendray bien à bout pendant que suis icy.

FIRST KNOWN WOMAN DENTIST PORTRAYED
Patient cursing swears, saying dentist wont get any more of his money or teeth. She
wearing an extracted teeth necklace as sign of her profession, pleads for permission to pull
more. She promises to be painless. — An old French medieval woodcut.

TEETH TEETH TEETH

35⁰⁰

THE INCREDIBLE WORLD OF TEETH

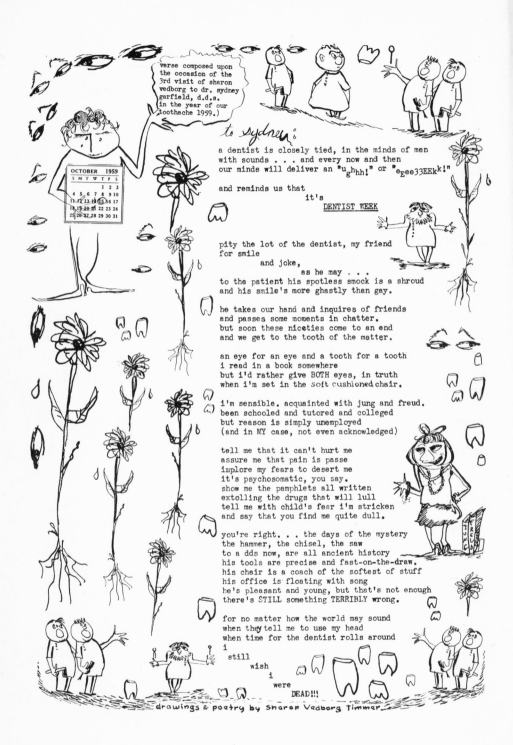

verse composed upon
the occasion of the
3rd visit of sharon
vedborg to dr. sydney
garfield, d.d.s.
in the year of our
toothache 1959.)

OCTOBER 1959
S M T W T F S
1 2 3
4 5 6 7 8 9 10
11 12 13 14 15 16 17
18 19 20 21 22 23 24
25 26 27 28 29 30 31

to sydney:

a dentist is closely tied, in the minds of men
with sounds . . . and every now and then
our minds will deliver an "u$_g$h$_{hh}$!" or "e$_{gg}$ee33EEk^k!"

and reminds us that
it's
DENTIST WEEK

pity the lot of the dentist, my friend
for smile
        and joke,
                as he may . . .
to the patient his spotless smock is a shroud
and his smile's more ghastly than gay.

he takes our hand and inquires of friends
and passes some moments in chatter.
but soon these niceties come to an end
and we get to the tooth of the matter.

an eye for an eye and a tooth for a tooth
i read in a book somewhere
but i'd rather give BOTH eyes, in truth
when i'm set in the soft cushioned chair.

i'm sensible. acquainted with jung and freud.
been schooled and tutored and colleged
but reason is simply unemployed
(and in MY case, not even acknowledged)

tell me that it can't hurt me
assure me that pain is passe
implore my fears to desert me
it's psychosomatic, you say.
show me the pamphlets all written
extolling the drugs that will lull
tell me with child's fear i'm stricken
and say that you find me quite dull.

you're right. . . the days of the mystery
the hammer, the chisel, the saw
to a dds now, are all ancient history
his tools are precise and fast-on-the-draw.
his chair is a coach of the softest of stuff
his office is floating with song
he's pleasant and young, but that's not enough
there's STILL something TERRIBLY wrong.

for no matter how the world may sound
when they tell me to use my head
when time for the dentist rolls around
i
    still
        wish
            i
             were
               DEAD!!!

drawings & poetry by Sharon Vedborg Timmer

Dedication

To those from the far past,
that first patched teeth and mouths and jaws   As Pioneers,
To Found the New Dental Profession Around the World.

To those Dentists who joined in the past
To form groups that became the American Dental Association,
Whose Members continue into the Present,
Improving Dental Education and Advanced Studies
Raising Dental Standards,
Using All Branches of Science and Research,
To Develop and Perfect Better Dental Materials and Methods
Valued Throughout The World.

The True University....is....Books
Thomas Carlyle

This Tome Tells of
The Incredible World of Teeth

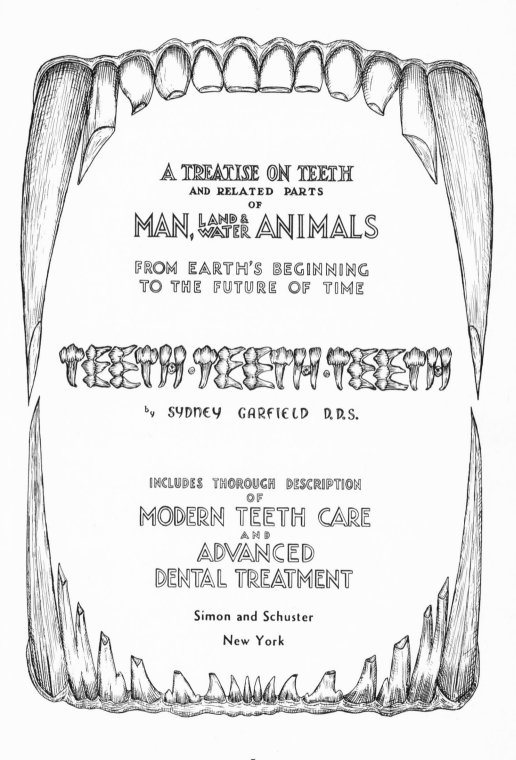

A TREATISE ON TEETH
AND RELATED PARTS
OF
MAN, LAND & WATER ANIMALS

FROM EARTH'S BEGINNING
TO THE FUTURE OF TIME

TEETH·TEETH·TEETH

by SYDNEY GARFIELD D.D.S.

INCLUDES THOROUGH DESCRIPTION
OF
MODERN TEETH CARE
AND
ADVANCED
DENTAL TREATMENT

Simon and Schuster

New York

ALL RIGHTS RESERVED
INCLUDING THE RIGHT OF REPRODUCTION
IN WHOLE OR IN PART IN ANY FORM
COPYRIGHT © 1969 BY SYDNEY GARFIELD

PUBLISHED BY SIMON AND SCHUSTER
ROCKEFELLER CENTER, 630 FIFTH AVENUE
NEW YORK, NEW YORK 10020

SECOND PRINTING
SBN 671–21097–1
LIBRARY OF CONGRESS CATALOG CARD NUMBER: 74–162711
MANUFACTURED IN THE UNITED STATES OF AMERICA

TEETH · TEETH · TEETH

A THOROUGH TREATISE

*TEETH was selected as a title of this book
for more than the name of the object it
identifies. Here it also represents the
especially important part teeth have played
in the lives of numerous lower creatures
and humans, since the beginning of time.
While presenting and revealing these biting
organ instruments to Man so thoroughly for
the first time, teeth are endowed with an added
role of romantic personal identity, being
capitalized several places within the text,
as though THE TOOTH had a soul of its own.*

THE TOOTH

*From the beginning THE TOOTH has been
one with man. He evolved with him from
the depths of oceans. From waters they
crept over the land. Bound to the surface
he lifted his head, then rising he spread,
and breaking bounds, entered the skys.
He's always been one with man — King and
peasant alike — through sufferings and
pains and agonies and death. And he
joined his pleasures and loves, and wars
and plagues, and orgies and feasts. And
now THE TOOTH enters other realm,
to moons and planets and the stars.*

Sydney Garfield

9

ACKNOWLEDGEMENT

Appreciation is expressed to all who helped make this treatise possible. Past and Present Professional Associates to whom the book is dedicated. Since the text was designed for Everyone, including those outside the dental profession, while being written to test its comprehension, random parts of the manuscript were submitted to young and old from wide ways of life. Gratitude is given to my Patients, and Strangers met along walks through public parks and in coffee shops, who were asked to read even the technical text for non-professional criticism.

Thanks to those that taught me at the University of Southern California School of Dentistry in Los Angeles. To Dean Dr. Robert W. McNulty deceased, who even while hospitalized for his fatal illness encouraged me to complete this book. To Dr. Wm. Pate Harrison, instructor of Dental Anatomy and Teeth-Bite-Mouth-Movements, who first interviewed me for admission to the school and accelerated my dental enthusiasm.

To teachers of Basic Sciences and Diseases of all the Body and Those of Teeth. To Drs. Solly Bernick and Robert L. Rutherford for the intimate nature of Development of Teeth. To Dr. Richard B. Tibby for Anatomy of our Bodies, fed by Teeth. To Dr. Lucien A. Bavetta for knowledge of all Nutritional needs and especially those of Teeth. To Drs. Rutherford and John.D. Soule for study of cause and spread of Diseases of the Body and of tissues around Teeth. To Dr. George S. Sharp for diagnosis and treatment of Tumors and Cancers in regions of the Head and Teeth. To Drs. Edward Brady and Harold Holt for Pharmacology of Drugs used to treat diseases of the Body, Mouth, Jaws and Teeth.

To Dr. Francis J. Conley, Director of Clinics, for application of Theory to Dental Practice. To Dr. Wm. W. Wainwright for X-Ray Diagnosis of Heads Jaws and Teeth. To Dr. Francis W. Summers for Knowledge of Children's Teeth. To Drs. Robert L. Reeves and Nathan Friedman for Peridontal Treatment of Diseases Around Teeth. To Drs. Dudley Glick and James V. Pianfetti for cure of Endodontic infections through the inside and beyond abscessed root tips of Teeth. To Drs. Arthur E. Smith, John E. Svoboda and Marsh Robinson for Surgery correcting diseases and deformities of Mouths and Jaws and Removing Teeth.

10

ACKNOWLEDGEMENT

To Drs. Guy Ho, Rene Eidson and Rex Ingraham for Skilled Technicalities of Cutting and Restoring Individual Teeth. To Drs. Donald E. Smith, Robert E. Willey and Henry Tanner, for knowledge of Permanently Attached Bridges Restoring missing Teeth. To Drs. Alan J. De Bre and Edward F. Furstman for design of Removable Dentures replacing Partly Missing Teeth. To Drs. Frank M. Lott and Stuart H. Vaughn for Full Removable Dentures supplying Entire Jaws of Lost Teeth. To Dr. Spencer R. Atkinson for basic Orthodontic principles used Straightening Irregular Teeth. To Others Deserving that may have been missed.

To Dean Dr. John I. Ingle and his Staff that continue Dentistry's Educational Progress.

Appreciation is felt for earlier past engineering associations, that probably helped provide a technically sensitive foundation for understanding dental structures. Study at the Cooper Union Engineering School in New York City, and several years of aircraft detail and major design experience, with the Convair Division of General Dynamics in San Diego and Lockheed Aircraft in Burbank California.

To Ursula Wasko my office assistant for random book helps in addition to her daily dental duties, and several clever suggestions.

Thanks to industrial contributors who helped produce the book. Rene Lamart whose Advance Reproduction Systems graphic arts company in Los Angeles with Larry Roberts and Bob Berry photographed all the original art, with extra effort to obtain high quality reproductions, for the cover and inside the book.

To the Roy and George Gore Brothers of Photo-Typehouse in L.A., for supervising typesetting the book with a new electronic computer combined photo technique. To Don Bannister who handled the bulk of the text. To Harry Winitzky for the finer detailed typesetting refinements. To Joe Kim for his precise page by page final finishing touches. I fondly remember while reviewing certain details with Joe, his comment concerning the last page of chapters that ended with an ornamented poem centered copy layout, "Yes doctor, it does look more elegant that way."

To Kingsport Press, Tenn. for printing and binding the book.

11

INTRODUCTION

Probably because dentistry is considered painful personal invasion, it is abhorred by many. Even during my early professional education, I had a misfit resentful instructor once say, "I hope you like spending the rest of your life working in filthy mouths."

Probably because prior to dentistry I studied and practiced engineering as a previous profession, I present other points of view. Each dental part must obey every physical and chemical law of nature, just like that of a bridge crossing a river, or of a flying machine. The aircraft designer must consider the function of his apparatus for take-off from hot tropical jungle, to arrival at the frigid antarctic, if that's where his craft is expected to go. The dental designer must consider the physical, and chemical, and biological environment of mouths. The problems are similar and sometimes extremely complex, though it is rare that any person's tooth is ever further than two inches from another. The dental environment is enhanced by the added complications of all the other organs and the mind of their living host around it.

Involved in this attitude, I would often explain their problems to patients who said, "Dr. Garfield, this is fascinating. Why don't you write a book." This is the book, for those who would like to know, and those dentists who would like to tell but don't have time to, and those others who practice their profession but somehow don't have the inclination to explain.

Here the book is presented. The first of its kind ever written. A treatise explaining dentistry and teeth to the world. Unknown by most till now. Some may say "Who's interested, Who cares to read about teeth." The aversion itself towards the subject, is evidence of strong personal involvement. This involved concern is captured, to trigger readers into a personal psychological stimulated search, to continue further, reading more. Opening to almost any passage, proves that vivid reality, of anything including dentistry, when dramatically presented to stir the senses, leads readers on and on, like that of other mysteries and intrigues.

The text begins with an exciting History of Dentistry. It ends with a stimulating science-fiction-like chapter predicting The Future of teeth's status in far tomorrows times. Between these boundaries is the bulk of the book, devoted to human dentistry. There are seventeen clinical chapters Explaining All Types of Treatment, easily understood by anyone, interestingly written in clear precise logical detail, relating the intricacies of Dentistry Through Life, from birth to child and adult and old age. One chapter analyzes deep Psychological Factors, sometimes sex related, of fearful patient's minds. Among what I call my six Romance Chapters, one discusses Teeth of Creatures of the Sea, another those of Animals that Live on Land. There is a chapter "Dentistry in Sports," containing personal interviews related to teeth, with world famous athletic personalities. One chapter written in the form of a Play, has a number of Acts From Real Life, portraying interesting and amusing dental related incidents, in the lives of patients.

There are over eighty full page art illustration plates, containing more than three hundred photographs and drawings. Most were made by the author. They picture modern dentistry as it is done and interesting teeth features of man, and water and land animals. Some show dentistry from ancient past. Most chapters contain one to several plates. Plates referred to in the text to help illustrate clinical information are identified by the number of the chapter they are in. The chapter plate number is followed by a dash number which identifies the numerical sequence each particular plate has in its chapter. Plate 15-4 is the fourth plate in chapter fifteen. Throughout the text, words of special significance are occasionally capitalized for emphasis.

Through long past years of ignorance, with pain re-enforced dental fears, knowledge of the subject has been avoided. With the Rapid Advance In All Science and the New Search For Knowledge, people are increasingly interested in causes of their bodies disorders. Patients pay several dollars and more for thorough dental examination. Treatment often costs hundreds of dollars, sometimes even thousands. Patients in ignorance do not understand and suspiciously wonder why.

This book explains the logic of dental treatment technicalities in a manner that stimulates interest even in the unconcerned. The head of a local library system told me, "Such a book has long been needed. I've had many requests, through my library years, from readers for books on dentistry. Nothing is really available."

Girls in training for Dental Assistants are taught and issued texts describing needs of their coordinated tasks. Time isn't available to explain the vast basic principles. Their limited education sometimes includes a few lectures by doctors. The assistant at work routinely performs expected duties without knowing reasons for many. Dental Laboratory Technicians, those that make missing teeth and other mouth parts, are taught to perform their particular tasks. Though capable at mechanical manipulation, their knowledge of the field is limited. The long experienced owner of a dental laboratory told me, "Doctor this book is fabulous. For the first time technicians will understand why they do the things they do. Every lab school will use it and you'll be swamped with sales from experienced technicians. I'll get one of the first myself."

Several medical doctors read part of the text and said, "Syd, medical students should and will be issued your book. Physicians are taught just about nothing of teeth. Your book explains the principles of treatment so interestingly, clearly, logically. Students will buy it. Many practicing doctors will too. I'm anxious to get my copy."

Like modern medicine, as dentistry grew, its procedures perfected to correct particular defects. Some developed into specialties preferred by dentists who limit their practice to them. Individual chapters are devoted to each professional phase of dental treatment. Since all dentistry depends on the same basic principles, in an attempt to make each chapter independently understandable, some information is repeated. Dentistry is sometimes very involved. Though each procedure is performed as described for the reasons explained, sometimes factors beyond the scope of this book lead the dentist to seek solutions other ways.

14

CONTENTS

CONTENTS

CONTENTS

THE HISTORY OF DENTISTRY

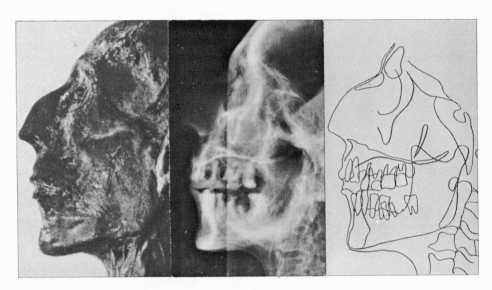

The above series is a side photograph of the mummified head of Ancient Egypts Pharaoh RAMSES II (1292-1225 B.C.?), an x-ray of Ramses head from the same side, and a diagnostic drawing of his dental disorders. Study indicates RAMSES II had lost teeth, decayed teeth, degenerated roots, abscesses, pyorrhetic gum recession and bone loss. His original bite relation was probably good. In the x-ray the dark-light contrast line passing vertically from above forward of Ramses eye down between his teeth is caused by the edge of his coffin through which the x-ray was taken.

Photographs through help of Dr. Mohammed Hassan Abd el-Rahman, chief curator Egyptian Museum, Cairo, Egypt, the University of Alexandria, Egypt, James Harris D.D.S. and Robert Aldrich D.D.S., University of Michigan at Ann Arbor, Michigan and LIFE Magazine, N.Y. N.Y.

RAMSES ROYAL DENTAL DISORDERS s.Garfield

TEETH TEETH TEETH

1

THE HISTORY OF DENTISTRY

In the beginning there was nothing. The earth was barren and void. And the Gods flashed lightnings and roared thunders and stormed torrents and rains. And from nothing came some things. And Animals were created and Man was created. And even in the beginning sickness came, to animals, and to man, and to his body, and to his teeth.

About one hundred million years ago, in the Cretaceous Epoch, towards the end of the Age of Reptiles, in a region now called the Red River District of Alberta, Canada, there was a grass eating dinosaur. He lived and he loved and he fought and he died. His skeletal remains can be seen at the National Museum in Ottawa. His teeth show evidence of decay.

About one hundred thousand years ago, while continents were rising through receding ice and waters, our Neanderthal ancestors learned to use caves and crude tools of stone. Then later in the Old Stone Age, about twenty-five thousand years ago, Cro-Magnon Man left primitive paintings and sculpture as signs of his culture. Skulls of these early humans reveal dental disease.

Then five thousand years ago, man had learned to use metals and write. As he gathered in growing groups mountains and water made nations. In Ancient Egypt there were Pharaohs, like the Ramses and Imhotep and Tutankhamen who worshiped the SUN GOD RAH. They were powerful and ruled supreme. Built Pyramids and Burial Cities, like Gizeh and Sakhara. Could get all the beautiful women they wanted. When they died, they were mummified by experts. And when their well-preserved remains were later unearthed, study disclosed a variety of diseases of the mouth. We've all had toothache!

Many early man made records indicate Egypt as the most ancient nation to develop civilization. Some of these records are sculpted clay objects, carved wood, stone tombs, and other architectural structures. Some of these records are in forms of hieroglyphic handwritings on papyrus, a plant the pith of which was placed in layers, crossed over each other, soaked in Nile River water, and pressed thin, providing man's earliest paper. Papyri have been found that tell tales, discuss morality, law, mathematics, and medical surgical and dental treatment. Papyrus records are named for the men who formed groups that found them. The Ebers and Hearst papyri concern medicine, including treatment of teeth and other mouth parts. The

TEETH TEETH TEETH

Smith papyrus discusses surgery including the mouth. Papyri are long rolled scrolls, about one foot high, written in adjacent sections following like pages. The Ebers medical papyrus is about 66 feet long, the Hearst 10 feet, and the Smith surgical papyrus 15 feet long. Egyptologists consider these manuscripts to have been written as early as 1700 to 1500 B.C., and contain material originating as far back as 3700 years before Christ.

Translation of the medical hieroglyphics discusses disease of the body, teeth, and gums. Prescriptions are given of substances like water, olive oil, honey, dates, onions, beans, dough and green lead, to be powdered and mixed. These are applied quote "against the throbbing of the bennut blisters in the teeth," and "to cure the bennut blisters in the teeth and to strengthen the flesh." References are made to painful swellings. Bennut blisters are mentioned for other parts of the body. They may have been pustules. Flesh described with teeth probably was gum tissue. Though there is mention of surgical body procedures, none is made concerning teeth.

The Smith surgical papyrus deals with diagnosis and treatment of wounds, like common injuries, and fractures from blows and falls. It is written in descending anatomical order, from the top of the head, going down. The papyrus is incomplete, stopping with injury at the middle of the back. Originally it may have gone on to the feet. The papyrus discusses bones of the jaws, and the ligaments tendons and muscles that attach and move them. One case describes in detail, treatment of a dislocated lower jaw. An Egyptian lower jaw has been found, dated by experts from 2900-2750 B.C., which contains two holes drilled through the bone to drain an abscess eroded under a first molar.

Keeping pace with the nation's social and industrial progress, Egyptian medicine reached high degrees of refinement. Records indicate Egyptian doctors practiced within narrowly limited specialties, and probably had an administrative medical system. Excavations near the Great Pyramid at Gizeh unearthed the tomb of a court physician Pepi-Ankh of the sixth dynasty (2600 B.C.). Translations of its carvings read, "The physician of the belly of the Pharao, the guardian of the anus, the surveyor of the physicians of the Pharao, the physician of the eyes of the Pharao." Translation of hieroglyphics involves interpretation of complex figures and symbols. Some of the phrases among others indicate to read, "physician for the teeth," "toothmaker," "chief of the treater of the teeth," and "chief of the toothers and physicians." Herodotus, a historian of the fifth Pre-Christian Era (500-424 B.C.) wrote, "The exercise of medicine is regulated and divided amongst the Egyptians in such a manner that special doctors are deputed to the curing of every kind of infirmity, and no doctor would ever lend himself to the treatment of different maladies. Thus Egypt is quite full of doctors: those for the eyes; those for the head; some for the teeth; others for the belly; or for occult maladies." Apparently even then in Egypt there were dental specialists, and practioners of supernatural magics.

Somehow the advanced pyramid-building civilization of the Egyptians declined and their medical knowledge with them. Most information of those early Pharaohs failed to reach other nations of the time.

Hebrews or Israelites were a small cultured group enslaved by the Egyptians for over four hundred years, until their escape to freedom about 1290 B.C. during Ramses II reign. They were fine physicians, yet left few written dental records. Their attitude towards teeth is seen in their bibles; "an eye for an eye and a tooth for a tooth."

Ancient led to Middle Ages. Cultures and nations grew. With Egyptian and Hebrew, Roman, Greek, Chinese, Etruscan, Arabian. Others were forming. Man's intelligence increased faster than his discovery of natural scientific knowledge. He had learned to talk and a few to write but little of his own body. In most of the world, few knew anything of inner anatomy or causes of disease. Searching for reasonable reasons, sickness was attributed to supernaturals, and evil gods and demons. Some claimed to be delegated priests and magicians representing the Divine, capable of cure with prayer and miraculous charms and enchantments. Others were considered Devil's agents, witches and sorcerers, attacking sickness with mysterious forces of evil. All were feared powers of society, well-paid for their services. When the sick recovered they often rewarded them even more, afraid otherwise their maladies might return. Treatment failure was claimed as proof the patient didn't deserve holy help.

Ignorance was rampant. Primitive people did not even associate the act of sexual intercourse with birth of babies. They believed both just happened to happen. Though such obvious things were eventually understood, other of their ideas completely accepted seem incredulous today.

Perhaps the oldest common belief of toothaches cause is the Toothworm. Clay tablets of ancient Babylonian and Assyrian Empires, shown in museums, have translations describing toothache caused by a demon that took the form of a worm and invaded teeth. References to the toothworm exist in old medical literature around the world. Perhaps the idea arose and persisted since close examination inside an extracted tooth reveals the soft inner pulp that looks somewhat worm-like. Also primitive dental hygiene was probably so poor, worms of fruit and other foods might have been found between teeth. The toothworm belief may even exist in primitive areas today. During the second world war, a military officer friend of mine was in China. He had heard the toothworm tale. While on the streets of Peking, he saw an itinerant medical-dental monger calling his wares.

TEETH TEETH TEETH

THE HISTORY OF DENTISTRY

Approached by a woman with toothache, my friend slyly-closely watching, saw the quack slip a tiny fly-maggot from a pocketed box to under his fingernail, and with sleight of hand, make a show of removing the worm from the tooth.

Ancient Chinese records reveal a belief dental disease was caused by excessive sexual intercourse. Luckily modern dentistry proves this isn't so. Those were days of darkness, fear of unknown magics and witchcraft. Teeth were treated by wrapping with tiny pieces of parchment containing written prayers. Inserting a live louse into a tooth cavity was another cure. In Germany it was believed kissing a donkey helped, and biting off the head of a mouse. The first urine of the morning was advised as a medical mouthwash, and urine of young boys was considered best. Little fellows paid for such substances may be ancestors of today's dentists. Babies first or milk teeth were actually believed to grow from the milk flowing from their nursing mothers breasts nipples as it touched infants bare gums. Rare children born with erupted teeth were sometimes killed as demons.

Intelligence burst forth through paths of philosophical concept. About four hundred and fifty years before anyone knew Christ would ever be born, Socrates the Greek (469-399 B.C.) established theories of thinking. Then his pupil Plato used these methods to reason of purity and goodness and beauty of soul beyond body. Then Plato taught his student Aristotle (384-322 B.C.) of advanced systems and logics. Progress demands even great teachers be surpassed by their students, and Aristotle used these methods to investigate further.

He proposed theories of ethics of good and bad, and happiness, which he used searching for knowledge around him. He described natural elements of earth and air and fire and water. He evaluated plant and animal forms, arranging them in higher and lower orders. Man was highest, and like other animals he declared, perpetuated from within themselves by reproduction. He believed lower forms like worms and flies generated spontaneously from nothing.

While some explored philosophies of mind, and plants and animals of nature, another Greek Hippocrates, now called the Father of Medicine, concentrated on the body. Few people ever traveled further than they could walk, yet Hippocrates journeyed Europe, Asia, and Africa, studying disease. He found sickness was not due to supernatural causes needing magic cures, but rather through faults of nature that could be corrected by physical and chemical agents. He and others of the time did no corpse dissection, since the human body was considered an inviolate, private, sacred entity. Most of his ideas of internal anatomy were inaccurate, made only by outer observation and deduction. Hippocrates wrote extensively prescribing heat and cold, and drugs of plants and earth, for use as

THE HISTORY OF DENTISTRY

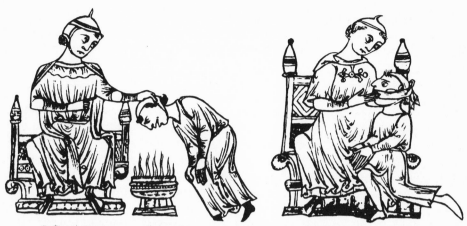

DRAWINGS FROM ANCIENT MANUSCRIPT

Probably originated by Ruggero de Frugardo, a Lombardy physician and surgeon in his manuscript CHIRURGIA written about 1100 A.D. (Trinity College, Cambridge, Eng.) In older times drawings and text were often stolen by writers from others. One treatment is by fumigation over fire. This was frequently given against the mythical toothworm believed for a long time to be toothaches cause. The other shows a bandaged swollen cheeked patient after the lancing of an abscess.

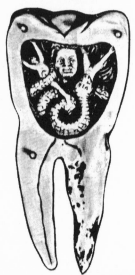 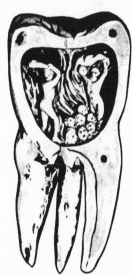

AN OLD IVORY CARVING
from southern France of later 1700's

The parts shown opened reveal inside the dreaded toothworm demon and its tortured victims. Closed together related by each halves guide pins and holes the tooth appears as any other hiding its inner pain drama. The toothworm tale was accepted for thousands of years and is probably still believed in some primitive places.

ARCHAIC DENTAL ATTITUDE   S. Garfield

TEETH TEETH TEETH

medicants against the symptoms of sickness. Knowledge was limited, and physicians of the body treated all the body including teeth. Division of healths arts into medicine and dentistry was not yet even considered.

Discomforts of dental disease were minor compared to the ravages of poor food, shelter, famines and epidemics of early times. Hippocrates' work was primarily medical though he also discussed teeth. He related body diseases to symptoms of the mouth, teeth, and gums. He described the treatment of lower jaw fractures, by tying rigid teeth adjacent to the break together, with linen cords. Yet even those brilliant men were so conditioned, that they failed to make personal explorative simple examinations, like looking inside the mouth. Hippocrates and Aristotle both left written records, indicating they believed men had more teeth than women.

The search for knowledge continued. Shortly before Christ was born, Celcus (25 B.C. to 50 A.D.) a Roman physician, applied science to dental treatment. He advised rinsing the mouth with fresh water in the morning. Pyorrhea was common in ancient Rome. Celcus described bleeding gums, loose teeth, gums separated from teeth, and ulcers around the teeth. He advised chewing unripe pears and apples, munching their juices into the area, washing with weak vinegar and astringents like nut gall and alum. If this failed, we quote his next treatment plan, "When this latter, however, cannot be obtained by drugs, the ulcer must be cauterized with a red-hot iron." For relief of pain he prescribed compounds containing mandrake and opium poppy. For toothaches and abscesses which even then "may be numbered among the worst of tortures," he prescribed emollients containing such narcotics and the application of hot water with a sponge held in the mouth.

Ignorance permeated knowledge. Communication was limited. Information spread slowly. Printing had not yet been invented. Doctors and other philosophers could only make records in individually handwritten books. Most influenced only the few people around them. Some with less intelligent analytical ability, but more convincing personality, through misguided ignorance or ill intentioned intrigue, won honors describing mysteries, bewitching those they could.

Pliny (23 B.C. to 79 A.D.) another celebrated Roman, advised prescriptions known to be ridiculous today. Pliny wrote, "to stop toothache bite on a piece of wood from a tree struck by lightning," and "touch the tooth with the frontal bone of a lizard taken during the full moon." He also recommended the use of juice extracted from plants grown inside human skulls. Dental quacks of those days probably misrepresented, selling wood which hadn't really been hit by lightning, bones of lizards caught during other moon phases, and extracts of plants grown in skulls of any animals they could find. Mind is such strong influence that some of these probably even worked for a while.

Archigenese (81-117 A.D.) a Syrian also left for Rome, then a center of culture, to become a famous physician and surgeon. He popularized daring amputations and trepannings. Trepans are surgical saw-drills used to enter and remove a portion of the skull for relief of internal pressures. Less logical surgeons drilled holes in heads for release of imprisoned evil spirits, believed to cause tooth and other aches. Archigenese made many contributions to dentistry. He demonstrated disease of the tiny, soft inner pulp of the tooth. He described dark hurting teeth sometimes undecayed outside, and invented a tiny trepan used to drill into the tooth for release of inner diseased substances.

Claudius Galen (131-200? A.D.) another Roman, is considered the greatest ancient physician since Hippocrates. He dissected lower animals including apes, making substantial contributions to the anatomical sciences. He corrected others earlier errors yet made personal mistakes, basing his own ideas of human anatomy, which had not yet been explored, on that of lower animals. Galen described anatomical and functional differences of human teeth, like the front biting incisors and rear grinding molars. He also wrote of the soft inner pulp and continued Archigenese' methods of drilling into teeth. He differentiated between toothache caused by disease within the tooth itself and that outside around the tooth. For painful tooth cavities, Galen prescribed fillings containing black veratrum, a plant with sedative properties. Yet limited in knowledge, he advised that the veratrum be mixed with sugary honey.

It is interesting that while most physicians increased knowledge of teeth treatment, little writing concerned the actual replacement of missing teeth. That may have been because chemical drug therapy involved unknown mystery. Whether magical or logical, either remedy commanded professional dignity. Doctors of distinction considered making and installing teeth a more obvious mechanical art, less intellectually inspired, less deserving of prestige. Probably because making teeth required personal intelligent artistic skills often demonstrated by craftsmen in those times, dental appliances were made which seem remarkable even today.

Archaeologists excavated excellent specimens identified as ancient Egyptian, Phoenician, Greek, Roman, and others. The greatest contributions to early prosthetic dental appliances were by the Etruscans, citizens of Etruria (1000-400 B.C.), a small nation that existed before neighboring Rome appeared (753 B.C.). Etruria occupied a hilly area along the central Mediterranean side of what is now Italy. Many examples of fine Etruscan dental appliances are in Italian museums. Few written records have been found of their medical or dental techniques. Many of the appliances were bridges, like present dental bridges, supporting missing teeth attached to adjacent existing teeth. Gold, man's first discovered metal because it is found pure, was then as it still is, the most common structural dental bridge material. Ancient skeletal jaw specimens have been found with such bridges in place. Some were discovered in tombs, others due to the hard resistance of teeth, and gold's high melting temperature, survived the fires of early cremations.

Replaced missing teeth were sometimes the patient's own lost, sometimes other peoples teeth, extracted from slaves, teeth of animals, or carved of wood, bone, and ivory. Some bridges were of gold wire twisted around natural teeth, also holding tied replaced teeth, sometimes passing through small holes drilled through the teeth. More rigid bridges were of thin gold bands like rings, made to fit around the crowns of rooted teeth, which after adaption in the mouth were soldered together outside the mouth. These supported other gold bands which held false teeth, sometimes with small gold rivets passing through them. Ancient Etruscan full tooth gold covering crowns also have been found. Such specimens of high dental refinement were available only to few. Most ancients probably did not even know they existed.

There was little knowledge of infection. No one imagined anything could possibly exist smaller than they could see. There was no thought of germs. Yet some ancients were concerned with keeping teeth clean. Pre-Semitic Sumerians were probably the earliest people to gather in cities, perhaps 8000 years ago. The University of Pennsylvania Museum has a gold vanity case considered Sumerian 3000 B.C. which contains tweezers, an ear scoop, and a gold toothpick. Toilet sets with gold toothpicks have also been found of Assyrian, Babylonian and old Chinese origin. An ancient Assyrian medical text describes cleaning teeth with the index finger covered with cloth, mentions the use of salt, and advises teeth cleaning to avoid bad breath. References to wooden toothpicks and mouthwashes are found in the old Hebrew Talmud, Greek and Roman writings. With medical progress concern for cleanliness increased. In the Old Roman Empire some noblemen had special slaves for cleaning teeth. They could be considered our earliest dental hygienists.

As man's searching intelligence grew, he found his existence explained in God and religions and Christianity. Later, in another part of the world, Muhammad (570-632 A.D.) was born in the Arabian city Mecca. He founded the Islam religion of Moslems, saying there is no God but Allah and Muhammad is his prophet. The Koran also showed its attitude toward teeth in Arabic revelations to Muhammad saying, "a prayer which is preceded by the use of a toothpick is worth seventy-five ordinary prayers," and "you shall clean your mouth for this is a means of praising God."

Islam spread as the Arabians invaded conquering parts of Asia, Africa and Europe. Spain fell in 711 A.D. Despite the killing and mutilation horrors of close-flighting wars of that time, the Koran like other religions also prohibited dissection of human bodies for study. Yet the Arabians made great contributions to chemistry, pharmacy, dentistry and medicine.

Albucasis, an Arabian physician and surgeon, is considered the dental surgeon of the Middle Ages. There is historical disagreement concerning his lifetime which probably was 1050 to 1122 A.D. He wrote extensively selecting material from earlier Greeks and Romans and adding much of his own. His work, "De Chiurgia" translated into Latin, Hebrew, Catalonian, and French, formed the basis of European surgical studies for several centuries. He first described the removal of stones from the bladder and several obstetric procedures. Albucasis made valuable contributions to dentistry. He wrote a chapter "On the Scraping of the Teeth" in which he declares absolute cleanliness is necessary. He described tooth deposits.

Albucasis wrote, "If a first scraping is sufficient, so much the better; if not, thou shalt repeat it on the following day, or even on the third or fourth day, until the desired purpose is obtained. Thou must know however, that teeth need scrapers of various shapes and figures on account of the very nature of this operation. In fact, the scalpel with which the teeth must be scraped on the inside is unlike that with which thou shalt scrape the outside; and that with which thou shalt scrape the interstices between the teeth shall likewise have another shape." He designed a set of fourteen peridontal scaling and curetting instruments which appear in his book. Drawings in today's few remaining volumes are poor and differ one from the other, yet it can be seen that their surgical tips possess features valued in modern instruments. It should be remembered this was before printing existed. Books were precious, written by the author, then copied individually, often by different handwriting craftsmen of the trade of writing book copies. Few could afford them.

For a long time physicians mentioned teeth removal but cautioned against it. Teeth were considered noble organs of the body. There were no satisfactory anesthetics and some thought the excruciating pains of extraction were a sacred rebellion against such unholy practice. When unbearable pain did lead practitioners to remove teeth, due to lack of proper technique and medications sometimes jaws were broken, more serious injury and infection resulted, even death.

Albucasis described several toothache treatments and advised that all be tried before removal. He discussed pain of the operation, and emphasized the importance of removing the proper tooth, since pain location could be misleading. He described ways of loosening gums around teeth for better vision before removal, so that less damage resulted to the jaws. He

TEETH TEETH TEETH

designed special instruments for loosening and extracting teeth, surgical elevators, forceps, saws and files and chisels. He specified that they be made of good Indian or Damascene iron. He stated a surgeon should be capable of designing instruments for individual cases if needed. He warned improper technique could disfigure the body causing deformities especially displeasing to women. He prescribed medications and recommended bleeding be controlled with powdered blue vitriol. He suggested post-operative mouthwashes of vinegar and salt.

Albucasis recommended that missing teeth be replaced with oxbone carved artificial teeth for better function and esthetics. Yet despite advanced thinking his writing shows belief in the toothworm.

Though science progressed continuously, superstitious ignorance persistently resisted. In early 1300's John Gaddesden a successful Oxford English doctor wrote an unusual medical book called "English Rose. The Practice of Medicine from Head to Foot." It isn't known what English Rose represented, it probably had significance as a title at the time. Gaddesden's book provides several ridiculous cures. If a tooth needed removal, he recommended the application of dried powdered crow dung, which he wrote would cause teeth to fall out. Among his treasured secrets he released information that the application of fat from a green frog was even better for the same purpose. In fact Dr. Gaddesden stated, green frog fat was so powerful as a tooth remover, that if a grazing ox unknowingly chews a little green frog along with grass its teeth instantly fall out. He recommended the brain of a hare or rabbit be rubbed on children's bare gums to help teeth erupt. He said hare brain was so strong it would even grow teeth again from the bare jaws of people who had lost them. Yet for some reason in the same book describing removal of teeth with crow dung and green frog fat, he includes several logical surgical procedures similar to those given by earlier doctors. Much evidence exists indicating many early writers would steal material copying from others.

Guy de Chauliac (1300-1368) a Frenchman, has been called the greatest general surgeon of the middle ages. The village he was born in near Auvergne adopted his name honoring him. His work "Chirurgia Magna" was a guide for teaching surgery up into the eighteenth century. It was hand transcribed into French, Provencal, Italian, English, Dutch, Hebrew, and even printed later in 1478. Much of his dental material was taken from Albucasis' work. De Chauliac critized earlier unproven methods of removing teeth writing, "the ancients had many medicaments which draw out teeth without iron instruments---these promise much and operate but little." He described human teeth anatomy details and correctly said they varied from twenty eight to thirty two which is the normal adult number including later erupted third molar or wisdom teeth. He wrote that dental

TEETH TEETH TEETH

THE HISTORY OF DENTISTRY

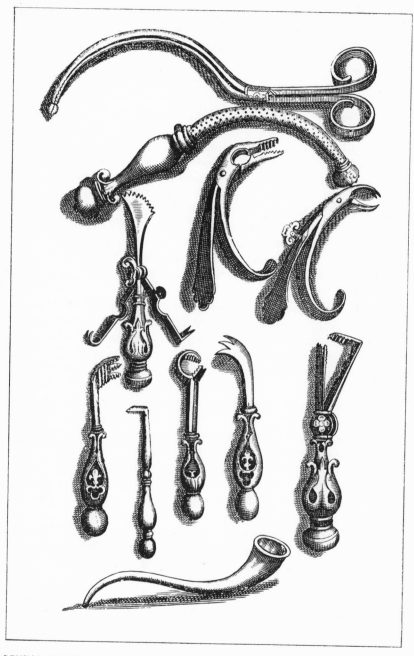

DENTAL SURGERY & RELATED INSTRUMENTS from ARMAMENTARIUM CHIRURGICUM an important text of the time by Johann Schutes 1595~1645 an Ulm physician

TEETH TEETH TEETH

operations were "particular" possibly defining dental surgery as a specialty. He specified certain instruments for such surgery and probably created the name Dentist. His early translated works use the names dentateur, dentiste, dentista, dentator.

Giovanni d'Arcoli (1412-1484), an Italian physician and surgeon taught at both Bologna and Padua. He seems to be the first to mention filling teeth with soft thin gold leaf. From the casual manner this is mentioned in his work and not seen in writings of others, metal fillings may have been common and omitted as ordinary knowledge.

Society was less organized. Crime less controlled. Police came later. This was before professional schools and license. Many physicians were sons taught by fathers. We wonder who taught the fathers. Some sincere wise men learned for themselves. Some were charlatans. Some searchers found access to books, some good, some bad. As knowledge of medicine and surgery increased many priests of religion seeing their value, attended both spiritual and surgical needs. During the first thousand years after Christ monks heads were shaven as a sign of distinction. Their servants and assistants acted as barbers and also attended other cares of the body. As civilization and its evils increased, religious leaders felt more time should be devoted to moral guidance. In 1613 the Pope declared operations that shed blood were incompatible with priestly performance.

Many physicians considered surgery or body cutting a manual thing like butchering, beneath their dignity. The torso was thought sacred, and the undignified slicing of one part not much different from another. To some hair cutting was like removing a thorn, or a toe's corn or opening a festering boil or pulling a tooth. Some preferred giving enemas which were quite popular, and doing embalming. Some applied leeches and let blood. There was a popular idea still believed in primitive places, that disease was caused by tainted blood which should be removed for cure. One technique was to apply starved blood sucking leeches to patients bodies, where they clung until they had sucked themselves full. Blood Letting was cutting a vessel and letting the patients blood drain splashing into a bucket. To advertise their services such barber surgeons displayed pails of fresh blood, which after congealing were considered less desirable exhibits, and poured to spoil stinking in the streets. In 1307 the City of London passed an ordinance, "no barber shall be so bold or hardy as to put blood in their windows, but let them have it privily carried into the Thames under pain of paying two shillings to the use of the sheriffs."

Some who prefered pulling teeth and specialized in such practice were called "Tooth Drawers." In those times trades were distinguished by dress. Toothdrawers wore pointed caps and necklaces of teeth they had pulled. Their necks were adorned with large unbroken curved long rooted

TEETH TEETH TEETH

specimens as signs of their skill. Toothdrawers are seen in paintings by several old masters.

Professional classes appeared and distinction bred antagonistic resentment and jealousy. Physicians looked down on surgeons. Trained surgeons looked down on those who also cut hair, and barber surgeons thought ordinary barbers beneath them. Each strove for position above others. They banded together to fight for their rights against trespass. Physicians united into the Guild of Surgeons, others formed The Masters and Governors of the Mystery and Commonality of Barbers and Surgeons, and the Master Barbers of London. Toothtreaters created other groups. Amidst all this dissention sympathy sometimes arose for the poor. Health services were rendered by the State in 1399 in England when Mathew Flint a barber surgeon was appointed at 6 pence per day, "to do all that pertains to his art to any of our poor subjects who shall at future time require it without receiving from them anything." I don't know whether "all" included cutting hair, perhaps it did. The plan wasn't successful.

With increasing progress man sought even more. An Age of Exploration for new lands, the riches of new fruits, spices, ivory, slaves and precious metals, developed colonies and continents. In 1492 Columbus discovered America. With distant explorations inadequate hygiene and dietary knowledge spread plagues and disease. Though some historical personalities are known to have lived longer most were less fortunate. The average life expectancy was thirty.

Ships set their sails into unknown waters for months even years at a time. Vessels left port overcrowded expecting some wouldn't survive the trip home. Their small size limited supplies to water dried beef and biscuit. The dietary value of fruits and vegetables were unknown. Navigational instruments were poor and wind power undependable. Old sea charts were half guesses. Ship captains needed special wisdoms, skills and often cruel strength. In unexpected storms and long windless waters, less motivated seamen suffered severe depression despondency and rebelled in mutiny. Confined poor mental and physical conditions aggravated their lack of vitamin C Scurvy, the occupational disease and scourge of the sailor. Starting in the mouth, its symptoms were much like pyorrhea, loosening and losing teeth and jawbone, with painful irregular overgrowths of bleeding gums. Even on land this condition was common though usually less severe and was also called scurvy. Treatment was limited to washing the mouth with urine which had slight antiseptic but little curative value. Many sailors in pain cut each others and their own gums away in gobs as it grew. Stranded in open seas with loss of supplies from lack of preservatives, men ate rotten meat, wormy biscuits, sometimes killed and ate each other. Rats were hunted as choice. They even drank their own urine. Scurvy from the teeth and mouth sometimes spread to gangrene of the limbs and death. Less than half crews sometimes returned. Some ships were left as ghost rafts of death, completely unattended, floundering, every man aboard gone.

Emperics were an ancient sect of physicians who disregarded theoretical study, basing their knowledge on practical experience alone. Until the 1500's medical and surgical progress was significantly emperical or practical. Little research had been done, body dissection was scorned and prohibited. Though even from earliest time there were some who sought analytical answers. The highly respected Roman physician Celcus (25 B.C.-50 A.D.), during Christ's time reported that Herophilus (335-280 B.C.) and Erasistratus (310-250 B.C.) dissected not only human corpses but also living men, criminals consigned to them by Kings of Egypt for study of the functions of living organs. Celcus' report of course, concerns events 300 years before his time, yet present historians and scientists from evaluation of Celcus works, consider him serious and reliable. If any records of such anatomical study were made by Herophilus and Erasistratus they've been lost, perhaps intentionally destroyed. There are early records of their dental contributions.

Claudius Galens' dissections of apes in the second century were the basis for human treatment well over the thousand following years. Man was influenced by a misguided lack of knowledge. Invading the human body with a knife for opening examination and study was sacrilege. Rebellion arose against ignorance by men of imagination. Bold intelligent pioneers who sought and fought for truth were considered mad by most of the masses.

Roger Bacon (1210-1293 A.D.) an Englishman, predicted powered ships that would cross oceans, vehicles moving without pull by animals, and others that would fly. Bacon preached "Cease to be ruled by dogmas and authorities, Experiment, Experiment, Experiment." Such strongly motivated searchers couldn't be stopped. Pioneering anatomists bought bodies from grave snatchers knowing that punishment if caught could be death. Italian Leonardo Da Vinci (1452-1519) was a multi-talented genius of the time of Renaissance, or Change from Medieval to New. In addition to his remarkable sculptures paintings and drawings, he was a scientist, astronomer, mathematician, engineer and anatomist. He first described the contact lens for eyes. He was an expert anatomical dissector and observer. Da Vinci was among the first to draw the human skeletal structure with its curved spinal column in technical excellence. Da Vinci saw art everywhere describing the "architecture of the beautiful instrument represented by the human body." He made probably the first accurate drawings of the skull, jaws, teeth and associated parts in various views and

THE HISTORY OF DENTISTRY

cross-sections. He described the forms of upper and lower teeth and their articulation or way of working together. Da Vinci was more a devoted artist and scientist than a personal publicist. He received little living recognition. His contributions to anatomy were not published until long after his death.

Advances made many directions. Copernicus (1473-1543) a Pole, analyzed the movements of heavenly bodies. At a time when Earth was considered the Supreme Center of the Universe, he shocked the world declaring our planet was only one among many others, continually moving around the Sun.

The greatest contribution to anatomical science was made by Andreas Vesalius (1514-1564) born in Brussels, Belgium. Vesalius has been called the Father of Anatomy. While young he studied in Paris under the famous anatomist Dubois, called Sylvius in Latin, then the language of education. Sylvius like others based his lectures on Galens' material derived from lower animal dissection. Vesalius displayed great brilliance and in 1539 was assigned the opportunity of editing a new Latin edition of Galens work. He was thoroughly scientific. At great personal danger Vesalius secreted corpses from Paris' Cemetery of the Innocents, and the hangmans gallows. He did extensive internal body dissections carefully recording his findings. In 1543 he published "The Human Body Construction," a thoroughly detailed treatise. His clearly presented findings disproved Galens accepted earlier erroneous work. Jealousy and resentment arose among his instructors and other physicians and surgeons throughout the world. Vesalius became famous and his services were widely sought. The Venitian Republic offered him a Professorship at the University of Padua where he founded the first anatomy school in Europe. His fame spread as he traveled lecturing. Most of Vesalius' work concerned anatomy of the general body, the torso and limbs.

Limited dental studies he made were similar to those of Leonardo Da Vinci. He declared Aristotle's theory of men having more teeth than women was wrong and easily proven by counting. Vesalius also counted ribs and disproved the notion of original creation that men had one less than women.

Vesalius' pioneering led others. Gabrielle Fallopius (1523-1562) his Italian disciple made added contributions. Womens fallopian tubes which pass from the uterus to ovaries on each side, providing passage for ovum and spermatozoa are named for him as discoverer. He wrote "Anatomical Observations" published 1562 in Venice. Fallopius also did detailed dental research. He disproved Vesalius' theory that permanent teeth develop from the roots of primary teeth and described the significance of the dental follicle in formation of teeth.

TEETH TEETH TEETH

THE HISTORY OF DENTISTRY

Bartolomio Eustachio, latinized Eustachius, (1520-1574) was another Italian anatomist who studied the head in detail. The eustachian auditory tube, from the tympanic cavity at the eardrum, to the nasal part of the pharynx bears his name. In addition to anatomy of other parts he recognized the importance of teeth. Eustachius complained of the low standards of dentistry and did anatomical research as a foundation for improvement. He wrote "Libellus de Dentibus" published in Venice 1563, the first book devoted to tooth anatomy. For his work he dissected aborted human fetuses, stillborn children, children that died when only a few months old and adult corpses. He also studied bodies and heads of lower animals. He thoroughly described tooth development. Eustachius is the discoverer of peridontal membrane which he described as "very strong ligaments principally attached to the roots by which these latter are tightly connected to the alveoli," or root sockets in the jawbone. His small ninety-five page volume includes tooth embryology, anatomy, blood and nerve supply.

While Italians Fallopius and Eustachius described dental anatomy, a Frenchman Ambrose Pare (1517-1590) pioneered dental surgery. Pare had little early education. His interest began as a boy with an older brother, a barber. Ambrose feeling limited, apprenticed to another barber who also leeched, bled, and pulled teeth. At sixteen he worked with a Paris "chirurgien barbier" further increasing his skills. He spent some years doing minor surgery at the Hotel Dieu clinic. Between 1537 and 1545 he was with the French Army. At the front in action he practiced surgery and dentistry. In those days battle wounds were treated with boiling oil and searing the flesh with red hot iron instruments. The torturous excruciating pains killed as many as battle damage. Pare gained great prestige and the resentment of other surgeons introducing soothing medicated emollients. He invented better methods for tying military wounds and improved bandage designs for hemorrhage control. He saved many lives.

Feeling need for further personal education, in 1554 at thirty-seven, he attended the Paris College of Surgeons and was awarded Doctor in Surgery. His proven ability and outspoken courage at proposing better methods, increased his reputation and the jealous antagonism of others. In 1562 he became Chief Surgeon to the Court of France. At a time when physicians and surgeons considered themselves distinctly separate professions, with resentments against each other, Pare saw the need for cooperative practice and combination. He insisted surgeons should have medical training and antomical dissection instruction. He organized schools. He wrote advanced treatises on general and dental surgery.

Pare stressed need for frequent thorough teeth cleaning. He designed improved oral surgery instruments, files, pincers, forceps, lancets,

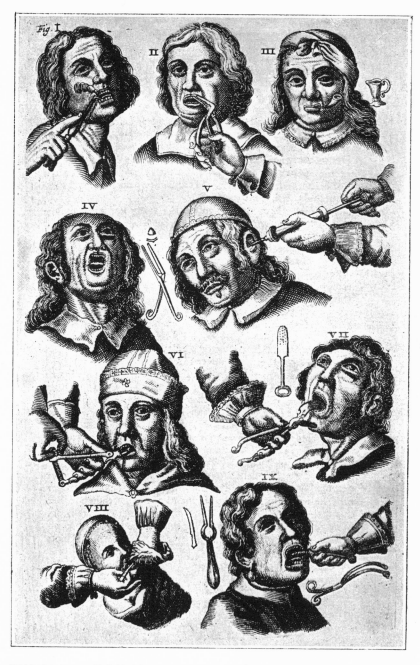

DENTAL AND RELATED OPERATIONS *from* ARMAMENTARIUM CHIRURGICUM an important text of the time by Johann Schultes 1595-1645 an Ulm physician

TEETH TEETH TEETH

elevators, others. He described superior oral surgery methods including teeth removal, and at this time when diagnostic technique was limited, cautioned that the proper tooth be removed. It was common then with their primitive methods, to tear large pieces of bone away attached to teeth. Jaws were needlessly fractured and faces deformed. Pare described ways of avoiding such surgical accident and wiring broken parts together until healed. For teeth that needed extraction and others incorrectly removed he proposed methods of replacement.

Pare also introduced the palatal obdurator, a comfortable removable appliance for closure of unnatural openings in the palate or roof of the mouth. Such imperfect biological passages which still occasionally occur were far more frequent in those times. They create great inconvenience to sufferers. Food while eating is forced awkwardly up through the opening into the nasal sinuses, disturbing speech and breathing. Such openings are caused in two ways. By lesions of syphilis, which uncontrolled was rampant at the time, eroding holes through the upper palate. Syphilis then was called the French disease, since Paris was a center for world travelers through Europe and to recently discovered America. Modern treatment of syphilis makes such perforations rare. Palatal openings are also caused by congenital or birth defects called cleft palates. They often accompany split or hare lips. They may occur in about one of two thousand births. Advanced oral surgery technique in modern countries, corrects such deficiency with tissue closure during infancy. Dentists rarely need to construct obdurators today.

Intelligent visions in discerned directions can accompany ignorance in others. Pare still believed toothache to be caused by a worm, that teeth grow throughout life, and like Galen 1300 years before him and others since, that certain fine taste sensations were felt through the teeth.

Progressive ideas in other fields of scientific endeavor were also temporarily retarded. Galilio an Italian, (1564-1642) discovered and demonstrated the law of gravity. Until then it was believed that a weight ten times as heavy if dropped would fall ten times as fast. Galileo dropped unequal weights as the same time from the Leaning Tower at Pisa, and amazed watchers as the objects hit the ground at the same instant. Yet many who saw for themselves wouldn't accept his proven theory. Galileo also helped perfect the telescope and added evidence to Copernicus' theory that the Earth moved around the Sun. Ruling powers blinded by ignorance, anxious to assert their own wrong ideas, and egotistically motivated to believe their Earth's self to be the center of all existence, despite his conclusive proof, destroyed Galileo's books and using personal and political pressure forced him to publicly renounce his discoveries. Truth can be hindered but can't be stopped.

TEETH TEETH TEETH

THE HISTORY OF DENTISTRY

In 1628 William Harvey announced the discovery of blood circulation. Added advances followed. Anton van Leeuwenhoek (1632-1723) a Dutchman, perfected powerful microscopes. With a magnification of 300 times he discovered what he called living animalicules, invisible to the eye, in human feces and swimming in a drop of water. He examined teeth scrapings and was first to see what looked like organisms living around teeth. He examined human teeth to discover dental tubules and wrote, "six or seven hundred of them are no thicker than the hair from one's beard."

Malpighi (1628-1694) an Italian anatomist of the same time, used the microscope studying tissues of the body in great detail. He started the science of histology, the study of the intimate microscopic nature of organic tissues.

THE ACCELERATION OF KNOWLEDGE

Ancient man first crudely, then bungling slowly began. Each step and stumble, fumbled, faltered and fast, led further and further forward. Social, spiritual, intellectual and technical improvement were on the way. Every increment of newly acquired knowledge provided more direct means for mans intelligence to increase the speed of his progress. With the eighteenth century and after, technological scientific development advanced more and more rapidly, and dentistry used and adapted each succeeding refinement to perfect its art.

In early 1700's Paris was a world center of culture and luxury. People of wealth from everywhere came for pleasure and extravagant excitement. They were anxious to preserve their youth and increasingly aware of the importance of teeth in such a role. It was there that Pierre Fauchard, considered the Founder of Modern Scientific Dentistry made his contributions. Pierre was a Frenchman, born 1678 somewhere in Brittany, died 1761 in Paris. His distinction is based on his book, "The Surgeon Dentist, a Treatise on Teeth" published 1728. It was by far the most complete book on dentistry ever written. Fauchard's title introduced the designation Surgeon Dentist or Dental Surgeon. Pierre Fauchard probably did most to give dentistry professional status. His preface makes early references to dental license and stresses the need for specialized dental education. He mentions a French law of 1699 which required a qualifying examination to practice dentistry. He complained that while government examiners were surgeons as they should be, they had little knowledge of dentistry.

Fauchard's book of 843 pages in two volumes was packed with valuable detailed theoretical and practical information selected from that of previous writers with additions and inventions of his own. He discussed Dental

TEETH TEETH TEETH

THE HISTORY OF DENTISTRY

Education, Anatomy, Pathology, Pharmacology, Orthodontics, Surgery, Caries or decay, and gold lead and tin Fillings, Operative methods of cutting or preparing teeth, Nervous related tooth disease, Pyorrhea, Making individual teeth, Fixed Permanent and Removable bridges and dentures, Replanting and Transplanting teeth, many others. He emphasized the importance of dental health to body health. He stressed the need for keeping teeth clean. His description of pyorrhea was so thorough, for a time it was called Fauchard's disease.

The most renowned physicians, surgeons, anatomists and scientists praised his work which created a new epoch in dental history. Many practitioners resented Fauchard. It was common then, for doctors to claim personal secrets and hold their work snobblishly sacred with an air of reserved professional mystery. They felt Fauchard's open presentation of dental information weakened their prestige, though many secretly benefitted from its contents.

Metal fillings at the time were made from pieces of thin soft metal sheet adapted and compressed into the cavity. Lead was least expensive and easy to work, the most popular filling material. Even today the French call any tooth filling "plombage" which means leadwork. The French word for lead is plomb.

Before the invention of modern adjustable dental chairs it was difficult to find convenient ways of getting at and into patients mouths. Dentistry was done with patients lying flat on their back, seated on the floor and in ordinary chairs, with dentist and patient contorting themselves for advantageous postures. Fauchard described practical dentist-patient operating positions best for the procedures performed.

Porcelain and plastic teeth had not yet been invented. Fauchard discussed tooth materials, how to prepare them and make teeth from them. He wrote, "human teeth, the teeth of walrus, hippopotamus and oxen, also bones of oxen, horses and mules teeth, teeth of the rhinoceros and the heart of oldest and whitest ivory." He preferred human and walrus teeth, "because they are covered by enamel and therefore last longer and hold their color better."

Fauchard knew nothing of impression materials for making exact working models of patients mouths. Those came later. Dentures then were handmade alongside the seated patient. Measurements were with instruments like rulers, pencils, compasses, and cut paper patterns tried in and out repeatedly. Bit by bit, appliances were built in parts, put together and checked for fit. It took long lengthy time and great skill. Fees of necessity were exorbitant compared with those today. Only the wealthiest could afford them.

Even the best dentures made could not fit as ideally as when molded over a precise mouth model. Proper adaption for suction keeping upper dentures from falling down was impossible. Fauchard designed, lower resisting against upper denture systems, connected with springs in the back which kept the dentures apart. In the mouth the springs reaction against the lower part kept up the upper. Closing the mouth overcame the springs forces against the lower jaw. They gave some reasonable service, though the continuous spring forces caused nervous tension when worn too long.

Pierre Fauchard was a man bold for his days in other ways. He married three times. First when young before coming to Paris. Little is known of that venture. The second time at fifty one, after his book was published, to Elizabeth Chemin the sister of Duchemin another famous Parisian dentist who had been his student. They had two children, one a son survived. After ten married years Elizabeth died. Pierre's third marriage in 1747 when he was sixty nine ended after four years in separation. He wrote, "for pecuniary reasons." Fauchard's daring transferred with his blood. His son Jean Bastiste born in 1737, intended to be a dentist instead became a counselor to the Parliament and the French Admiralty. At seventeen he married a sixty year old woman. It didn't last long. Tiring of law, he changed professions and used the name Grandesmil to become a famous Parisian theatrical performer at the Comedie Francais, more celebrated than his father. Multi-talented he changed again to become the first Professor of Elocution at the Institute of France.

Fauchard described and recommended replantation and transplantation of teeth, which had been earlier described by others and was practiced at the time. Replantation is the replacement of a tooth into its own jawbone socket from which it was accidentally or intentionally separated. Restoring a decayed tooth properly inside the mouth was often especially difficult in Fauchard's time. He recommended in certain cases, carefully extracting the tooth, filling it and replanting it to place. Replanting gave some reasonable limited satisfaction, and with modern dental methods is successfully accomplished today, primarily with teeth that have been knocked out accidentally. Transplantation was the placement of an extracted tooth into a tooth socket other than its own. Usually the tooth of a person of limited means was transplanted to a mouth of wealth. Materials other than human teeth were sometimes shaped and tried.

Transplanting teeth became popular. The procedure was entirely surgical not needing the fine detail of precise complicated metal restorations. It was easier and tempting to try during a period when dental follow up care was not as closely attended as today. Periodic medical and dental examinations were rare. It was especially tempting to quacks. The immediate result seemed satisfactory and practitioners made exorbitant claims that they may even have thought sincere.

TEETH TEETH TEETH

THE HISTORY OF DENTISTRY

The primary problem was getting proper teeth. They had to match, at least reasonably their neighboring teeth, and weren't easy to find. Of course in those days when pyorrhea was more prevalent more were loose and available. Yet matching teeth was tough. Teeth may seem to some, to be rather alike, though they differ far more in size, shape, and shade, than most imagine. No two roots are ever exactly alike. Transplanting dentists advertised in newspapers describing teeth they sought. "Wanted by Doctor Phumf, one strong bright, long two rooted molar, for a man of means who will pay well." Higher prices were offered for live ones in the mouths of prospects in poverty who came to the office for inspection. If a deal was made, an appointment was arranged when the selling donor sat on one side of the dentist and the wealthy receptor at the other. The tooth was extracted and transplanted. Results were better with front teeth, having only single roots easier to fit, usually with reshaping as needed. Teeth with more than one root, especially molars, were tried but hardly lasted at all. Larger selections made better results more likely. Some advertisers offered to buy any teeth with the intention of building up large assorted stocks for dental availability. Teeth were extracted and collected on battlefields and stolen by gravediggers. They were sold to some of our earliest tooth supply dealers. There were even toothnappers who roamed streets watching mouths of talkers. Armed with forceps, instead of or in addition to a gun, they would attack and extract, creating a black market in white teeth for sale to shady dentists. Novelist Victor Hugo, in his masterpiece of early 1800's France, Les Miserables, tells of beautiful unfortunate Fantine selling two of her incisors, extracted for forty francs. [Readers are asked NOT to appear at the author's office offering teeth for sale.]

Teeth transplantation was popular. The New England Colonies had itinerant medical-dental doctors traveling from town to town. They placed ads in newspapers preceding the announced date of their intended arrival, with described services and fees. Many of these men carried a box of teeth for transplantation. As transplants failed, more and more in time, they were suspected of being a source for transmission of syphilis. Teeth are rarely transplanted today.

In 1765 in Pennsylvania, the College of Philadelphia organized the first medical school in the New Americas as its Medical Department. There were about 3500 physicians in that English possession, soon to become with the Revolution in 1776 the independent United States of America. Only 400 of these men had a medical degree which had been studied for abroad. The others taught themselves with books and assisting other doctors. Many also practiced dentistry. A popular dental treatise for those who could read French or its German translation was Fauchard's "Surgeon Dentist." Fauchard's book was followed by others. In England John

TEETH TEETH TEETH

Hunter a physiologist, physician and surgeon, Professor of Surgery, and Surgeon General to the English Army, wrote "Natural History of the Human Teeth,"London 1771, and "Practical Treatise on the Diseases of the Teeth," London 1778.

While much of Europe was torn with political discord, overcrowded, stagnant and poverty stricken for lack of work, the new United States was growing. Emigrants came in search of opportunity. James Gardette, a French medically trained dentist who first practiced in Plymouth Mass. 1778, and then settled in Philadelphia in 1784, wrote on March 30, 1791 to his brother an engraver in France. "Let me invite you, my dear Spiritow, to come to America, where I will make a dentist of you and make your fortune. I will undertake to teach you and within a year to put you in a position to earn as much in an hour as you did in a week scratching copper in France. If you decide to come and join me you should be provided with books upon my profession and I would recommend: 'The Surgeon Dentist,' by Fauchard 2 vol." This was sixty three years after Fauchard's book was published. Gardette also suggested other books. He didn't mention that prices and wages were also soaring in the new world.

DENTAL MOUTH MODELS

The increase of dental knowledge improved its quality, while improved dental services spread the demand for them. A great early technical advance was Mouth Models, models made to exactly duplicate peoples teeth and jaws. Several examples of ancient dental appliances have been found which indicate they may have been made from impressions and models of the mouth. If so, nothing is known of the methods or materials used. Ancient artisans who made them left no records of their making. Mattaeus Purmann (1648-1711) a German surgeon of Breslaw, left early writings indicating he worked with wax to make models of mouth parts. Purmann's work isn't clearly explained. It seems he may have formed and carved wax into models to fit the missing parts, and then used these wax models as guides outside the mouth to copy, carving restoring parts like teeth and jaw fitting bases to hold the teeth, from ivory, bone and other material.

This led to added advances. Philip Pfaff (1716-1780) another German, wrote the first significant German treatise on dentistry. Pfaff was dentist to Frederick the Great, King of Prussia. Pfaff used heated softened wax to take impressions of the jaws. He mixed plaster of Paris, named for the city near which it was first found, with water, and poured it into the impressions where it soon hardened. Removing the outer wax, left rigid hard working models of the patients mouth. Pfaff also tried to introduce

1

THE HISTORY OF DENTISTRY

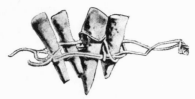

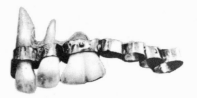

ANCIENT GRECIAN APPLIANCE - within 1000 B.C.
Archaeological Museum - Athens
Gold wire tying teeth together
Sometimes also supported replacements
of human or animal teeth, or carved, wood, bone, ivory

ANCIENT ETRUSCAN APPLIANCE ~ 700 B.C.
from an old tomb - Civic Museum, Corneto, Italy
Made of gold band soldered rings & rivets to hold
replacements. Specimen has 2 natural teeth
& riveted ox tooth & 4 spaces for others

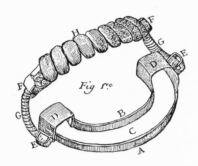

Fig 1.e

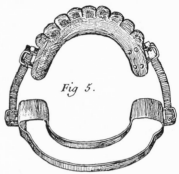

Fig 5.

DESIGN FOR AN UPPER TEETH DENTURE - STABILIZED BELOW COMBINATION

The teeth often carved of ivory or hippopotamus tusk as a unit were riveted to gold brackets
attached each side to coil springs to keep them up reacting against the lower
enclosure which surrounded the lower natural stabilizing teeth.
from LE CHIRURGIEN DENTISTE by Pierre Fauchard 1723 A.D., Paris, France

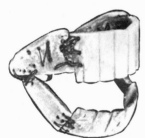

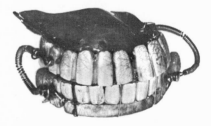

A 1500 A.D. DENTURE
from an excavated Swiss tomb
Parts carved from femur of an ox. Joined
by tying wire. Upper & lower kept apart
by a spring strip. Such dentures were
available only to wealthy yet functionally
useless. A French source says they were
removed at dinner for eating & reinserted
for conversation between courses.

A GEORGE WASHINGTON DENTURE
mid-later 1700's
The U.S. first presidents letters indicate
he had dental problems. This one denture
of many was probably made by John Greenwood.
Its teeth were ivory. The upper base of swaged
gold was kept above by coil springs reacting
against the heavy lead lower base for keeping
the wire tied lower teeth weighted down.

DENTURES THROUGH TIME *S. Garfield*
several of many

TEETH TEETH TEETH

44

artificial teeth carved from mother of pearl. Mouth models revolutionized dental appliance manufacture. Dentists no longer were limited to step by step construction inside the small dark awkward opening of the patients head. Models permitted more accurate working in open space and light, faster better and cheaper. Dentists who didn't care for the actual making of dentures, if they chose, could have others do that part of the job for them. The mouth model created the new trade or profession of Dental Technician In time it was realized plaster hardened and kept its size and shape more accurately than wax. Dentists learned to use plaster of Paris to take impressions of the mouth. These precise impressions were then used to make more accurate plaster models of the mouth. Dentistry was improving and available for more people.

It was probably about 1760 that mouth models were first used to make denture bases of gold sheet formed in sections soldered together. With soft gold coins being used for money they were available and beaten thin as a material formed to make dentures. Bases were also carved of ivory, bone and hard wood. These bases made to fit the jaws held false attached teeth which could be human and expensive, or animal teeth or carved of mother of pearl, or any other practical thing. Sometimes dentures were all one piece, base and teeth the same substance.

DENTAL PORCELAIN

In 1774 at St. Germaine, a French town near Paris, there was an apothecary or pharmacist named Duchateau. His dentures were hippopotamus ivory. Duchateau was disturbed by their absorptions of stains, foul odors and tastes. Grinding his drugs in a porcelain mortar he noticed it kept clean despite heavy use and thought better dentures could be made of porcelain. Confident of his ability but lacking knowledge, he consulted porcelain manufacturers and artists that worked with porcelain. He tried to make porcelain dentures for himself. Deficient in dental information, and because of difficulty controlling the shrinkage of porcelain during firing, he was unsuccessful in several attempts. He sought the help of Chemant a Parisian dentist. Together after several failures they finally made a one piece all porcelain denture that Duchateau could wear. Encouraged and anticipating a fortune from his discovery, though not a dentist, Duchateau tried to make several such dentures himself, for people of high rank. They failed and Duchateau's interest in dentistry diminished.

Dentist Chemant continued and developed a complicated technique for making all porcelain dentures. They fit reasonably, were difficult to manufacture, extremely expensive and broke easily. Only the wealthy could afford them. Falsely claiming complete credit for a porcelain denture invention, Chemant after court disputes was awarded a patent. He made all porcelain dentures. The French Revolution against royalty arose and Parisian workers guillotined King Louis and Marie Antionette. Chemant fled France to England. In London his dentures were welcomed at first, then diminished in demand, as imperfections became evident. All porcelain dentures were abandoned during the 1800's.

Although porcelain shrinkage in firing, created fit difficulties in large pieces like an entire denture, which was also subject to easy fracture, small pieces of porcelain can be size controlled and are strong. Porcelains immaculate cleanliness and color integrity are valuable dental qualities. Several men tried to perfect its use. It was Guisseppangelo Fonzi (1768-1840) a dentist from Italy practicing in Paris, who perfected the first porcelain individual artificial teeth. He was also an artist, a poet, interested in the sciences, and an author in fields outside dentistry. After much experimentation Fonzi developed a porcelain tooth containing a platinum hook, projecting from its back, for soldering to gold denture bases. He became famous, successful and wealthy. His patients included nobility around the world. In 1815 Fonzi was called to the Bavarian Court at Munich, where he made dentures for the King and other palace notables. In 1823 he was asked to St. Petersburg, Russia, where after making dentures for the Czarina, wife of Alexander the First, she frequently said, "Fonzi has given me a new life." At the Royal Court in Madrid he treated the King of Spain. Porcelain teeth were used more and more. At first most dentists made their own, for less expensive cases in blocks of two, three or four. As porcelain teeth popularity increased improvements continued and commercial ventures for making them began. In early 1840's in Philadelphia the S.S. White Company began manufacturing porcelain teeth for home and export on a large scale. Today porcelain teeth are inexpensive and can be made undetectable from natural teeth.

DENTAL EDUCATION

The increase of knowledge and improvement of materials attracted more men to the dental profession and created a need for organized education. With feelings of professional pride dentists were printing publications of their own and forming groups of their own. In early 1800's, New York City and its large port was a center for cross ocean commerce with Europe. Its new Society of Dental Surgeons of the City and State of New York, probably the first formal dental society organized, discussed the need for a school of dentistry. Petty controversies with members of the New York State Board of Education delayed its formation.

In 1827 in the town of Bainbridge Ohio, John Harris a medical doctor interested in education, with the help of a small staff taught his profession. Alert to the importance of teeth in health they included dental treatment. John's brother Chapin A. Harris another physician, became especially interested in dentistry. Chapin traveled through the South practicing medicine, and dentistry which he preferred. He later moved to Baltimore.

In the small city of Baltimore Maryland, Horace H. Hayden a dentist and lecturer to medical students of the University of Baltimore for a long time realized the need for a dental school. He proposed repeatedly that the school add a dental division. Some medical faculty liked the idea, but many resented the intrusion of a new professional status arising alongside their own. They claimed dentistry was mechanical, not to be considered a branch of the healing arts. Chapin Harris met Hayden and both studied dental problems together. Mutually motivated they joined professionally and appealed to the medical faculty for establishment of a school for scientific dental instruction. Their request was refused. In 1839 they organized the Baltimore College of Dental Surgery which was granted a charter February 1, 1840 to become the first dental college in the world. Its first class was five of which two finished, and received the degree "Chirurgiae Dentium Doctor" translated Doctor of Dental Surgery, D.D.S. The profession was finally firmly founded.

ANESTHESIA

The greatest objection to disease is not always its physical damage, often its pain is of even greater concern. In ancient times it was discovered correcting sickness surgically was a valuable means of treatment, which unfortunately often caused pain more severe than the disorder itself. Surgical pain can be controlled by induced insensibility, which the Bible first described when "the Lord God caused a deep sleep to fall upon Adam, and he slept; and he took one of his ribs, and closed up the flesh." Early man himself also sought and found anesthetics to control pain. Ancient Indian writings describe "Sammohini" the fumes of a burning hashish hemp, marijuana, the inhalation of which permitted medical and dental operations. Others of early and middle ages used juices of opium, mandrake, and certain hemlocks. For some reason such use did not spread. Ether, a gas, was discovered early in the twelfth century by an Arabian chemist, Yeber. For a long time it was considered a laboratory curiosity which created exhilarating affects when inhaled, like alcohol. In 1842 Dr. Crawford W. Long a physician in the small town of Jefferson Georgia, discovered ether also had anesthetic value. He successfully performed several minor surgical procedures using ether, but did little to publicize his work. He may not have realized its potential values. Because of the absence of strong anesthetics major surgery was rarely possible, considered, or performed. Surgical techniques were held back, retarded. Body cutting was limited to minor procedures, only simply corrective and patch, and when demanded by accidents like those of the battlefield for amputations, and sewing of large body tears and lacerations.

In 1773 the brilliant English minister and chemist Priestly who discovered oxygen, synthesized nitrous oxide later called "laughing gas," for its mood elevating and laughter creating affects. Inhalation of nitrous oxide stimulated many to laugh, sing, dance and often enjoy wild exciting ideas. Its reactions were unpredictable, some became aggressive wanting to fight.

On December 10, 1844, the Connecticut Courant, a Hartford newspaper, advertised a public lecture and demonstration of nitrous oxide affects. The gas would be administered to all who wished to inhale it. Admission was twenty-five cents. Dr. Horace Wells a Hartford dentist attended with a friend named Cooley. When volunteers were called Cooley inhaled the gas and instead of laughing or dancing like most began fighting. Struggling, his foot caught behind a bench and he fell heavily forcing his leg over a sharp projection. As Cooley rose Wells noticed a wide bleeding gash yet Cooley seemed to feel no pain. Wells, alerted to the event's significance, before even going home, that same evening visited and discussed it with a dentist friend Dr. Riggs. Wells was determined to try the gas on himself.

The next day he bought some from the lecturer, and seated in his own office inhaled the gas to insensibility, until as his arms fell on December 11, 1844, Dr. Riggs painlessly pulled one of Dr. Wells' molars. Riggs said "a grand discovery was born to the world." Wells used laughing gas successfully in his office and felt it should be available to all.

He went to Boston where he knew Wm. T. Morton a dentist. Morton induced Dr. S.C. Warren a prominent physician and surgeon at the Massachusetts General Hospital to permit demonstration at the hospital surgery amphitheater. Dr. Warren introduced Wells, with implied sarcastic ridicule to the audience of students and physicians, who were skeptical that anything constructive could be contributed by a dentist. Wells nervously sensitive in the unfriendly atmosphere had difficulty administering anesthesia to the patient who wasn't inhaling properly. As the crowd jeered impatiently, Wells, nervously uncertain, removed the anesthetic bag and told the surgeon to operate. The patient screamed. With the audience yelling "fake and impostor" Wells left in shame. His expected triumph was a failure. He returned to Hartford, disappointed. Being an emotional man he couldn't work for some time. He later resumed practice using nitrous oxide successfully and told neighbors of it. In those days dentists could obtain invention patents on treatment methods, though not today.

TEETH TEETH TEETH

Urged to seek a patent Wells replied, "No, let it be as free as air." In a short time, brooding again, resented and ridiculed by neighbors, his nervousness brought sickness which closed his office for several months. Returning Wells again successfully used gas for surgical anesthesia but his enthusiasm was gone.

Meanwhile in Boston, Dr. Morton acutely interested probably heard of Wells' successful continued use of the gas in Hartford about 100 miles away. On June 20, 1845 a Boston newspaper had published "A dentist in Hartford Connecticut has adopted the use of nitrous oxide in tooth pulling. It is said that after taking this gas the patient feels no pain." Wells' name wasn't mentioned though it couldn't have been anyone else. Morton consulted a Boston physician Dr. Jackson who had special chemistry interests for instructions in making nitrous oxide. Rumors concerning anesthetics were increasingly heard and Jackson suggested ether, with which he was more familiar and had materials available for producing. He made some for Morton. That same evening Morton used ether to successfully extract a tooth. He consulted an attorney about an invention patent never mentioning Wells. The attorney suggested he get a release from Dr. Jackson who signed one, since in those days it was already considered unethical by some doctors for a physician to profit from treatment inventions. About two weeks later Morton again asked Dr. Warren of Massachusetts General Hospital to demonstrate, this time his own use of inhalation anesthesia with ether. Warren was still skeptical, but being friendly with Morton under his persuasive persistence set a date for October 16, 1846. Morton administered the anesthetic to his patient who inhaled deeply. Warren himself was the surgeon. As his knife entered, the patient kept comfortably still while a small neck tumor was removed. Warren's assistant Dr. Bigelow said, "I have seen something today that will go around the world."

Morton different from modest Wells, exploited his opportunity becoming famous and wealthy. Dr. Jackson left out, now resented Morton's success and claimed honors for himself. He wrote to Paris for recognition in Europe as the sole discoverer of inhalation anesthesia. Wells' friends tried to inform the public and the controversy entered the newspapers. Morton now in a powerful position claimed all credit for himself. On January 24, 1848 in Hartford Connecticut, Dr. Horace Wells ended his own life. The New York Evening Post called it "Melancholy Suicide."

Sincere practitioners of both the dental and medical professions insisted on a thorough investigation. In 1864 the American Dental Association protested the injustice, and declared Horace Wells of Hartford Connecticut deserved the credit and honor for the introduction of anesthesia in the U.S. In 1870 the American Medical Association also credited Horace Wells a

TEETH TEETH TEETH

dentist for the discovery of practical anesthesia.

Today ether inhalation is considered impractical for dental surgery while nitrous oxide serves a valuable role. Modern general anesthetics have been so perfected that major surgical procedures of many hours duration are comfortably performed safely.

Most dental operations use Local Anesthetic Injection penetrating the flesh through a hollow tubed needle into the area desensitized while the patient remains conscious. Many thousands, perhaps millions of years ago, anesthetics were injected through fine almost microscopic hollow needle stings by wasps which immobilized other insect victims. Hollow bee stings and snakes fangs also deliver paralyzing poisons. The hypodermic syringe (hypo means under, dermic, skin) was invented by Dr. Rynd a Scot 1844, in Edinburgh, for the injection of medications. Rynd probably never thought of using it for anesthetics. His syringe was crude and bulky. Soon syringes were used for morphine injection to relieve severe arthritic joint pains.

The first injectable anesthetic was cocaine, a constituent of the coca leaf chewed by South American Indians as others chew tobacco. Cocaine in the leaf was a stimulant, and anesthetizing the stomach lining also lessened hunger. Chewing coca leaves also anesthetized the tongue and mouth. In excess the leaves were habit forming and poisonous. In 1860 in Vienna, Dr. Albert Nieman isolated cocaine from the leaf. Later in Vienna, Karl Koller a medical student, discovered cocaine painted in the mouth acted as a topical anesthetic to stop gagging and permit deep throat examinations. Dilute solutions helped eye examination.

The first injection for local anesthesia may have been during the U.S. Civil War of 1865. A soldier's face was shattered. The surgeon couldn't apply a face mask for general anesthesia and used his medical syringe to inject the narcotic morphine locally into the area needing operation. The anesthetic worked while the patient was awake. In 1885 Dr. Wm. Halstead a Baltimore dentist injected cocaine, blocking nerves of the jaw permitting painless anesthetic surgery. The National Dental Association awarded him a medal. Cocaine was available as powder which the dentist freshly mixed with boiling water for syringe use. The solution was unstable in air.

During World War I, Dr. Harvey Cook of Indiana was annoyed by the inconvenient preparation of repeated fresh small batches needed for military surgery. He conceived the idea of sealing solutions against contamination in individual cartridges from which they could be ejected by an inner sealing end moving through as a plunger. He first tried empty clean brass army rifle cartridges. Then he cut lengths of glass tubing and sealed their ends with rubber pencil erasers. As injection anesthesia increased

TEETH TEETH TEETH

cocaines harmful quality became more evident. It irritated tissue and sometimes sloughed or eroded flesh at the site. In 1900 Alfred Einhorn had researched cocaines molecular structure trying to separate if possible the anesthetic from the poison. In 1905 Braun introduced novocaine (novo for new). Novocaine satisfied cocaines anesthesia and eliminated its toxicity. The drug has been even further refined and synthesized now using the name Procaine. Other fine injectables have since been developed. Some combine with procaine. Hypodermic syringes, needles, and anesthetic carpules, have been perfected and are available sterile, so low in price, fresh ones are used for each patient and discarded.

DENTURES FOR THE MASSES

Anesthetics permitted the removal of diseased teeth which previously undermined health, yet had been left in the mouth because of the fears of painful extraction. More such teeth were now removed and more dentures needed to replace them. Artificial porcelain teeth were available and accurate models of the mouth, but making denture bases for holding teeth to fit such models and the mouth, was time consuming procedure.

Claudius Ash, founder of the English dental materials company that still uses his name, was a skilled silversmith, who in the nineteenth century was famed as a fine London dental technician. His services were sought by the best dentists. It often took Ash six weeks of his full time to complete a single denture, fitting the parts he made by hand, meticulously, step by step, to the patients mouth model for a satisfactory fit. Dentures were very expensive, proudly prized by the few who could afford them, like jewels, even more. People especially women who couldn't indulge in dentures wore Plumpers, ivory balls carried in the mouth to fill their cheeks where teeth were lost. Girls that wanted to look good couldn't talk.

During the time Wells discovered anesthesia and later, Charles Goodyear found interest in a new material made from juices of certain tropical plants. Small pieces were used to erase marks from paper by rubbing. It was called rubber. Rubber was unstable and soon decomposed. Since rubber was waterproof, Charles Mackintosh a Scottish chemist, learned to apply it in layers over cloth coats which became rainproof, and for a long time a raincoat was called a Mackintosh, in some parts of Britain they still are. Charles Goodyear learned to stabilize and harden rubber giving it the trade name "Vulcanite." Patents of invention were obtained in 1851 and in 1858 further improvement patents were issued to Nelson Goodyear, his brother. At first rubber was used primarily for thin layers or coatings as by Mackintosh. In time methods were developed for manufacturing rubber products in molds. Many new articles could be made accurately cheaply

THE HISTORY OF DENTISTRY

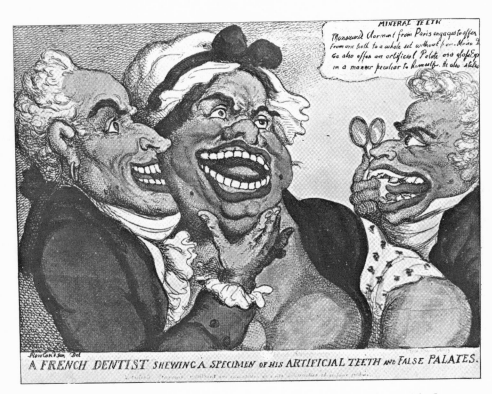

AN ENGRAVING BY THOMAS ROWLANDSON 1756-1827 LONDON, ENGLAND

The popularity of mouth problem subjects portrayed by many artists of earlier centuries is evidence of the greater dental needs in the lives of many during those times. Here Rowlandson shows a dentist proudly displaying the superior result of an advanced technique to a prospective patient who is obviously suffering pyorrhea tooth loss which was a prevalent problem. *S.G.*

TEETH TEETH TEETH

THE HISTORY OF DENTISTRY

this way. Fortunes were made in the new rubber business.

Vulcanized or hardened rubber was a found miracle to dentistry. It could be easily molded against the patients mouth model more accurately than a base made by the finest hand fitting technician. Anyone mechanically adept could learn to process vulcanite dentures in a short time. Their use spread making dentures available to people who couldn't afford them before. It was a time of new-found teeth.

The rubber-mold dental discovery spread. Many who expected the inevitable fate of toothless later life, could now proudly present their broad smiled dental display as a symbol of successful social distinction.

Vulcanite forming wasn't quite free, patent rights of use had to be paid. In 1868 Josiah Bacon, a businessman, gained control of the dental molding process. He demanded fees for individual office rights, varying from 25 to 100 dollars a year depending on the size of the practice, plus one dollar for each denture replacing up to five teeth, and two dollars for dentures with six teeth or more. He claimed the right to examine each dentist's records. About five thousand dentists accepted his terms. Since the process was simple some infringed his rights. Some resented his attitude and despite the value of vulcanite dentures wouldn't make them.

Bacon had spies traveling the country probably working on commission. Some were tough and intimidated dentists including the innocent. Bacon advertised in newspapers threatening to sue and prosecute any dentist who violated his rights. He was hated. On April 13, 1879, Josiah Bacon was found shot to death in a San Francisco hotel. The police were baffled at first since robbery didn't seem to have been a motive. Investigation disclosed Bacon was resented by many San Francisco dentists. Several had been heard to threaten him. Some days after the shooting, Dr. Samuel Chafont a dentist, surrendered to the police. He claimed Bacon with a court order, had stopped him from using vulcanite in Wilmington Delaware. When Chafont moved to San Francisco, Bacon followed him and again started legal proceedings, threatening him with prison. Chafont claimed he only intended to frighten Bacon, that his pistol fired accidentally. The case was publicized throughout the country, even in Europe. Many dentists, physicians, and the public sympathized with Chafont. Many contributed funds towards his defense. Dr. Chafont was convicted of second degree murder and sentenced to ten years imprisonment at San Quentin. Quite a character, after three years he escaped and was recaptured to serve his full term. Dentists seem to get involved in all sorts of intrigue, though I've never heard of any that killed his abandoned mistress who might have been blackmailing him, by secreting a black widow spider in her tooth cavity. In 1881 the patents expired and dentists could make dentures as they chose.

TEETH TEETH TEETH

THE HISTORY OF DENTISTRY

FILLINGS

The earliest fillings used were just that. They were soft materials, did little to strengthen the tooth, yet often stopped pain merely by insulation and keeping air from the open cavity. Often, decay wasn't even removed before they were put in. Some early dentists inserted fillings into hollow decayed tooth crowns, before gripping them with forceps for extraction, just so the crown wouldn't crumble. Pure gold prepared in soft forms like gold leaf and foil, has been for a long time and is still used today for filling teeth. Such gold if kept immaculately clean, and carefully put into the cavity bit by bit, with great pressure, as each small portion is applied to place, will weld to itself as a mass. They are superb dental restorations. The process requires special skills and often took hours for one filling. Such fillings were extremely expensive, available to very few. They are especially difficult to place in the back of the mouth. Contamination by the slightest saliva or other debris could cause unexpected early failure.

The first metal fillings of any significant value were made of bismuth, lead, tin and mercury, mixed and melted. The alloy was called Fusable Metal. The combination was used for its low melting point, just under 212°F., the boiling point of water. Held in a small container, inside another of boiling water, after melting it was actually poured through small curving long stemmed funnels and tubes, through the patients twisted head opened mouth, into the tooth cavity where it solidified. Perhaps upper teeth were filled while patients hung head down. Fusuable alloys were popular for a while in France and the U.S. Later a combination was found that melted as low as 140°. Small solid pieces were placed into the tooth and touched with hot instruments to melt, adapt and fill. Dentistry included dangers of mouth and face burn hazard.

Filling teeth value was questioned. Failure was frequent. Skillful dentists saved teeth successfully yet some said fees were high. It seemed simpler to most to tolerate pain until extraction if unbearable.

SILVER AMALGAM—Mercury named for the God with wings on his heels is a constituent of all amalgam alloys. The only metal liquid at ordinary temperature, mercury is fascinating. Silver in color, impossible to pick up evasively slipping through fingers, for a long time mercury has been called quicksilver. It hardens or freezes solid like any other metal at 37.96° below zero Fahrenheit. Any alloy or mixture of metals one of which is mercury is called an amalgam. The most common dental amalgam is silver amalgam, used to fill most teeth today.

M. Taveau, a Parisian dentist in 1826 used powder filed from silver coins, mixed with mercury into a soft putty like mass. He called it "silver paste." Placed into a cavity it hardened or amalgamated as the silver powder and mercury mutually dissolved into each other. It was inexpensive and worked well but had disadvantages. The filling often expanded inside the tooth splitting the crown apart. Sometimes it swelled to raise above the tooth causing improper biting and pain.

Some of the new silver paste fillings were satisfactory. Differences depended on factors dentists were not yet even aware of. The science of metallurgy was young. Some silver coins contained a small amount of copper for hardening which actually had some value, and in those days silver itself as used in the mint varied in refinement. The mercury was relatively pure. The particles of powdered silver varied in size and the proportions of mix. Generally the silver mixed with mercury expanded, yet the use of silver fillings spread.

To a large extent the success of silver fillings depended on individual dentists skills. Today the intimate nature of dental materials and tooth structure that holds them is known. Students are taught to cut a tooth, so that the particular filling material it holds and the tooth structure remaining to hold it, are stronger as a completed unit. In those times it depended more on the judgement of each individual practitioner. Some did well, others not so good. News of the new silver fillings spread through the world, increasing in popularity. Some complained their silver fillings failed.

In the 1830's two Frenchmen, the Crawcour brothers, came to New York City, selling with lots of publicity what they claimed was a new remarkable filling material scientifically developed in Europe. They called it Royal Mineral Succedaneum a fancy term for royal mineral substitute, gold. They had a charming, warm, winning manner, and demonstrated their products with samples that looked good outside the mouth and in their own. They sold lots of succedaneum. It was really a rather poor grade of silver amalgam. In a short time it was obvious the new discovery wasn't much good. The Crawcour brothers left a lot of damage and took a lot of money. The wide use they created for silver amalgam started an even greater rebellion against it. Controversy within the dental profession began, becoming so strong it has since been called the Amalgam War. Some of the most prominent dentists, previously conservatively doubtful, declared vehemently against the use of any silver fillings. Some said silver amalgam was poisonous, detrimental to patients health. Some physicians agreed. They were men of high office in the new "American Society of Dental Surgeons" formed in 1840. Feelings led to an official declaration "the use of amalgam is malpractice." The society demanded that its members sign a pledge certifying, "any amalgam whatever is unfit for plugging teeth or fangs and I pledge never under any circumstances to use it in my practice as a dental surgeon." It was stated members must sign the pledge or be expelled from the society. The Amalgam War raged. Opposing groups formed and resentment spread. There are no records of bombs thrown, but dentists against amalgam may have prohibited their sons from courting daughters of dentists who used silver fillings. Many resigned from the society.

During all this a few dentists experimented independently. In 1848 Thomas Evans in Paris tried an amalgam of mercury and tin. Instead of expanding it shrank loosening inside the tooth, and tin amalgam was soft. Dr. Evans found adding cadmium reduced the shrinkage. In Philadelphia 1855, Dr. Townsend after several trials used four parts of silver whose expansion he counteracted with five of tin and mixed that combination with mercury. This made a significant improvement. It was becoming evident a more scientific approach was needed. During the 1870's Dr. J. Foster Flagg organized a group devoted to amalgam research. Scientific investigation proved silver amalgam was harmless to health. Silver and mercury, each of which are used in several beneficial medical drug compounds, unified in the amalgam filling to form an inert mass that has no biological affect on the outer body that surrounds them.

G. V. Black (1836-1915) born in Illinois, probably the leading American contributor to dentistry, did more to perfect silver amalgam than any other man. First he designed an instrument he called the gnathodynanometer (jaw movement measurer) for measuring movement forces of the jaws. The profession was amazed to learn one hundred and seventy five pounds was often exerted in hard chewing, and some sometimes applied as high as three hundred and twenty five. Normal eating action rarely uses more than was 1/5 of the force available. He found that metals used in amalgams must be pure or the mixes they made would be undependable. After years of experimentation, Dr. Black formulated an amalgam combination that was strong and kept its shape and volume in the tooth, neither expanding or contracting. Continuing research since by the American Dental Association and the U.S. Bureau of Standards has added refinements but today's formulas are similar to Black's.

Dr. Black used a microscope to study the intimate structure of the tooth, just as a sculptor seeks to find the nature of his marble. He designed new instruments for cutting teeth. He created new principles of internal cavity design so that the tooth would best support the filling and the tooth and its filling combined would best resist forces upon them and invasion by germs.

Like many brilliant men Black's activities extended beyond his profession. He participated in musical and dramatic arts. He wrote papers several of which entitled, Inflammation, Typhoid and Scarlet Fever, the Basis of Morality, Rain and Storm, and The Earthworm, indicate the great range of his interests. He became involved in the politics of his community and later devoted himself to education becoming the Dean of Chicago's Northwestern University Dental School.

THE DENTAL DRILL

The first drill was probably a small piece of hard stone fractured to a fine point that could be twisted into the tooth. Next came drills made of thin metal rod also turned by turning the hand, or rolled between the palms. Though strong lights and small mirrors were not yet available, a short drill could be used further back in the mouth by revolving between the fingers. Such drilling was of limited value. Access and light were poor, and direct hand and finger turning couldn't twist drills with much power or speed. The tooth's tiny details were not thought of much yet and teeth were more usually removed.

One of man's earliest inventions was the Bow Drill. Created before formal dentistry began, bow drills were used to make holes in all sorts of things, and later by early dental and bone surgeons. As recently as 1962, I saw a primitive jeweler on a street of Marakesh Morocco, bow drilling small holes through gold. The drill consists of two separate parts each held by a hand. One, a bent bow, delivers the motive power. The bow is like the bent bow of an arrow, with a string tied across its opposite ends. The other section has a handle, like a piece of broomstick of round hard wood or metal, long enough for holding in the fist. The handle is hollow like a tube and is closed at one end. The open end has a hole which enters going into along the center axis to the closed end. The drill itself is a long straight thin round metal rod, of such diameter to freely enter and rotate in the handle. The drill rod is longer than the handle. One rod end inserted inside the handle is smoothly blunt. Its opposite end sticking out is the drill sharply wedge pointed for cutting a hole. To drill a hole the operator encircles several turns of the bowstring around the outer drill rod. With one hand directing the handle he presses the drill point into the work being penetrated. The other hand strokes the bow back and forth like that of a violin, while the encircling string winds, twisting and reversing the turning drill being pushed in, drilling a small hole through. For a long time the need for drilling teeth was not thought of. Later when such treatment was done bow drills were awkward for use in back of the mouth.

As technological progress increased, gears were invented for man's more complicated machines, like agricultural equipment and steamships. Gears, which are wheels with driving teeth around their edges, transferred rotating motion inside the machine from one location to another. Dentists adapted gears to hand drills, like those for going through wood, which were held in

TEETH TEETH TEETH

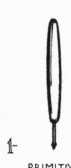

1~
PRIMITIVE
HAND DRILL
turned in one hand
or rolled between palms

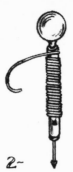

2~
TOP DRILL
one hand holds knob
other pulls string
wound to turn
Described by Hippocrates

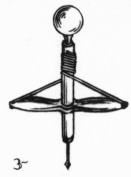

3~
CROSS DRILL
one hand holds knob
other pushes crosspiece
down wound to turn

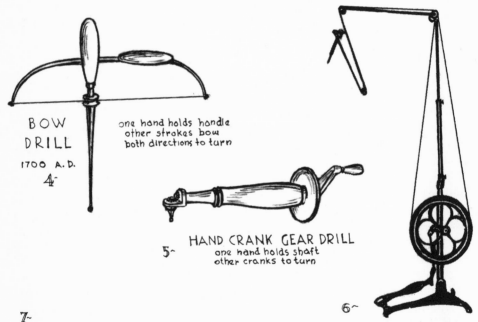

BOW
DRILL
1700 A.D.
4~

one hand holds handle
other strokes bow
both directions to turn

HAND CRANK GEAR DRILL
5~ one hand holds shaft
other cranks to turn

6~
FOOT PEDAL POWERED DRILL
Pulley-cord transmission drives small
handpiece for easier mouth access
Angle drilling attachments also available

7~
MODERN ELECTRIC MOTOR DRIVE
& AIR ROTOR ULTRA SPEED
MINIATURE DRILL PRECISION HANDPIECES

EVOLUTION OF THE DENTAL DRILL S. Garfield

TEETH TEETH TEETH

one hand while the other hand turned a crank around a small arc circle, more convenient than stroking a bow. Next a greater advance was made when dentists learned to adapt bevel gears from the industrial machine industry; they transmitted forces at an angle, so that drills placed into the patients mouth could drill up into upper teeth and down into the lower. Such an appliance was called a Contra-Angle and still is. They're now much smaller and finer. Their bearings are miniature, as precise as those of gyroscopes which direct missiles at the moon. In 1829 James Nasmyth a Scottish engineer tried to conserve dentists energy by applying a coiled wire spring to be hand wound in an assembly for driving small dental drills. The power was low and constant rewinding needed. In 1864 Harrington used a speeded clockwork mechanism with similar results. Though James Watt perfected the steam engine in 1769, I doubt anyone tried adapting steam power to drive dental drills, though it could have been done. The equipment was huge, awkward and expensive. I can see the dentist struggling to drill through an especially hard tooth, yell to his pretty assistant shoveling coal into the mouth of a steam furnace, "More! More! Faster!"

A letter has been found dated November 14, 1860, written by Isaac John Greenwood the son of John Greenwood, dentist to General George Washington, first president of the United States. Isaac describes the use by his father in 1790, of his grandmother's old wooden foot treadle driven spinning wheel, to operate a dental drill.

Dental improvements continued while other events occurred. In 1865 the U.S. Civil War was fought during which for the first time bombs were dropped on other men from balloons.

Later Singer and Howe developed the sewing machine also powered by feet. In 1871 Dr. J.B. Morrison, a dentist, adapted the foot driving portion of the sewing machine to efficiently operate a drill, leaving both dentists hands available for other things. Some busy dentists used seated Assistants feet with signals "start" and "stop." When electric motors appeared they powered sewing machines and dental drills. Dr. Morrison was especially inventive, a year later in 1872, he introduced an improved dental chair. In 1880 the first dental school in France was founded in Paris. In 1881 as the U.S. expanded its western boundary to the Pacific Ocean, the College of Dentistry, University of California, was established in San Francisco.

X – RAY

Medicine and dentistry were advancing. The microscope was available to detect several discovered disease germs. Certain bio-chemical diagnostic tests had been found. It was not yet known that a way could be created for seeing from outside through flesh into the unopened body. Earliest references to penetrating rays are found in Ancient Asian Indian literature, which tells of a tree Bhisajya Raja, whose rays gave an illuminating picture of deep body structures. The log of this tree was reported to contain a gem so powerful, that when placed before the patient his insides were revealed as a lamp shows all objects inside a house. Such logs were said to have been used in 600 B.C. by Jivaka the cranial surgeon. Nothing is known of such a tree today.

Some semblance of such phenomena appeared in Paris 1902, when the intensely radioactive metal radium was discovered by the Curies who extracted compounds of the element from pitch-blend uranium ore. Radium emanates rays which can be seen in the dark and will penetrate solid substances to affect photographic film.

Several years earlier in November 1895, William Konrad Roentgen, a German Professor of Physics at Wurzburg University, while in his darkened laboratory discovered another similar ray. It came from an electrified vacuum tube completely enclosed in a black cardboard box. The invisible rays penetrated the box, moved through the dark room, and struck a phosphorescent barium screen causing it to visibly glow. Roentgen amazed, soon found the rays also penetrated wood and many other materials which stopped passage of ordinary light. He called them "X-Rays." They are also identified as Roentgen Rays. They were stopped best by metals especially platinum and lead. One time, while working, Roentgen's hand came between the ray emanating tube and the phosphorescent screen. He was astounded to see the distinctive forms of his internal skeletal bones while the outer surrounding flesh hardly showed at all. He flexed his hand and saw his finger bones bend on the screen. Motivated scientifically and curiously interested in photography he placed his hand over a photographic plate and after developing had the first x-ray every made. He took a similar picture of his wife's hand showing a ring on her finger. News of his findings astounded the world.

Not understood at first, x-rays started all kinds of stories. The magazine Photography published a poem, "The Roentgen Rays, The Roentgen Rays, What is this craze - the towns ablaze - I hear they'll gaze, through cloak and gown, and even ladies corset stays - These naughty naughty Roentgen Rays." London newspapers advertised x-ray proof underclothing. Cartoons were popular of clothed women seen nude through their covering garments. Assemblyman Reed of Somerset County, introduced a bill to the New Jersey State Legislature prohibiting the use of x-ray opera glasses. A New York newspaper reported, "At the college for physicians and surgeons, the Roentgen Rays were used to reflect anatomic diagrams directly into the brains of the students, making a much more enduring impression than the ordinary methods of learning." Roentgen's wondrous discovery was not fully appreciated by many at first and even skeptically evaluated by others. The president of the British Physical Society declared, "I do not see how the x-ray can lead to results of any significance."

Early apparatus was crude and slow. Exposures took as long as twenty minutes and more. During that entire time the part of the patient being pictured had to be held perfectly still. In December 1895 only two weeks after Roentgen announced his findings, Otto Walkhoff in Braunschweig Germany, took an x-ray of his own teeth using twenty-five minutes of exposure time. Though crude it revealed his inner dental and jaw anatomy. Such pictures had never been seen before except as anatomical drawings sketched by artists from dissected dead. The first significant application of x-rays was during the Spanish American War of 1898 when they were used for locating bullets, previously groped for by blind exploration with serious surgical damage to the body.

In 1897 the College of Dentistry of the University of Southern California was founded in Los Angeles. In the same year at a charity bazaar in Paris, 126 prominent persons were burnt to death within ten minutes. About thirty unfortunates destroyed beyond any other means of recognition were identified by dental records.

As news of x-ray spread, Dr. C.E. Kells in New Orleans became perhaps the first dentist in the U.S. to use them. The dangers of excessive x-ray burns was not yet known. Dr. Kells in ignorance, year after year, with his same own hand held film plates positioned in patients mouths for thousands of x-rays. Each time his old slow apparatus emanated its rays they also penetrated Dr. Kells' hand. The dental profession as a group like the medical profession, was slow to appreciate x-ray value and knew nothing of its early dangers. After ten years in 1906, Dr. Kells transported his equipment from New Orleans to Ashville North Carolina, for demonstration to convince the Southern Dental Society. Like other x-ray pioneers, Dr. Kells devoted attitude and ignorance sacrificed him to science. First he lost three fingers, then his whole hand. His continued suffering led to suicide.

X-ray equipment has since been so perfected and film made so sensitive that today far more accurate pictures can be safely taken in fractions of a second. Modern dental x-rays reveal diseases of the mouth undetectable by the most thorough eye examination.

STRONG PRECISE DENTAL STRUCTURES

Continued invention and perfection of equipment, materials and methods, lowered costs increased dental services and led to further improvements. Until then teeth were restored with soft pure adhesive gold foil, and silver amalgam fillings. Such materials served well to restore teeth by filling cavities as their name Filling describes. Like tooth itself these substances have compressive strength, or the ability to resist forces applied directly upon them like clay brick used in building. They have little tensile strength tying them intimately together and from continued prolonged use, individual particles of such fillings may tear crumbling apart. A better material would also have tensile strength like steel, so that in addition to replacing missing tooth parts it would strengthen the tooth with a man provided tensile quality, better than tooth enamel or dentine. Such material can help hold teeth together. Hard gold alloys had already been used this way by forging and bending and soldering. These processes are time consuming, expensive, and difficult to do with the precision needed in dentistry. Metals when melted liquid can be easily directed into precise forms, which after they cool solidifying hard as castings, have superior compressive and tensile strength. It would be easy if molten metals could be poured into tooth cavities to harden. Earlier, tin, lead, mercury, all soft, weak, low melting point metals, were tried this way and abandoned. Gold alloys molten to a liquid for precision flowing are at red and white hot temperatures of 1600 degrees and higher.

On January 15, 1907 Dr. Wm. Taggart a Chicago dentist, read his scientific paper in New York City entitled "A New and Accurate Method of Casting Gold Inlays." His work of many years consolidated and adapted various art and industrial Lost-Wax processes to the production of especially precise castings as needed for dentistry. Dr. Taggart's process involved the use of soft wax in the mouth, to carve models of the missing tooth parts needed, and a technique outside the mouth for replacing the wax model with an identical precise gold structure casting.

These castings finished in the dental laboratory were placed or laid and cemented in place inside the tooth and called Inlays. They have tensile strength, so that when hit by even hardest foods and opposite chewing teeth, they withstand forces being transferred to their adjacent natural remaining tooth parts. All this is telling of what may seem tiny things. Such details though small are of great value to the preservation of teeth. Dr. Taggart's process quickly spread. More gold inlays were made. Improved methods permitted larger more complex castings. Today gold and other metals are precisely cast for structural parts of large dental bridges and other oral appliances. Materials perfected by dentistry for precision casting have since been so refined that other industries now use them.

TEETH TEETH TEETH

INSIDE AND BEYOND THE HEART OF THE TOOTH

In the technologically expanding United States, with the spirit which accompanies progress, more efforts were made to save teeth and more bridges to replace lost teeth. Wealthy Europeans came to see America and for what was considered modern dentistry. Even the fastest drills were slow. Tooth cutting was shocking to the teeth they cut. Teeth for supporting bridges replacing missing teeth needed especially heavy work. Such severe operation was agonizing to the tooth's live inner heartlike pulp and nerve. It was common practice before cutting crowns of such teeth to drill a hole through into the soft live pulp contents and pack in arsenic. This penetrated killing the nerve. After several days of pain subsided, heavy tooth preparation could be done. Arsenic is a deadly poison. It is used to kill vermin. Yet in trace amounts arsenic may be necessary to life. It is found in all plant and animal cells. Certain arsenic compounds have been used as a tonic. Certain of its compounds kill germs. Ehrlich's salvarsan 606 treatment used arsenic to cure syphilis. The dental theory was that the arsenic confined inside the hard strong root walls was an antiseptic reservoir within the tooth keeping the area germ free. Many bridges were built on such teeth foundations, supporting replaced false teeth and served well for years.

In 1911 William Hunter an English physician with a wealthy London practice, lectured to the Medical Faculty of McGill University in Montreal Canada. He accused "American dentistry" of contributing to poor health. Hunter referred to cleverly constructed precise bridges as "Mausoleums of gold over a mass of sepsis." To some extent he was right. This was before today's revealing blood infection tests were known. In London Dr. Hunter had noticed unhealthy looking tissues surrounding the bridges of several of his patients and suggested they be removed. The patients objected. Their bridges were expensive, kept them looking younger and chewing better. At Dr. Hunter's persistence some sicker people were convinced. The bridgework, supporting teeth, roots and all were removed. Foul smelling pus followed and many patients recovered feeling better. Teeth became considered a source of "Focal Infection" and the theory of focal infection took hold and spread. Teeth were extracted in great numbers, many unnecessarily. Though x-rays had been invented, the equipment was crude, very expensive and not used much yet. Dental x-rays involved tiny details the interpretation of which was not yet known. All sorts of disorders were blamed on teeth, rheumatism, poor eyesight, kidney pains, almost everything.

Infected teeth did undermine health and much had been caused by the arsenic. Unknowingly the arsenic ate its way through the tooth root tips

TEETH TEETH TEETH

THE HISTORY OF DENTISTRY

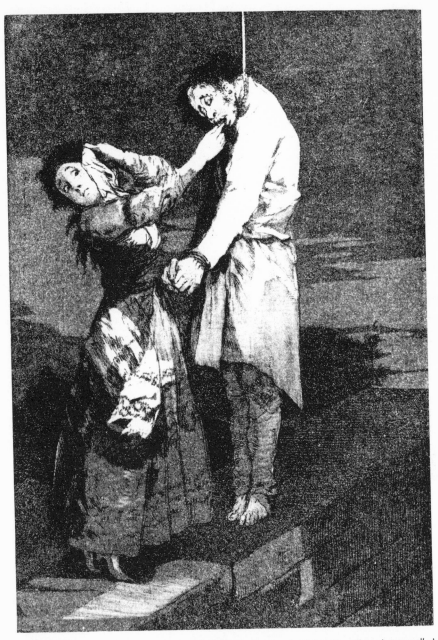

An aquatint etching by the Spanish artist Francisco Goya. 1746-1828. The above called A caza de dientes or TOOTH HUNTING portrays custom of his time. Teeth were stolen from the dead and extracted alive for sale to dentists for transplanting into other peoples mouths. There was common superstition that toothache could be cured by touching teeth of the dead

TEETH TEETH TEETH

destroying the weaker surrounding jawbone beyond them. After the arsenics ability to counteract germs was spent, the deep eroded bone was especially subject to severe germ invasion.

During this time, while some dentists were concerned with inner causes and treatment of dental disease, others became interested in the affect of substances from outside the body on teeth. In 1914 a Dr. Cook discovered different ratios of tooth decay in different parts of the country which he felt was due to differences in the quality of drinking water. He made no reference to fluorine or fluorides. In 1925 a Dr. Bunting found evidence in a survey at Minonk Illinois. Children born and raised there had less decay than others who moved to Minonk after their teeth had developed. Bunting also felt it was the water but didn't know the active agent. Later Minonk water was found to contain 2.5 parts per million of fluoride.

In the U.S. meanwhile concern for hidden dental infections continued. Dr. Edward Rosenow of Rochester's Mayo Clinic campaigned against such focal infection into the 1930's. Physicians, unfamiliar and hardly concerned with dentistry before this time, ordered boundless teeth extractions. Teeth were removed for headache and stomach problems. In some cases it helped. In many the teeth were lost but the inadequately diagnosed disease remained. It was an era of mass needless teeth extraction losses and full removable dentures.

The dental profession alerted, concentrated to correct its own deficiencies. X-ray techniques were improved. Methods were devised for treating the inner pulps of teeth without arsenic, using harmless beneficial drugs for sealing root tips, so that x-rays showed that even bone which had been lost before by abscess infection actually grew filling back in healthy. Tooth cutting equipment has been improved so that virtually no shock is experienced by even heavily cut teeth. Nerves remain alive, healthy and functioning, in teeth that support bridges replacing many that were missing.

Dental advances seem endless. Further improvements are yet to come the nature of which we do not even know.

A HISTORICAL TOOTH OF GOLD

While researching for this chapter, "The History of Dentistry," in several of the more thorough texts I discovered an old story of a very special Golden Tooth.

In 1593 in Schweidnitz, a small town near Silesia in Germany, a seven year old boy Christoph Muller the son of a poor carpenter, was found to have erupted a golden molar tooth, the last in his lower left jaw. The tooth in front of it was missing. At that time nothing was known of such things around the countryside. It was the age of alchemy, when the sought for philosophers stone would turn everything it touched to gold. The astounding news traveled fast. People came from diverse distances to see the wonder. Among them was Jacob Horst, Physician and Professor of Medicine at the Julius University in Helmstadt. These were times of little logic and long sought for miracles. In 1595 Dr. Horst wrote a book about the tooth. Printing not long invented was rapidly increasing. Reading spread as a new life experience. All sorts of things were published and bought including Dr. Horst's book. Many copies were sold.

Dr. Horst said the tooth was a sign from heaven. He made astrological analytical calculations which declared Christoph's birth and tooth resulted from both natural and supernatural causes. On his birthday, December 22, 1585, the Sun was in conjunction with Saturn in the sign of Ram. Dr. Horst said the coincidence had special significance. Nutritive forces at the time had a particular strength, causing a great heavenly increase of heat, so that the boy's tooth instead of becoming hard bone continued forming into gold. This he said, like phenomena of earthquakes, eclipses and comets, was a sign of great events to follow.

He presented complicated biblical interpretations of his own which he used to make predictions. Since the tooth was on the left side of the lower jaw, the events would begin with calamities of war, famines and pestilences. The Golden Tooth indicated a new Golden Age. The Roman Emperor would sweep the Turks from Europe. An epoch of happiness would follow. Christianity would rule and since the golden tooth was last in the jaw it indicated the Golden Age would be perpetual beginning Judgement Day. Horst's writings created sensation. He gave many university lectures which caused serious discussions and controversies.

For years others also wrote concerning the tooth. Horst was famous. Studies began in what was a new Science of the Golden Tooth. Many people completely accepted the validity of the tooth being gold but differed with Horst's interpretations. Many devoted, defended his precise position. Some considered Horst a fool or faker, and the tooth a fraud.

Christophs' father permitted examination of the tooth for payment. He wasn't quite as poor now. Gold tests were made and passed. At times however, the boy went into fits of apparent madness making inspection impossible. It was noticed this happened when learned investigators approached.

Duncan Liddel a Scottish professor visiting Germany, years later wrote a book revealing the truth. He noted the tooth was larger than the others, and had none in front or behind. Liddel deduced a thin plate of gold had been fashioned to cover it. One day a doubting nobleman with a dagger, forced the boy's mouth open. Thorough inspection revealed the gold had worn

TEETH TEETH TEETH

through and natural tooth showed around its borders. Many resented the disclosure and attacked Liddel preferring to believe Horst's Golden Predictions. The story of the tooth persisted. Reports of another golden tooth appeared of a boy in Poland. Like Scotlands Loch Ness Monster and Flying Saucers, mysterious romantic intrigues seem to persist. A hundred years later in 1695 still another dissertation was written interpreting the Silesian tooth of gold.

RECENT GOLDEN TEETH INTRIGUE

I was recently told of a self styled preacher who could cure defective teeth with gold inlays by devoted prayer. As a result of discussion with my informing patient who is interested in metaphysics, my name and home address were given to the evangelist reverend of what he called Advanced Understanding. I asked not to be identified as a dentist. In 1966 in the Los Angeles area, I received correspondence through the mail from the reverend who used the title Doctor stating he had gold inlays appear in his mouth initiated purely by what he called Spiritual Energy. He declared no dentist had put them there. They were available for inspection but not by dentists or others who doubted. Offerings to keep his work going were not demanded but appreciated. I was informed all such offerings were tax deductable.

Knowledge that follows this dental history
Explains, Informs, Clears Earlier Mystery

TEETH TEETH TEETH

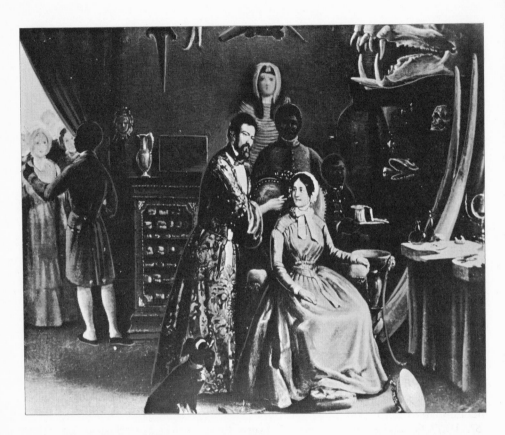

AN EXTRAORDINARY DENTIST ∾ Dr. Georges Fettet practiced in Paris during the reign of Louis Philipp and Napoleon III. He would have been an unusual man for any place or time. This painting by E. Pingret of Dr. G. Fettet in 1850, shows the distinguished doctor in his distinctive office. He adorned its walls with teethy anatomical specimens and other rare curios. Claiming a superior denture making technique he advertised extensively, using many pictures of himself in popular publications. He rode Paris' streets driven by elaborately harnessed horses pulling his beautifully appointed denture-shaped carriage, accompanied by blaring trumpeteers.

2

AN ORDINARY DENTIST

I'm a dentist, a bachelor. Not quite content. At one time I was married to the most wonderful girl in the world. She was beautiful, bold, sexy, sensitive, graceful, well formed, occasionally blond, intelligent and generous. We had happy years. As with others in these troubled times unfortunately, discord replaced our bliss, our love lost, we rebelled and parted.

My wife a former professional dancer and I, were walking along Hollywood's Sunset Blvd. when she guided me into Schwabs Sunset Drug Store. Schwabs Sunset is rendezvous for artists actors writers, and aspiring artists actors and writers, of canvas screen T.V. and theater. Gertrude saw at a far corner Laslo Vadnay, a friend of Pre-Sydney Garfield Days. Before coming to this country Laslo a Hungarian, was renowned as a writer in Europe. He's been called the Mark Twain of Hungary. Laslo's written many successful T.V. and motion pictures.

"Lutsy" she cried, "Gertrude" Lutsy replied. After greetings I was introduced. "Lutsy" she said, "It's wonderful seeing you again. Surprise, I'm married and would like you to meet my husband Syd, he's a dentist." "No" Lutsy said, "Please - No - Gertrude - No -please not a dentist. I can write a story about a lawyer, a politican, a doctor, cowboy or Indian. I can write about anything, a banker, a crook. But no Gertrude, no, please not a dentist. I can't write a story about a dentist." "But Lutsy" Gertrude said, "You don't know Syd. He's not an ordinary dentist." [Laslo Vadnay later became my dental patient. I hadn't seen him for several years until on Feb. 27, 1967 he visited my office for dental treatment in preparation for a trip he was taking within a few days to Hungary. I showed him part of this book's almost completed manuscript and reminded him of his statement at our first meeting. Laslo said, "Syd, I've just changed my mind. I could write a story about a dentist." I will never see Laslo Vadnay again. He died in Budapest, April 18, 1967.]

Several divorced years later, noontime, I left my office on Camden Drive Beverly Hills, for a lunchtime stroll as I often do. Turning left I walked north to Little Santa Monica Blvd. Across the street I saw what might have been a blonde angel. I'm partial to blondes. My eyes widened. She was graceful, well formed, tastefully simply dressed, walking west. I crossed for a closer look. She was gorgeous and continued walking. I followed.

TEETH TEETH TEETH

She crossed Rexford and stopped at windows of The Flea Market. The Flea Market, no longer there, was an art and gift shop at the north-west corner of Little Santa Monica Blvd. and Bedford Drive. I crossed Bedford and with shy courage stopped near. Moving closer I spoke. Surprised delight, she answered, friendly too. Voice soft, sweet, warm. I could hardly believe. We exchanged comments concerning the objects in the shop window. It was wonderful that she had such sensitive appreciation, liking the same things I did. Thrills. She called my attention to a small Italian black wrought iron square topped table, covered with alternating little black and white tiles. "It's a pity" she said, "the designer did not realize if he had used only another row of tiles each way across the top, the table could also serve as a chess or checker board." I hadn't noticed or thought of this clever deduction and told her so. I was tempted to be bold and ask to meet her again, but lacked courage. Meekly I left and crossed the adjacent parkway to Santa Monica Boulevard another street without the Little in its name that runs close and parallel. Longfully I looked back regretting my lack of daring. I've reacted this way before.

From the distance my following eyes saw her get into a parked car, and from alongside the seat take a package which she opened for lunch. This was more than I could possibly resist. I returned, and through the auto's open window said, "Pardon me miss, but when I first saw your beauty I was overwhelmed, and hearing your sensitive remarks concerning the art was wonderful, and your brilliant analysis of the table top. You're marvelous. But because of personal feelings of inadequacy I lacked the courage to ask to see you again. However after leaving, looking back when I saw you, sweet, beautiful, clever as you are, so down to earth as to take your lunch with you to have in your automobile, parked in Beverly Hills, that was too much. I had to come back." She gave me her name and telephone number. We soon dated. First once then twice a week. I was soon seeing Dolores every day. After we'd known each other for perhaps two months Dolores said, "Syd, remember that first day I met you, and when you came back to the car to talk with me. I liked you, but when you said you were a dentist I thought - Oh My God - Not a Dentist. But Syd, really, now that I know you I must tell you, you're not an ordinary dentist."

A DENTIST

The degree is D.D.S. D.D.S. means doctor of dental surgery. Some dental schools give the same training for the same profession but issue the D.M.D. degree which means doctor of medical dentistry. There's really no difference in license or practice. By ancient definition a doctor was a learned man and teacher. Today doctor is also an academic title, and a doctor is any person upon whom a college, university, or other accredited institution, has bestowed the doctorate degree. There are many kinds of doctorates awarded to those who study the particular material needed to earn them. Often the few letters designating the titled degree are the first of the modern name, such as M.D. for medical doctor and D.V.M. for doctor of veterinary medicine. D.D. is doctor of divinity. D.C. means doctor of chiropractic and in states that recognize such degrees chiropractors may call themselves doctor. Many doctors have the Ph.D which means philosophy doctor or doctor of philosophy. Philosophy is an old word for knowledge or wisdom. Ph.D is awarded in many branches of knowledge. The degree is more commonly held by psychologists, physicists, other scientists and members of schools of higher learning like college professors. Many people ordinarily think of doctors as those that treat the body's ills.

AN ORDINARY DENTAL EDUCATION

In the United States for dental school admission to earn the dental degree, students must complete the same preparatory college material needed for admission to medical school. In addition, dental students today are subjected to tests of manual skill. Dental education takes four full years of intensive study, just like the medical, and contains much of the same material studied by medical doctors. Since dental disease affects the entire body and the surrounding body affects mouth health, dental students are taught basic human medicine. In Italy, dentistry is a specialty of medical practice and the dentist must first complete his medical education before studying dentistry, just as in the U.S. where psychiatry is a specialty of medicine, the psychiatrist must first complete his medical education.

Dental students study the human organism thoroughly. In the anatomy laboratory, in small closely supervised teams, each student dissects human cadavers, young and old, male and female. The entire body from skin outside, through the muscles to the ligaments that hold them attached to bones and support vital organs, heart, liver, kidneys, lungs, brain and others, each are examined closely and discussed. Students must pass examinations given directly on such human bodies and written examinations proving such knowledge. Special attention is given to structures of the mouth and head. Students also study the skeletal structures, bones of the body and the bones of the head. Opportunity often exists to purchase personal specimens. It is sad, though interesting, that most, probably all human skeletal material comes from poverty stricken India, where commercial enterprises exist in which living workers are employed to clean bones of the dead which are sold as biological specimens. And even at this level skulls with fewer teeth, are considered less desirable and are lower priced.

Dental curriculum includes physiology, the function of each organ and its tissues and how they coordinate contributing to the function of the entire body. Histology is studied, the microscopic nature of human tissues and their characteristics in each organ, skin, ligaments, lungs, kidneys and all others. Biochemistry, the intimate chemical biological changes which occur in organs and tissues and cells, blood and lymph and body secretions. Embryology, the development of tissues and organs from their first beginning when the mother ova or egg is fertilized by male sperm. Then on as they specialize, changing to each organs full mature functioning form at adulthood. Dental students study all the body's glands, thyroid and parathyroid, and adrenals and pituitary, and the sex glands, and what they do, and secrete, and what those secretions do. And through all this study of the body special attention is given again to the affect of those things on mouths and teeth.

In addition to normal body functions, Pathology, the study of disease is undertaken. Parasitology, the sicknesses caused by mans larger invaders like worms, and the habits of those parasites. Bacteriology, the nature of germs and invisible viruses, how each appears under the microscope and as they attack our tissues causing their forms of disease. Again wherever disease is evidenced in mouths they're given concentrated attention. Dental students also study Tumors, benign or harmless and malignant deadly Cancers of the body and in greater detail again those that grow in regions of the mouth, jaws and throat. They're taught to take biopsy specimens when in doubt. Anesthesiology is taught so that procedures may be perfomed without pain. Pharmacology is included, the nature and chemistry of natural and synthetic medications and toxins and anti-toxins and anti-biotics and drugs and narcotics so that dentists can properly prescribe. Nutrition is studied, the body's feeding requirements, food values which best satisfy them in good health and vitamins and other supplements for deficiency diseases.

Dental education of course centers around teeth. These are studied from every biological aspect, starting with their formation in the uterus embryo, through successive stages as disclosed by dissection of deceased human specimens. The intimate chemical physical nature of teeth are analysed and the way they attach into jawbones. The muscles that move those bones, the circulatory blood vessels that feed teeth, bones and adjacent tissues, and the sensory nerves that send brain signals to move all those things and how they move.

The dentist is taught the pathology or diseases that attack hard outer tooth substance like enamel and dentin and soft inner live contents like pulp and

TEETH TEETH TEETH

nerve. He studies the intimate nature of diseases that destroy the attachments of teeth to their surrounding soft gum and hard bone supporting tissues. He's taught medical, surgical and mechanical treatment of those diseases. His education includes basic engineering sciences and qualities of the physical materials used and the technical training for operating the hand and power tools used to work them. Artistic concept of how teeth should look for best personal appearance and psychological factors related to teeth and the people that chew them.

Each dental school has a clinic in which students under examining control of dentist instructors must complete minimum amounts of many types of dental treatment. This is similar to the practical experience medical doctors get during their internship. Students x-ray patients, examine them, make models of their mouths, discuss treatment plans and procedures. Under guidance every phase of dentistry ordinarily expected later outside, is performed by each student in school. They clean teeth, apply anesthesia, first injecting each other for practice. Fillings of all kinds are made, plastic and porcelain, silver and gold and inlays and fixed bridges and jackets and removable bridges and full removable dentures. Extractions, pyorrhetic and other surgical procedures are performed and endodontic saving of abscessed teeth. The program is tough. Students are in school all day, not only two semesters of each four years but most of summer vacations between. Time is spent studying at home. Some of the work may be pleasurable but the heavy schedule seems torturous at times. After graduation with the dental doctor degree the government submits each student to an examination which must be passed for license to practice. This is all endured becoming an ordinary dentist. Many continue with advanced or post-graduate training. Some study further techniques for individual specialized branches of dentistry and limit their practice to such work.

These dentists or ordinary dental doctors like physicians or ordinary medical doctors are sometimes unreasonably expected by some to be very extraordinary people. Each as a human born of ordinary sired women can only be the ordinary person he is. Doctors of Divinity may be considered by some to be emissaries of God but doctors of health should only be expected to be people.

All doctors, even those who present an air of apparent aloof austerity are quite human under the skin. As Gilbert & Sullivan's opera says, "Things are seldom what they seem, skim milk masquerades as cream." Some dental doctors are humble, some are proud, some reserved, some are loud. Some are shy, others bold. Some hot, warm, cold. Some successfully are rather content. Some have trouble with children, wives and related relatives. Many have the same occasional ordinary feelings of insecurity felt by other ordinary people. Some are especially capable. A few may be incompetent. Most like most others sincerely do the best they can and render satisfactory services.

Even the finest die from ordinary causes and also make occasional errors. People indignantly feel a brain surgeon can't afford ever to make a mistake. It's more reasonable to realize surgeons, medical and dental can only do what humans can. Professional services they receive for their own bodies selves sometimes fail and supreme efforts performed by them even to their most beloved may not succeed.

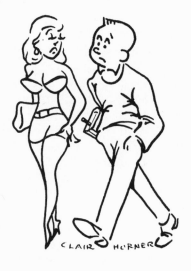

You only say you love me. You date me cause I have so many cavities you can take tests with.

TEETH TEETH TEETH

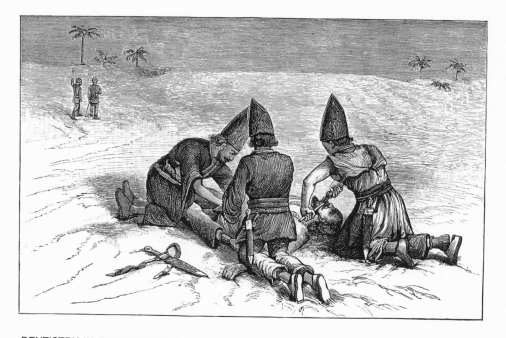

DENTISTRY IN THE DESERT—Drawn by A. Locher during an early 1880's caravan trip from Bombay to Constantinople. Described in his book ''With Star and Crescent,'' published 1888. Assistants holding the patient were needed to keep him controlled.

TEETH TEETH TEETH

PSYCHOSOMATIC PSYCHOLOGICAL PSYCHIATRIC DENTISTRY

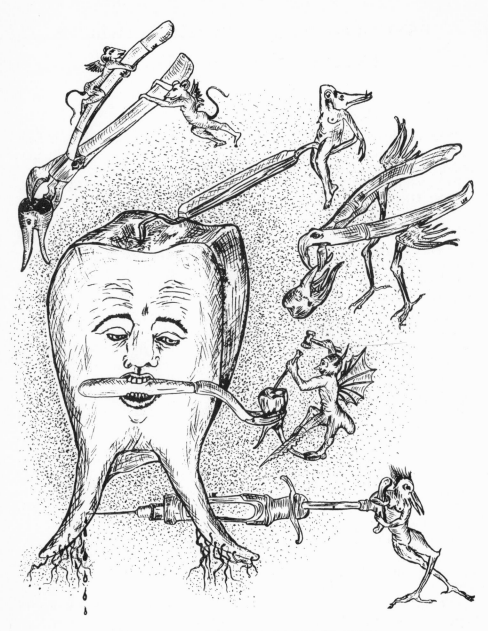

MENTAL DENTAL by RICHARD LEE

TEETH TEETH TEETH

3

PSYCHOSOMATIC PSYCHOLOGICAL PSYCHIATRIC DENTISTRY

PSYCHE is the mind. SOMA the body. Psychosomatic is the mind and body combined as a unit. The word psychosomatic is popularly used relating the minds emotions to affects they cause on body health.

PSYCHOLOGY is a science of the mind of man in all its aspects. PSYCHIATRY is a specialty of medicine dealing with mental disorders.

This chapter describes various mental phenomena related to dental problems from those of simple significance to some of such severity that psychiatric assistance may be needed.

The basic unit in dentistry is the tooth. I looked up the word in the giant sized Webster's New International Dictionary, Unabridged, and found the word tooth occupied two and one half columns of a full three column page. The tooth is very important to man. Over a full half column gave the somatic or physical anatomical and physiological definition of the tooth as it occurs in man and other animals. Two columns devoted to other uses combining the word tooth with other words. Many of these definitions involve emotional applications.

If something is "toothsome" it is tasty or delicious. A "tooth" for fruit or sweets indicates preference for such things.

And then, things could be, "as clean as a hounds tooth."

There are "teeth" that go around the gears of apparatus for the transmission of power in intricate mechanisms like that of a tiny fine precision watch and mammoth mountain moving machines.

To ride in the "teeth of a gale" or in the "teeth of danger" is being intimately involved with such a situation.

And to get a really tough job done we have to "sink our teeth" into it.

Or seeing a beautiful girl though those who find her "toothsome" shouldn't sink their teeth, they might like to take a little bite or at least a nibble.

Also, important international laws governing relations between powerful nations are of little value unless these laws have "teeth in them."

And the military might of such nations are fully prepared for battle only when they are "armed to the teeth."

Teeth are related to emotions and often to strength and virility.

TEETH TEETH TEETH

PSYCHOSOMATIC PSYCHOLOGICAL PSYCHIATRIC DENTISTRY

Primitive tribes in many parts of the world hunt and kill their enemies and wild animals. They often remove and use their teeth as bodily adornments feeling that this way they can transfer to themselves the ferocity, bravery, virility and strength of their conquered prey. Generally we think of people that are toothless as being rather harmless.

DENTAL PSYCHOLOGY

Let's study the psychology of some dental patients who'd rather not be a patient at all. Who would want to be. It's even bother brushing teeth; it's nuisance getting closely between them and far behind those back tooth corners and a couple of minutes every morning may not sound like much but it's lots of trouble when you have to do it. So "Don't bother me Teeth and I won't bother you." But it won't work that way. Teeth demand loyal treatment and if you're not true to them they will become false to you. Those who avoid facing reality can foolishly try to forget, but then at a party there's a slight pain--, well, it passed away and it's easier thinking it's nothing at all. Last week while at work it came back worse. It left again thank God. But tonight it's murder - unbearable - I can't possibly stand it. I hate going to the dentist. But that's not as bad as this P-A-I-N I'll pay anything to stop.

We resent being forced to go to the dentist. In these days of competitive aggression, with an expanding search for freedoms, we rebel at being forced to anything. Our lives have been so eased by increasing comforts we resent intrusion by any diversion from our expected paths of ease. We resent the failure of a light, a radio or television set, the plumbing leak and an automobile's sudden unexpected lack of performance. We resent the failures of continued comfort but it's wonderful receiving the benefits of proper restoration. We prefer not having to pay for such services though they're worth the price.

FEAR ∞ Many psychological factors affect dentistry. Perhaps the foremost is fear. Fear is a powerful deterring emotion. President Franklin D. Roosevelt, at a time of great national and world crisis said, "We have nothing to fear but fear itself." Many fears are based on misconceptions caused by ignorance. Entering a strange dark haunted house one is instantly alerted with fright. A wisp of cobweb felt in the dark against skin of arm or cheek could terrorize as a squeeking creak magnifies alarm. Turn on the light - remove the dark ignorance to see. Sigh, relief, perhaps even laugh, at understanding unwarranted fear. The strongest emotion keeping most from dentistry is fear. Fear of pain, magnified by dreaded

TEETH TEETH TEETH

PSYCHOSOMATIC PSYCHOLOGICAL PSYCHIATRIC DENTISTRY

expectancy, exaggerated beyond proportion by ignorance of what really happens.

Some fears are begun by causes that are real and even natural. The child initially feels tooth pains when his first are forcing their way through. Parents at this time who've similarly suffered themselves, and had other real toothaches, and been misguided by their own parents in alarm, themselves now alarm frightening their children. Children and parents today live in a time of scientific dental revolution. A period when memories of pains that needed suffering for the performance of earlier treatments, invade the beginning of an era when dental therapy and cures need no longer be felt. To say that modern dentistry is absolutely painless is untrue. It is true however that modern dentistry can perform all its needed functions with little pain discomfort and often with none.

A middle aged unfortunate woman was my worst patient for years. She had many emotional problems and a dread of dentistry. Half her teeth were gone, and those remaining ugly and unattractive and most needed treatment. They always seemed to hurt. It was only when she suffered unbearable pain that Mrs. Tumolt would make an appointment. She'd come to the office apprehensively fearful, often crying ashamed. She may have needed psychiatric help for reasons other than dentistry. In the dental chair she always sat frightened, closely watching every of my moves. Mrs. Tumolt was aware of her own problem and when she felt forced to come for help would often say, "I'm better today Dr. Garfield, can't you see I'm a better patient today." It was sad. Seated for treatment she was almost unmanageable, poor soul. An assistant had to stand by assuring her, holding her strongly to get anything done.

One day Mrs. Tumolt came to our office for the removal of two teeth, she was terribly frightened. Coincidentally, I had with me the original manuscript of this book's chapter "Oral Surgery." I suggested that she read while waiting, a portion describing in vivid detail the extraction of teeth. She said she would. Later peeking through a communicating window into the reception room, I saw Mrs. Tumolt sitting restlessly afraid. The written pages were lying unopened on her lap. Nervously she said she'd read them later. I demanded that she read the material immediately, emphasizing that concentrating and understanding its contents was part of her treatment. Peeking through the opening I saw Mrs. Tumolt slowly reading attentively, turning page after page. As I later entered the waiting room she said, "Gee Dr. Garfield, this is interesting, I didn't know it was anything like that." We waited till she'd read it all. That was the first time in all our years that Mrs. Tumolt responded cooperatively while her dentistry was performed.

TEETH TEETH TEETH

PSYCHOSOMATIC PSYCHOLOGICAL PSYCHIATRIC DENTISTRY

Associated with fears based on ignorance are fears of body invasion and loss of personal control. The bodies we own are very private and we resent their being entered without willing invitation. It is an intrusion of our rights of self and ego. The dentist is in the peculiar position of being a better informed legally accredited authority, with such a right and power. We resent it, especially since in ignorance the patient doesn't know what is being done, may wonder whether the right thing is done, has little control of what is done, and in this age of increasing personal rivalry many resist such loss of control.

THE NEEDLE ∞ Lets study some aspects of the injection of a hypodermic needle, inside the mouth into deep beneath the tissues, for administration of anesthesia as it may affect some fearful people. The dentist is in power now - in complete control. He is making a very personal invasion. He enters the patient through the mouth, a very special place. The mouth is the patients primary source of communication. A major means for guiding his life. Through it he talks conveying his ideas, and tells of his strength and conquests and loves, and does love, and aggressively expresses hate, and often uses it to earn and eat his bread. And in this personal controlling place of his own he is made utterly defenseless. The patient feels weak and frightened as the mouse helplessly held by the clawed paw of a cat. He is at the mercy of the dentist.

And now an especially intimate invasion takes place. In some ways more intimate than any other in life. Through a fine hollow needle, which seems to get sharper longer as it comes closer, and in a way is a sneaky approach, the dentist through the mouth is penetrating and entering his very flesh. He objects, and seeking every excuse even magnifies pain in objection. And all this is done so critically close to the brain, the controlling mechanism of his very being. And just beyond reach of his eyes. He cannot see or understand or affect these things. Even those who do, might still suffer vestiges of inherited fears. Some dentists themselves undergo similar reactions while being treated by others. They are also human, believe it or not.

Even after anesthesia is administered many people are apprehensive about the work. I've had significant success with such patients saying, "I don't expect to hurt you. I will proceed slowly in such a manner that even if you were not anesthetised it would first not hurt at all and then only slightly like this," at which time I slowly gently increase the pressure of a finger pinch. I continue, "If it should hurt you at all, raise your free left hand." This is the opposite side from where I usually work. I see that the left hand is free of any covering. "Now I do not want you to be brave and cooperative, and try to bear even slight pain if you should feel it. I don't

TEETH TEETH TEETH

want you to feel any pain at all. If you do feel even the slightest, raise your left hand and I will stop. In fact, even if you don't feel any pain, you can test me by raising your hand. I will stop." If the hand raises, I stop. The patient soon feels in control and losing fears of the unknown unexpected, gains confidence. Work is always accomplished. The hand is rarely raised. Work stops if it is, yet rarely ever has to. With a few such appointments stopping isn't needed any longer.

SEX

An ancient practice concerning teeth and sex was told me by an Arab. Though investigation disclosed it was common knowledge in some areas, I could not document its origin. The details are that Mohammedan princes and sheikhs in addition to emasculating or removing the masculinity of selected males, by castration of their sex organs, for conversion to eunuch guardians of harems of women, would often also extract their teeth.

Psychological analysis relating teeth to strength virility and sex, have been made by important contributors to the mental sciences. Hermann Rorschach M.D. the Swiss psychiatrist, created and perfected the Rorschach Ink Blot psychological testing technique. Ink blots with random designs and patterns are studied for imagined recognition of common object forms within them, like seeing images in the sky's clouds. What the person tested discerns as objects in the blots, is valuable clue to his psychic situation. According to the diagnostic standards established by Dr. Rorschach, recognition of teeth in ink blots is indication of aggression. Aggression is often related to virility and sex. Seeing the mouth in ink blots is also evidence of sexual symbolism. Sigmund Freud M.D. the father of psychoanalysis, makes several references relating teeth to sex and the loss of teeth to castration. Strong healthy teeth indicate feelings of sexual security. Dreams involving fears of the loss of teeth often relate to fears of castration and the loss of sexual prowess.

ANIMAL PSYCHOLOGY EXAMPLE ∾ The following story told me by Earl Chumley a former animal trainer with the Los Angeles Zoo, and a many year experienced animal dealer is significant. In the early 1950's at the L.A. Zoo they had an especially vicious eleven year old male African baboon. He attacked all others caged with him, young and old, small and large, male and female. He was especially active sexually, regularly raping all the female baboons. He terrorized the other males and the entire cage. He would lift his lips, baring his teeth, showing his fangs. He had long upper canines often used in ferocious attack on the other animals. He was hard to handle. The zoo veterinarian decided to extract them. Immediately his personality changed. He lost all aggression and his virility ceased. He sat regressed now in a corner browbeaten. Perhaps he needed an animal psychiatrist. Even old females started picking on him and he would retreat rather than fight back. His spirit was gone. He lost weight and his coat became shaggy. For two and a half years this former bully now afraid kept shyly to himself. Perhaps veterinary-dentist-made false fangs would have helped. As a result of his declining condition special medical help, food, and vitamins were administered. For the first time at the age of thirteen and a half he started making feeble sexual advances again. He never returned to his former vigor or virility and died a few years later. To quote Earl,"You've got to have teeth to be a fighter and you've got to be a fighter to be a lover. You can't have one without the other."

HUMAN EXAMPLE ∾ A strong, handsome, well dressed, intelligent, successful stock broker patient whose front teeth I had restored and improved with porcelain jackets once told me, "Whenever I feel low and depressed I look at these beautiful virile teeth in a mirror and feel a sense of well being returning."

Our bodies are the only thing we really own and the loss of any part including teeth are a loss of part of ourselves. I believe many people with paining teeth avoid dentistry for fears including the possible loss of those teeth, subconsciously relating this to aging and the loss of attractiveness and sexual virility. Such psychological knowledge can be of value in planning dental restoration.

Lets consider the case of a patient all of whose upper teeth are missing except for the two cuspids, eye teeth or canines, right and left, one on each side. All teeth behind the cuspids are missing. The four front incisors between the cuspids are missing. I will describe three possible restorative treatments. The simplest least expensive, would be to extract the two cuspids leaving the upper jaw completely toothless covered with bare fleshy gum. Without a denture in the mouth, the patient's lower jaw moves far upward flattening the lips forward, aging the face. Many hate being seen that way by friends and mates. Many shamefully hide such mouths with hands. Wearing a well made denture helps while it is worn, though full removable dentures without rooted teeth to hook on to, are sometimes hard to handle.

The second treatment would be first restoring the two cuspids if they needed treatment, and providing a removable denture which supplies the four front teeth between the cuspids, and the back teeth on each side behind them. With the denture out of the mouth, the two upper toothed person is still not very attractive to friends, but doesn't look quite as weak or meek, and himself feels the confident added presence of those two natural parts, even for the short time his denture isn't worn. The more properly related lower jaw, which can't overclose, also provides more natural personal feeling. When the upper denture is worn the two supporting cuspids supply far better side grinding control, giving the wearer greater security and personal confidence. He can enjoy eating better. This treatment costs more than the first and is worth it.

The third possibility is best. This involves making a fixed front bridge, restoring the four front teeth between the cuspids, permanently attached undiscernibly to each cuspid right and left for support. It helps strengthen each tooth mutually, can't be taken from the mouth and doesn't need be. It looks and feels like the patient's own. All front teeth feel naturally grown giving more confidence while kissing, talking, smiling, selling, laughing and eating. They can bite much better. The remaining back teeth are now a smaller removable denture easier to handle and chewing better. The patient is awarded with greater self value and a stronger feeling of security. He can better face friends and lovers and probably feels more desired by both. Unfortunately some people think a whole man is worth more than a part. This treatment is most expensive. It's better dental and psychological therapy, worth its price.

PSYCHOSOMATICS

Psychosomatic symptoms are seen in both dental and medical experience. Many suffering physically needing the sickbed often also find psychic or mental relaxation in such seclusion. Some find that poor health provides an excuse for avoiding the responsibilities of life's trials. Its a way out. Although sorry to suffer the sickness when forced to stay home or enter the hospital for physical care, the automatic accompanying release from daily frustration is welcomed. Some yield to temptations subconsciously creating psychosomatic signs, or pseudo-symptoms of suffering, as an excuse for avoiding duty and obligation. Some such may occur often, sensed as diseases of the body. With advances of dental technology, treatment, and thought, they're seen as increasing symptoms of dental disease.

Mind, to matter or the physical body relations, are easily demonstrated. Simple acts of either can cause reactions in the other. Sudden alarm from the stick of a sharp pin, and awe at sight of beautiful flowers are obvious, also gooseflesh from fright and blushing from shame. Diarrhea can occur from emotional disturbance and frequently heart palpitations. Toothaches stop as patients arrive for treatment. Sometimes physically demonstrated psychosomatic symptoms are serious. The sufferer senses such excessive mental anguish that extreme physical signs are needed to detract them. For some subconscious minds it seems easier that way.

In the 1930's appendicitis was in style. It was talked about and many sufferers felt its symptoms. Appendicitis operations were popular. Anybody who was anybody had an appendectomy. Walter Alvarez M.D. an eminent physician pioneering psychosomatic aspects of gastro-intestinal problems, wrote a paper in The Journal of the American Medical Association 1940, Vol. 114, Pg. 1301, demonstrating how the psyche or mind led to all these appendicitis operations of the soma or body. Three hundred and eighty five patients were the subject of this study. All had their appendix removed. One hundred and thirty of these were operated on after an acute or sudden attack. Two thirds of these were cured. Two hundred and fifty five patients had suffered chronically. They had no acute attack but had experienced appendicitis symptoms for a long time. They also had their appendics removed. Only 2 of these 255 were cured. The other 253 seemed to continue to suffer from appendicitis even though they had no appendics in their bodies. Surgery of the mastoid bone located near the ear was another fad suffered which has since been abandoned.

Psychosomatic symptoms are sometimes the basis of dental dissatisfactions. In some cases the problem may be difficult to solve. In some cases the physical faults have been corrected, and continued complaint could be caused by deep psychological disturbance. Psychiatric help may be necessary.

Perhaps because the physical defects of simpler dental diseases like teeth decay are readily discernible with modern diagnostic methods, they're less frequently claimed as psychosomatic symptoms. Its easier to substitute mental for physical faults with factors harder to find. Bruxism, the excessive gritting teeth grinding together, is a significant psychosomatic symptom. It may carry over from primitive man's threatening teeth gnashing, as still seen today among aggressive lower animals. Bruxism, done unknowingly by those who do, is often a physical demonstration against life's frustrations. As a doctor I've been surprised to discover my own teeth gnashing during critical difficult dental procedures. Men and women who brux in sleep can't believe mates who wakened by their noises complain. Surprised, in personal defense they deny such gritting, though analysis by psychotherapists usually reveals conflict causing conditions. Women gnash more than men. Some bruxing is considered an expression of resentment against the sleepers companion. Perhaps it is a more considerate way of rebelling less violently. Some sleepy gritty gnashes, are reactions to acts being dreamed. Unfortunately, in addition to its raucous noises, bruxism wears teeth away, loosens them, loses them, and causes other dental problems. Sometimes the fault is a dental defect, difficult to detect that can be cured. Sometimes deep initiating psychic problems may need psychological assistance.

Removable dental appliances, as false replacements for lost body parts, provide more opportunity for complaint. Most people enjoy their dentures, participating in all lifes comforts they provide. Others seem impossible to satisfy. Removable dentures replacing teeth, act as evidence of the loss of complete original more youthful existence. They must be tolerated, and resentfully are by some, for the very replacement they perform. For those who are never satisfied, dentures provide maximum opportunity for dental psychosomatic symptoms. Such unfortunates go from dentist to dentist to dentist, for equal numbers of dentures and more, all of which carefully made and adjusted never seem to work.

Some subconsciously resent their own neglect as personal guilt, leading to the loss of their teeth. Some prefer to transfer that guilt as dentistry's fault for permitting such loss. Some, whose lives have been preserved and prolonged by the removal of arms and legs, resent surgeons they feel could and should have saved them. Its a tough situation that sometimes seems unsolvable. Psychiatric or other psychotherapy may be needed.

SELF SACRIFICIAL PSYCHOLOGY

And now some psychology of sacrifice, of giving up and paying money for dental services. Dentistry has to be paid for. That money represents an expenditure that could have been used to acquire material goods and pleasures. Its annoying to consider exchanging by sacrifice, potential pleasures, for associations involving pain. So who wants to visit the dentist. I've found that patients who repeatedly neglect themselves and only seek treatment when painfully forced to, resent payment most.

Those who have learned the values of modern dentistry willingly undergo extensive more expensive restorative treatment and willingly pay for it. They're not only paying to relieve and prevent pain, but far more are receiving personal material comfort, health and pleasure. They will look better, feel better, and be rewarded with more confidence and success. Dentistry is a practical, profitable investment in one's self.

Understanding Mind, and its Fear
dispels decline, Brings Progress Near

TEETH TEETH TEETH

PSYCHOSOMATIC PSYCHOLOGICAL PSYCHIATRIC DENTISTRY

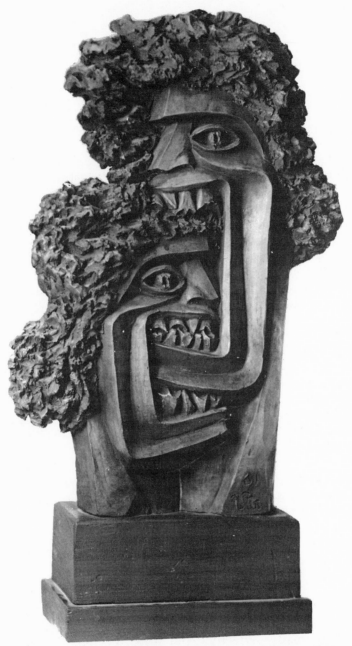

**SCULPTOR VITO PORTRAYS POWERFUL JAW DRIVEN TEETH
AS SYMBOLS OF AGGRESSION**
oto maxmilian foto

TEETH TEETH TEETH

4

KEEP TEETH CLEAN

Many people consider cleaning teeth necessary nuisance. More than few foolishly feel it unnecessary. Even among some of intellect and culture, though most won't admit it, there sometimes exists a psychological deterrent to cleaning various personal parts. They may be disgusted with themselves and right to feel that way. Some dislike bathing, yet enjoy picking ears, nose, and toes. These seem to supply with the thrill of hunt, an intimate exultation when particular elusive pieces just beyond reach, are captured and retrieved. Laziness is a factor, it's work and bother.

Practically all dental disease starts with dirty teeth. In the warm moist mouth environment dirt harbours germs, causing bad breath, tooth decay, peridontal disease, loosening and loss of teeth and health. Keeping teeth clean helps keep them healthy. A popular concept that teeth must be lost with age is wrong, with proper care like other organs, teeth can be kept, usually for life.

TRAFFIC OF THE MOUTH

Food passing through the mouth, around the mouth parts that chew and move them, could be considered sort of a traffic of those things as they pass through. Along this passage dirt and debris collect in particular places while other areas keep rather clean.

To some extent even ordinary mouth movements clean teeth. Outer surfaces are wiped by lip and cheek motions, inner by the tongue. While biting and chewing, teeth passing through food get sort of scrubbed, better with rough tough stuff. This is however superficially inadequate. Also, unfortunately, some of the same biting that wipes dirt off, drives debris deep into almost inaccessible crevices. That's where toothpicks enter.

CLEANING

Casual cleaning even with the toothbrush is of little value. Proper thorough cleaning requires detailed care. You know how difficult it is to clean even fingernails perfectly. And there are only ten. And each is separately controllable, on a single readily accessible side of a single available maneuverable finger. And we can see what we're doing as one hand manipulates an instrument, cleaning the fingernail on a finger of the other, while all fingers of both hands coordinate moving to cooperate. A person may have as many as thirty two teeth, all out of sight. No one in the world has ever been able to see their own live teeth. No mirrors please. A few can see the tip of their tongue if they try. And some teeth are far back, tough for even dentists to see in other mouths with mirrors. And each tooth has five surfaces needing cleaning. And surfaces between teeth far back are practically inaccessible. It's not easy. That's why many teeth are lost, especially towards the rear, where they're harder to reach. It can all be done with proper, intelligent, regular, careful cleaning worth the effort. It's better to save teeth, keeping them attractively chewing in mouths, although those who prefer lazy ease and are sentimental can save their teeth in an old coffee can.

Cleaning teeth is peridontal treatment, or the care of conditions around the outside of teeth, to which another clinical chapter is devoted. Keeping teeth clean is so important, however, that this do-it-yourself phase of peridontal treatment was given this chapter of its own.

The dirt trapping crevices are our cleaning objectives. The word dirt according to Webster's New International Dictionary originates from Old Norse, Middle English and Dutch words, drit and dreet which mean excrement. In Old Anglo Saxon dritan meant to void excrement. These may only seem foul and offensive. Dirt around teeth damages and destroys. Get rid of it.

One time while examining a patient I was surprised to find growing from amidst dirt between his upper right first and second molars a tiny sprouting seed. Being a nature lover I was delighted. Being interested in the patient's welfare, and because despite the dirt's fertilizing value the lack of regular sunshine would yield a poor crop, I removed the tiny young plant and cautioned the patient concerning dental care.

DENTAL HYGIENE DETAILS ∾ The fine crevice between tooth and gum edge where teeth leave the gum, which runs like a collar around the neck of each tooth, is called the Gingival Sulcus or Sulcus. The fine crevices at depths of the tiny, hilly projections on the chewing surfaces of back teeth are called Fissures. The places where adjacent teeth touch are called Contact Points. They're really so close there's no space at all. The small spaces between adjacent teeth around the contact points are called Contact Areas or Interproximal Spaces. All these close confines are choice sites for germs, probably the cause of most teeth decay and other dental diseases. All these places must be cleaned. It requires constant care.

A TOOTHBRUSHING METHOD ∾ Various toothbrushing methods are recommended. Some dentists prefer one over another. Some prescribe different procedures for patients' different conditions. No toothbrushing technique or any other technology will accomplish its intended purpose unless properly performed. To clean teeth all dirt must be removed from their deep entrapment. The following toothbrushing method will clean well where applied.

Systematic procedure should be used on each jaw starting fully back on any one side, moving forward, missing no area, towards the front, then on and around to the far back of the other side. Outside the teeth, under the cheeks and lips, then inside towards the tongue. Upper jaw and lower. Any sequence may be followed as long as all tooth surfaces, outside and in between, are covered. None may be omitted, give special attention to the far rear. Details are described for cleaning upper back teeth since these are usually most difficult. Similar method should be followed all around the remaining upper and all lower teeth.

In toothbrushing it is best to think not only of the brush as a whole but also visualize, imagining each bristle as a toothpick or arrow, directed at the crevice it enters to clean. Start choosing either upper side. Place the brush bristles up, inside the cheek, back into the mouth, to slightly past the last tooth. See that the bristle tips are directed up in towards the teeth and adjacent gums covering the teeth, gum margins and above. Direct the brush, pushing the bristle points in like an arrow, lightly several times, feeling the ends into the flesh gently stimulating. It is important to feel bristle tips go into the gingival sulcus, between gums and teeth. This is a vulnerable dirt collecting area. Continue pushing gently in and out and turn the brush, sweeping down. As it sweeps down pushing, bristles now also enter the interproximal contact spaces between teeth. Continue sweeping on down past the teeth. Sweep a full stroke. Always try to push bristles individually, directed as arrows or toothpicks deep into all crevices. That's where most germ damage is done.

If severe bleeding occurs, dental treatment is needed. A small amount at first is considered normal. After teeth are treated by professional cleaning, some bleeding may still be seen the first few times they're brushed this way. This thorough method soon strengthens, toughening the tissues, so that bleeding stops. A small amount of hemorrhage from removal of dirt between teeth is worth it, will soon stop.

Dirt left deep, avoiding bloody damage, will eventually disease severely. The worst tooth infection is a tooth decayed internally, abscessed deep into the bone. Doing nothing won't cause bleeding, though the infection increases dangerously. Proper tooth extraction treatment removes the deep

TEETH TEETH TEETH

infection, usually with heavy bleeding. Only after such surgical cleaning removal of the dirt infected tooth body part, normally accompanied by bleeding, will the area heal healthy. Removing deep dirt at home, with similar simple bleeding, can be considered a very minor personal surgical procedure also beneficial.

The same pushing brush up, in, sweeping down action, should be repeated for about six total strokes. Six should be similarly applied up along the inner tooth surfaces. Every area, inside and out, should be brushed treated this way, around fully back to the opposite side of the jaw. The same must be done to the lower jaw, brush now pointed down, sweeping up, all around outside and in.

Reaching those deep crevices also automatically brushes the prominent tooth faces. Chewing surfaces of back teeth are easier. Any sort of thorough brushing, scrubbing action up into the uppers and down into the lowers will do. With acquired proficiency all teeth can be brushed in three minutes.

FREQUENCY ∽ Damage starts as soon as dirt deposits. It's best brushing after every meal. Deposits also originate from materials other than food, tobacco, salivary substances and natural mouth tissue debris. Quantity varies from person to person, and with it the need for cleaning. Teeth should be cleaned at whatever frequency is necessary to keep them that way. Despite thorough home care, dirt somehow collects, needing professional cleaning treatment called Prophylaxis at the dental office. Dentists themselves need such periodic care to keep their own teeth clean. The doctor can best determine the proper prophylaxis frequency for each patient.

TEETH CLEANING THINGS

There is large variety of teeth janitorial supplies and equipment, powder, paste, liquid cleansers, hand and power tools, though I don't know of any teeth vacuum cleaner. The dentist may prescribe particular products for personal conditions.

TOOTH PASTES ∽ Like soap and other cleansing agents they all do the job if applied thoroughly. Select the substance with the feel and flavor preferred. Added fluorides probably have extra value especially to growing children.

MOUTHWASHES ∽ Help clean soft debris when swished and pumped between teeth. They briefly refresh breath.

TEETH TEETH TEETH

TOOTHBRUSHES ∾ Toothbrushes come with bristles of standardized rigidity, soft, medium, hard. I prefer the stiffest that won't damage tissues. Both nylon and natural bristles are available and satisfactory. Nylon, being synthetic, is more dependable for each standardized stiffness. Brushes with fewer bristles, like three row and two row brushes, can reach deeper into crevices, cleaning more thoroughly. They don't last as long. Multi-tuft brushes last longer. Their numerous bristles crowding together cannot enter close spaces as far. They're good for gum massage. Good practice is to alternate daily with use of few row and multi-tuft. This gives the bristles a chance to recover and benefits with values of both. Brushes are useful only while their bristles are rigid, erect. You can save the price of toothbrushes at the expense of your teeth. Some brushes have at their handle end a small soft rubber tip, helpful for gum stimulation.

DENTAL FLOSS ∾ is a valuable between teeth cleaning tool. Stretch the floss or thin tape between opposite hand fingers and force drag the tape between adjacent teeth. Strop across back and forth like shining shoes.

TOOTHPICKS ∾ I like toothpicks, always carry one in my pocket, leaving restaurants I often take three or four. When needed to reach that maddening spot they seem worth a thousand dollars. Needed in emergency by a stranger, they may make a valuable friend. Some think toothpicking damages tissues. Any gum bleeding from dirt removal is insignificant, well worth the cleaner result. Healing rapidly follows. Men of distinction used to use soft gold personal toothpicks, with a flair of style, including elevation of the small finger. One time traveling through Mexico at a small souvenir shop in San Luis Potosi, I saw a mens leather wallet containing a long, narrow, sewed pocket. I asked the thin pocket's purpose. "That Senior," I was told, "is for the toothpick." Soft wooden toothpicks home poked deep between teeth are also good tooth root gum massagers. [Unlike an unfailing faithful friend, toothpicks may slip and stick you in the end, though I wouldn't call such a pick a traitor. Once toothpicking deep, before an important Sunday social appointment, a long piece broke buried wedged tight, hurting between my upper left second and third molars. Even I, a skilled dentist couldn't get the darn thing out of me. After desperate telephoning and a troublesome trip to a professional friend, I survived. Still a picker, perhaps I live too dangerously.]

POWER TOOTHBRUSHES ∾ Ancient Chinese invented the toothbrush which has since been serving long. Modern electric motor driven brushes have added value. Their powered strokes, while they throw the toothpasty stuff sloppily around, remove dirt some human brushers might miss. For those unwilling or unable to exert themselves, electric brushing helps. Here too, however, power brushing won't do the job unless the operator applies his apparatus thoroughly to all places.

HYDRAULIC TEETH CLEANING ∾ Hydraulics is an engineering term for the use of fluids, usually water, often under pressure in motion. Advances in teeth cleaning have been made with small powered hydraulic home appliances, that force jets of water or washing solutions under adjustable high pressures, through a fine nozzle held by the hand directed between the teeth. There's a slight splashy mess, well worth the result. Liquids this way, pressurized between teeth, are the first real approach to washing dirt forcefully out from the inside. It's like tiny, powerful, between teeth enemas. Results are especially beneficial where deep inside cleaning is important, in pyorrhetic areas, under bridges, and into detailed hardware of orthodontic apparatus. Such cleaning serves a need unsatisfied any other way. Dental sciences are conquering its problems. Ideal care combines toothbrushing with hydraulics.

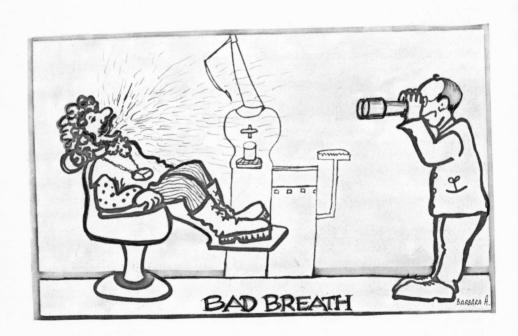

TEETH TEETH TEETH

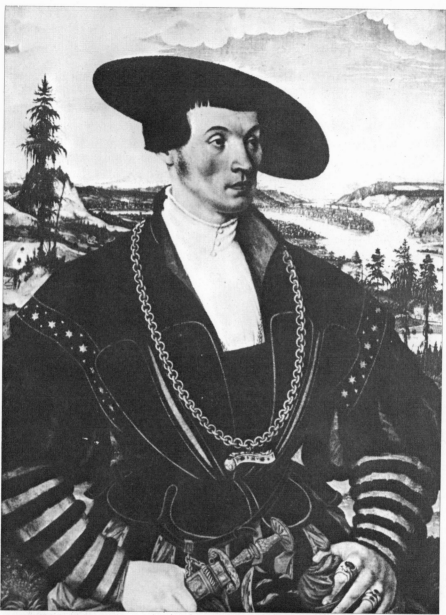

MAN WITH A TOOTHPICK∾This painting of Florence Italy Nobleman Sammlung Marcuardi by Hans von Shonitz, about 1500 A.D., was typical of his Renaissance time. His neck chain carries an ornate case containing a soft pure gold toothpick. These were freely used even at court dinners by the best mannered, while pieces they picked were spit out with gusto. Times have changed.

TEETH TEETH TEETH

5

EXAMINATION

People visit the dentist as a doctor specializing in diseases of teeth and surrounding mouth parts. The mouth contains a collection of small, important organs supplied by arteries, veins, nerves, lymphatics and other glands, connected by major and minor vessels to the head and brain above and the larger body below. Anything affecting any part affects the body as a whole. Dental disease affects general health which also influences conditions in the mouth.

I was told this story by a dentist who prefers I don't use his name. I will call him Dr. Alberti Firenzi. About 1938 in Chicago Dr. Firenzi had patient Steve Pulaski, a young man of Polish heritage. He had known Steve two years. One day Steve asked, "Dr. Firenzi, could you extract a tooth for my mother? She has a terrible toothache." "Of course," Dr. Firenzi replied, "Bring her to the office whenever you like." "That's impossible, Dr. Firenzi, my mother is paralyzed and can't move." Steve offered to pick Dr. Firenzi up Saturday noon, take him home to treat his mother and return him to the office. In those days Dr. Firenzi's fee was one or two dollars per extraction. Dr. Firenzi got all information possible concerning Mrs. Pulaski's physical condition, made prearrangements, and assembled his home treatment kit containing instruments, injectable anesthetics, medications, and a powerful flashlight.

Saturday noon Steve took Dr. Firenzi to their walk-up tenament apartment. Steve's mother was stout, about 56 years old, sitting immobile in an overstuffed chair, head rigidly fixed, staring wide blank eyed. Mrs. Pulaski, through hardly moving lips, spoke slowly, groping for broken words. She had little mouth, lip, control. Dr. Firenzi found her teeth horribly infected around both jaws. There was pus from between heavy deposits and the gums were festering swollen. He was amazed to learn Mrs. Pulaski hadn't left her chair for over two years except to be taken to the bathroom. Fed like a child by spoon, she could hardly move arms or legs. She even slept sitting up in the chair. No x-rays were available and this was before antibiotic therapy. Dr. Firenzi soon saw the long neglect demanded, that not only the seemingly single pain causing tooth be removed, but all. He told this to Steve and his mother. Both agreed.

Carefully, Steve holding the flashlight, Dr. Firenzi cleaned the area, applied anesthetics and medications, and extracted the tooth. Healing was

EXAMINATION

satisfactory. Every Saturday, guarding against infection, Dr. Firenzi cautiously removed another tooth. On his third visit Dr. Firenzi was amazed when Mrs. Pulaski, with her eyes and a slight nod, directed his attention to the fact she could move fingers of her left hand. With these fingers she gestured towards her extracted teeth. Regularly every week, Dr. Firenzi told me, it seemed as if by magic, as each additional tooth was removed, Mrs. Pulaski would demonstrate another moving part of her body. First fingers of the left hand. Then the right. Then the left arm and shoulder - and a foot - and a leg.

"It was," Dr. Firenzi said, "as if mysterious electric wires of nerves ran from each organ to the particular defective teeth that had been crippling each individual appendage of Mrs. Pulaski's body." Paralyzed Mrs. Pulaski started mobilizing, tooth by removed tooth - finger by hand - by right foot, by right molar - by left leg. She got better and better. After years of hopeless paralysis she could slowly get up with assistance and stumbling walk with a cane in each hand. She soon fed herself. She was born again. Within a few weeks, happier healthier Mrs. Pulaski's mouth healed. Delighted, excited, Steve brought a photo to Dr. Firenzi showing his mother standing with canes by herself in the street in front of their house.

This case is exceptional. It often happens, however, that teeth appearing normal outwardly are diseased internally, undermining body health. To find the fault and properly plan treatment, thorough examination is necessary.

DENTAL EXAMINATION

To examine is to inspect carefully in detail, investigate and test with the object of discovering the real nature of the thing. Dental diseases are sometimes elusive. Using every available means at his disposal, the dentist, like a detective, seeks the solution. Every clue could be important and must be investigated. The patient's medical history is taken. His physician may be consulted. For diagnosis of some dental diseases, body tests also used by medical practitioners may be ordered.

CLINICAL EXAMINATION ∾ Clinical examination is important and though limited is sometimes the only examination needed. Clinical examination is the investigation of disease by sight and touch. Using visual observation or sight, the dentist looks directly into the mouth using a strong light and a small mirror to see inside from behind. Touch includes palpation to feel texture and hardness and resiliency of soft tissues and the rigidity or looseness of teeth. They're all clues.

The dentist may see what seems to be perfect teeth, dirty teeth, irregular teeth, broken teeth, teeth slightly or grossly decayed. Several, many, or all,

TEETH TEETH TEETH

may be loose or missing. He may recognize inflammation or infection of gums or advanced peridontal disease. There may be signs indicating internal bone disorders like abscess. There may be surface lesions of minor or major severity, even cancers. Signs seen above the surface are only limited indications of conditions below. Some symptoms might be obvious to any observer. When detectable this way, they've often reached advanced stages of degeneration.

X-RAY EXAMINATION ∽ Dental disease is common. Few have the fortune to avoid its damage. Most can be detected in early stages with x-ray examination. X-rays disclose internal disorders not visible from outside and help plan proper treatment. Ideal dentistry can't be done without them. I myself a dentist, demand x-rays of myself before permitting any significant dental therapy. Some people resist x-rays. Some doubt their value, want to avoid the cost and may have fear of x-ray damage. Such fears have been proven to be beyond the logic of modern diagnostic x-ray need.

I tell an old appropriate story. Three men were arguing, each claiming the honor of being the most stubborn man in the world. One man made his claim based on dental experience. He said, after both before him had told their tales, "You guys think you're stubborn. Now let me tell you. My teeth always looked good and rarely bothered me. Yet, one night I felt a terrible toothache. Next morning I went to the dentist to have it pulled. He asked, 'Which is it?' I replied, 'You're the dentist. You should know.' He asked, 'Which is it?' I said, 'You should know.' He pulled one wrong tooth and another asking which it was. I said, 'You're the dentist.' The stupid doctor pulled every tooth in my head. Well I ask you who is the most stubborn man in the world."

International events and news releases from World War II to recent past, make it reasonable that intelligent ordinarily informed people, be concerned with possibility of x-ray exposure danger. The atom bomb horrors of radioactive explosion and fission fallout at Hiroshima and Nagasaki have never been approached by any preceding and are hoped will never be repeated. This catastrophe and following bomb testing initiated a fright of any energy radiation. Some sincere, well intended scientists and philosophers recoiled from these mass misfortunes. Understandably, in haste appraisals were made causing fear of exaggerated dangers of rays from several sources including diagnostic x-ray.

Rays are naturally radiating all around us all the time. Cosmic rays from outer space unceasingly enter our world and probably helped man's natural evolutionary changes from the beginning of time. They are an uncontrollable part of our environment. We may not be able to live without them. Mankind never has. There are natural mineral radioactive substances in and on Earth's surface emanating constantly. There are radioactive elements like potassium forming part of our body and necessary to the body, radiating within us all the time. These were all radiating before man ever knew radiation existed, and he developed from primitive forms to the complex biological organism he is, in that radiation environment. And the measured total of all natural radiation that reaches a person's body, over any reasonable period, is greater than that received by dental x-rays.

Earlier in our century x-rays for examination were radiated in dangerous quantity. Not to patients that needed them often, but to x-ray technicians, physicians and dentists, who unknowingly stood in radiation paths many, many times, of every many days, treating many patients many years. It was those x-ray workers that suffered. With advanced high speed equipment, film, and intelligent care, diagnostic x-ray danger is gone. Some communities exert civic control to insure safety. Recent studies reveal these facts but haven't been given the great attention that caused radiation fears when United States and Soviet Union were involved in the dares of atom bomb testing contest. The problem is complicated and as with others has different points of view. The collection of conflicting data by different authorities is so overwhelming it becomes bewildering, amusing, and confusing.

The most radio-sensitive organs are the gonads, ovaries of women, testicles of men. Radiation upon them in excess dose produces mutations or unpredictable inheritable changes in their newborn. Testes of men are more susceptible since they are not as deep inside the body. Radiation effect on organs is greater with temperature increase. The anthropologist and geneticist Ashley Montagu in his book Human Heredity, Signet Science Library 1963, Page 334 refers to Swedish investigators Ehrenberg, van Ehrenstein and Hegdran who reported a 1957 study of the scrotum temperature of nude and clothed men. The scrotum is the sac surrounding testicles. They found the scrotum of clothing covered men to be 3.3° centigrade higher average than of nude men. I don't know where the men were in Sweden when their testicle temperatures were taken. Such temperature rise, according to the researchers, would increase mutation rate by 85%. According to Montagu's book, such natural increase is probably more dangerous to future generations than fallout from hydrogen and atom bombs. It could be. Montagu suggests a clothing design change for men to open skirts like women. These reports and others of more and less significant scientists lead me to submit a solution of satire.

I offer an invention for which I ask no profit or royalty. I make it available free to any trouser or appliance manufacturer. It is a small, thin apparatus, worn inside a trouser strapped to the leg. It would obtain energy from walking, to generate and store in a miniature battery as electricity, to operate a motor driving a small fan to keep testicles cool. It could be adjustable. On the same page of Montagu's book another scientist, Webster, is seriously stated to prove, it would require 250,000 x-rays measuring 14 by 17 inches and 300,000 head or skull x-rays to reach a radiation dose equal to that from men wearing pants. My calculations show 50,000,000 dental x-rays to approximately equal a pair of pants. This should include underwear.

For recent authentic material I had several phone and personal meetings with Dr. William Ward Wainwright, my radiology professor in dental college. Dr. Wainwright is a specialist. He's been Professor of Radiology heading those departments at several dental universities. He was Director of the Radioisotope Laboratory, University of So. Calif. School of Dentistry, and has done biology radiological research at the National Los Alamos Scientific Laboratory. Under a science grant, Dr. Wainwright wrote "Dental Radiology," McGraw Hill 1965, probably the most modern comprehensive presentation of the subject. His book covers all phases of dental x-ray including danger possibility. According to Dr. Wainwright, after making allowances for cosmic radiation, other natural sources, fallout, industrial and other man made origins, and including an expected amount of medically needed x-rays, there is a balance of radiation that may still be safely tolerated. This, according to Dr. Wainwright, permits a person from birth to the age of 30 years to safely take a total of 500 sets of 20 dental x-rays each within that 30 year period. That is 16-2/3 sets of 20 films per year, an amount far exceeding any imaginable need.

X-RAY ACTION ∞ X-rays were so called by their discoverer Roentgen, since he didn't know what they were. They are similar to ordinary light rays with the added unique ability to penetrate opaque substances like wood, bone, and even very thin sheets of metal, things light cannot go through. X-rays affect photographic film just as light rays do. The affected film itself or x-ray picture is also called an x-ray. They are sometimes called roentgen rays and the pictures roentgenograms. X-rays are also called radiographs. X-ray is valuable for diagnosis not only because it penetrates solid substances, but especially because its penetrability or passage through varies with the density or hardness of the substance passed through. Through very hard, dense things like silver or gold fillings no rays will pass. Through hard outer tooth enamel hardly any rays can pass. Through hard, thick, compact bone not many rays will pass. More go through soft bone. Through less substantial substances like flesh most or all rays easily get through. Hard, dense, thick things stop x-rays; softer stuff lets lots through. That's how X rays. If x-rays are radiated through an object containing materials of different densities or hardnesses, beyond to film on the other side, different amounts will get through the different places depending on the density of the substances penetrated, and the film will be affected in different degrees in those different places.

TAKING X-RAYS ∾ Most dental x-ray film is small, measuring 1-1/4 x 1-5/8 inches with corners rounded to lessen digging into the mouth. Each comes in a separate sealed little paper envelope, light tight black inside, called a Packet. Within the x-ray packet next to the film on one side only there is a highly polished sheet of lead called the Backing. Outside the packet is marked to show the lead backing side. To take an x-ray the operator places the film packet inside the mouth behind the tooth area to be rayed, with the lead sheet side away from the teeth towards the back. He tries to get the film packet deep beyond around the tip or apex of the tooth roots. It could be uncomfortable. Such x-rays are called Periapical x-rays. Periapical means around the tip. Most dental x-rays are periapical. Outside the patient's mouth the x-ray machine is aimed towards the face at the film, with the parts to be x-rayed between. While patient and packet hold still, the timer switch button is pressed, and the machine radiates its rays for a small fraction or seconds.

X-RAY DYNAMICS ∾ In that short time all the following happens. X-rays from the machine pass through the cheeks, gums, teeth, jawbone, the outer paper of the film packet on in and through affecting the x-ray film. They hit the polished lead backing sheet which reflects them back like a mirror, again affecting the x-ray film. This permits radiating rays only 1/2 the time otherwise needed to expose the film. An x-ray may be needed for only a single tooth or taken as a series all around both upper and lower jaws. Each packet is placed within the mouth most advantageously for the teeth within its range.

As the rays radiate the soft flesh cheeks and gums have little if any ray stopping ability. The x-rays go right through. Metal in the mouth like silver or gold fillings, stops all rays in their path from reaching the film. Around the outer crown of each tooth, enamel the hardest, densest body substance, yet less dense than metals, stops most rays. Inside the enamel, hard dentin yet a little softer, lets a little more rays through. Centered in each crown and along inside each root, the soft pulpal nerve contents let more rays penetrate to the film. Around the teeth the surfaces of the jawbone have a harder, thin outer layer, letting less rays pass. Inside the bone, like inside a piece of beef bone, the bone is spongy with little, soft, fat filled vacuoles or spaces. This lets rays through according to softness or hardness at each spot. The varying amounts of rays reaching the film affect it that much.

TEETH TEETH TEETH

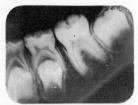
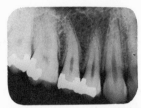
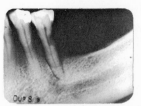

primary teeth followed by developing adult teeth

Normal teeth with metal restorations in normal bone

adentulous or toothless jawbone behind remaining diseased teeth

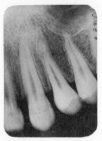
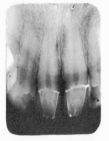
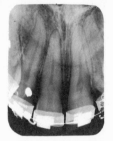
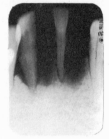

Fractured cuspid crown other teeth and supporting bone normal

Porcelain jackets cemented over central incisors

orthodontic apparatus stainless steel bands & wires moving teeth

Extreme pyhorretic bone loss hidden by gum. Teeth about to fall

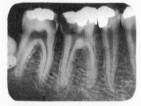
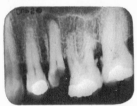
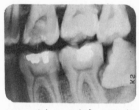

severe inner decay under fillings & invading the pulp chamber. unseen outside

Bicuspid crown decayed thru canal with abscess at root tip pyhorretic deposits between molars

Horizontal impacted 3rd molar erupting into & destroying the second molar root.

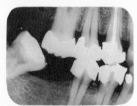
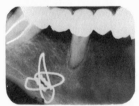
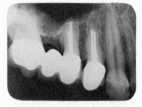

Inlays wrongly overextended from teeth hidden under gums should smoothly blend into contours of tooth surfaces. correct examples shown elsewhere

Surgical wire joining severed jaw now healed together. Porcelain covered metal structure bridge replaces missing teeth & also helps strengthen jaw

Endodontic treatment sealing of both bicuspids root canals. single jacket & 3 tooth metal bridge structure covered with natural looking porcelain

SEVERAL DENTAL X-RAYS & DIAGNOSES
s. Garfield

MORE SIGNIFICANT FEATURES ARE DISCUSSED - X-Rays reveal harder natural & other materials. Soft tissues such as cheek & gum are invisible. X-Rays sometimes have artifacts, unrelated small marks accidentally created during processing, identifiable by the doctor. Edge lettering is the film manufacturers mark.

PLATE 5-1

TEETH TEETH TEETH

Each exposed packet is removed from the mouth with patient relief, spit wet. Its intact outer sealed covering paper still protects it from ordinary light. Its inner x-ray exposed film is affected with the contrasting amounts of rays that penetrated the different tissues.

BITE-WING X-RAYS ∾ Bite-wing x-rays, in addition, are also often taken of the back teeth. The film packet is placed in a small bite-wing paper or plastic bracket, with a thin tab protruding directly out along from the center of the x-ray packet, dividing it into equal halves. The packet is placed inside behind the back teeth, with its tab towards the cheek between the teeth. As the patient bites the tab, it is held securing the packet in place. The upper half of the bite-wing film covers the upper teeth crowns. The lower half covers the lower teeth crowns. Bite-wing films give good pictures of both upper and lower back teeth crowns together, without showing their roots. They're valuable examination aids, especially for cavities where the roots are not involved.

PROCESSING X-RAYS ∾ Exposed film is processed in the dark room laboratory which is sealed to keep out ordinary light. Its dim amber reddish safety light permits working without affecting the film. In the darkroom the packet is opened, the film removed, developed, fixed, washed and dried. Fixing stabilizes the picture so it can't be affected by light any more. It can be examined anywhere.

X-RAY DIAGNOSIS ∾ The x-ray is a negative. It is viewed before a light that shines through. Where all x-rays were stopped as by metal fillings, the film is seen clear, whitish. Between and around teeth where the rays easily passed through soft cheeks and gums, areas are black. Harder enamel around tooth crowns stopped most rays, showing almost as white as metal. Where decay existed within enamel, invisible to the eye inside the teeth, soft decay replaced the hard, healthy enamel and x-ray penetration shows dark, revealing infection invasion. If decay enters dentin internally, towards or invading the pulp, that also shows deeper, dark, soft. If the infection has abscessed or cysted, completely invisible to the eye without x-ray inside the bone around the root tip, that also shows dark or soft, the bone has been lost indicated replaced by soft decay. If supporting bone under gums is gone from pyorrhetic disease, that soft gum area permitting rays to pass, shows the shrunken lost bone level. If a tooth is blocked or impacted completely invisible inside the jaw, its harder tooth form is clearly defined showing its position surrounded by softer jawbone. If the expected normal bone pattern is irregular, inside in a local area whiter or darker, indicating possibility of a harmless bone tumor or even a cancer,

TEETH TEETH TEETH

that could show. X-rays are valuable examination tools, dentistry shouldn't be done without them. Plate 5-1, SEVERAL DENTAL X-RAYS & DIAGNOSES demonstrates the interpretation of thirteen different dental x-rays.

For detailed examination the dentist may prefer to study his patient and films together, referring back and forth one to the other. He often uses a long, thin, pointed instrument called an Explorer or Probe to pick and stick into deep, doubtful recesses. That's how the pick probes.

Sometimes examination of a critical tooth requires even more than clinical and x-ray study. Like an Exploratory Operation for major medical surgery, the dentist may need to remove all decay and even what looks like good existing dental restorations, before deciding whether he can save a tooth and how.

PANORAMIC X-RAY ∾ Patients ask why dental x-rays can't be taken without film held annoyingly deep inside the mouth. Recently they can be. Equipment has been designed attached to a floor platform on which the patient sits in the machine's chair. The chair contains an adjustable bracket to comfortably stabilize jaws keeping them accurately related to the film and radiating x-rays. Behind the patient, rising from the platform, is a vertical beam structure which goes up and forward high above the head. From this beam above, there is suspended a horizontal swingable turret arm, extending forward from behind its rotation center. At the rear arm end behind the patient at jaw level an x-ray tube is mounted. The forward arm end, in front of the patient, carries the unexposed mounted x-ray film. The arm swings so that the film moves around in front of the patient's face. Behind his head, coordinating with film movement, the x-ray tube also swings, following radiating its beam from the back, through the head and teeth on to the film outside in front. It only takes a few seconds for a single, large panoramic picture of all upper and lower teeth and jaws. There are several advantages. It's easier on the patient. It gives an excellent appraisal of anatomy spacial relationships. It's especially valuable for far back third molar regions, hard to get to inside the mouth, and even gives a good picture of the rising ramus part of the jaw. There are some disadvantages. The equipment is expensive. X-rays passing through the intervening rear head structures result in less accurate detail, despite the fact that the rays are focused at the teeth location. Fine details for any individual tooth or area are not as clear. Conventional x-rays may also be needed for detailed study of particular pathological parts.

MOUTH STUDY MODELS ∾ Much dentistry involves dental apparatus for replacing lost teeth and other mouth parts. Sometimes visual and x-ray examination though valuable are not enough for designing the necessary dental appliances. Upper and lower models of the patient's teeth and jaws are made, which the dentist can relate as they are in the living mouth, for study.

OTHER EXAMINATION AIDS ∾ In pace with dental advances, other examination aids are used as needed. Sometimes electrical instruments are applied to measure the vitality response of the live pulp inside teeth. Sometimes biological smears are taken for germ culture to identify bacterial infection. Sometimes biopsy sections of suspicious lesions are removed for microscopic pathological examination. Sometimes photos of suspicious lesions are taken for identification. Some dentists take photographs of teeth before treatment to help plan their improved appearance. These can be compared with happy surprise when treatment is completed.

Search Explore — to find The Cause
Examination Helps Cure the Flaws

A Surprifing Cure for the Tooth-Ache.

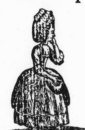

I am come to you to get Relief for a moſt violent Tooth-Ache.

My Letter, that ſmells ſo very pleaſant, when delivered, is your Relief.

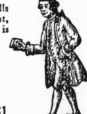

WHICH

Has never been known to fail.

TO the Nobility, Gentry, and Others. If the Pain be ever ſo violent, and if the Teeth are rotted away below the Gums, nay even to the Stumps, the Patients are ſure to get rid of the Pain, cauſed by the Tooth-Ache, and that in leſs than two Hours, after I have delivered to them a ſmall Letter (ſealed up).

This Letter ſmells very pleaſant, when delivered, which the afflicted are to put into their Pocket, and as the Tooth-Ache leaves them, this agreeable Smell leaves the Letter. But if not the Tooth-Ache, this reviving Smell will not leave the Letter.

Any one that is not ſatisfied in their own Opinion of the above Cure, and think it impoſſible, I beg leave to mention thoſe Families I have cured, and I believe that will give them the greateſt Satisfaction. I have cured ſeveral Thouſands of the Tooth-Ache, for above theſe Twenty-three Years. But I ſhall only trouble you at preſent to read theſe few Names, and where they live, which are as follow:

Mrs. King and her Daughter, No. 19, Old Bailey.

Mr. and Mrs. More, No, 42, St. James's-ſtreet.

Mrs. Griffiths and Mrs. Richards, Tufton-ſtreet, Weſtminſter.

Mrs. Crowder, No. 9, Queen's-Head-Court, Pater-noſter-row.

Mrs. Jordan, No. 100, St. Martin's-Lane.

Mrs. Salt, No. 21, Panton-ſtreet.

The two Head Cooks of St. George's Hoſpital.

If not cured, nothing is expected; but I am ſure, with God's Bleſſing, to cure every one that comes to me with the Tooth-Ache; and before they go from me, they are deſired to return the ſmall Letter to me again, and on telling me they have no Tooth-Ache, I then leave it to their own Generoſity to ſatisfy me for their Cure.

My Patients often get rid of their Tooth-Ache in leſs than One Hour after coming to me. but I am deſirous that every one who comes to me to be cured, will ſtay at leaſt Two Hours with me. This great Secret is not known to any one but myſelf.

Removed from No. 9, YEOMAN's-ROW, BROMPTON, to No. 100, ST. MARTIN's-LANE, oppoſite MAY's-BUILDINGS, near CHAIRING-CROSS. Where I attend at my Apartments every Day, from Eight o'Clock in the Morning till Eight in the Evening, except Sundays.

☞ For the Good of Mankind, it would be a Charity to let this Bill be put up in ſome Part of your Houſe, that this Cure may be made as public as poſſible to thoſe who have the Tooth-Ache.

N. B. The pooreſt Sort of People cured gratis, from Eight till Ten every Morning. [1757.]

EARLY UNIQUE TREATMENT TECHNIQUE

TEETH TEETH TEETH

6

DIAGNOSIS AND TREATMENT PLANNING

The mouth like any other piece of frequently operated complicated equipment, with continual use often eventually breaks down. As with automobiles and washing machines failure could occur for numbers of reasons.

POOR ENGINEERING DESIGN ∿ Examples are crowded irregular or improperly shaped teeth, or teeth developed with roots too short to support them.

POOR ARTISTIC DESIGN ∿ This is primarily failure of visual satisfaction, though usually teeth that look better are better. Beauty is important, but tooth standards vary with people's attitudes. Some like big ones, others like them small. Some like them fat, some like them thinner, rounder, darker, most like them lighter. Some don't care what their teeth look like.

POOR MATERIALS ∿ Some people unfortunately are born and grow with soft weak teeth and supporting bone, more susceptible to decay. Fluorine and good diet might have helped.

IMPROPER FIELD OF OPERATIONS ∿ Automobiles are designed for the part of the world they're used. The average auto will not function in severe frigid Antarctica. Similarly the surrounding body should be kept healthy for teeth to work well.

OVERLOADING EQUIPMENT FAILURE ∿ Excess tonnage causes trucks to break down. Heavy chewing is good but excessive grinding in sleep or daytime nervousness loosens and wears many away. Cracking too hard a nut will fracture, and opening a bobby pin.

INADEQUATE MAINTENANCE ∿ Any automobile will soon fail if its regular oiling needs are not satisfied and minor repairs neglected. Teeth too need regular care.

CONTINUOUS NORMAL USE AND WEAR ∿ This is the common cause of eventual failure of practically everything in the world, including the oral machine, teeth and mouth.

ANCESTRAL LINEAGE ∿ This is a less mechanical more biological feature some may be proud of. Since heredity is a dental factor it would be wise to guide the courtship between one's prospective parents. Select a good looking father and mother to be, with the sort of stuff you like and healthy attractive long rooted teeth. Yours will most likely be that way probably accompanied by other nice things too.

TEETH TEETH TEETH

TREATMENT PLANNING

After examination and diagnosis of defects, treatment is planned. Some people want no more than emergency removal of a painful tooth. They prefer limiting their dentistry to such loss until following emergencies demand removal of more. Such neglect may be limited to teeth, though it often extends to other of life's endeavors.

Mouths suffer many disorders. The teeth may need only cleaning. Conditions may require a special diet or consultation with a physician. There may be mouth lining soft tissue lesions, of outer or inner diseases of supporting gums and bone. Peridental or other oral surgery may be indicated. There may be teeth not involved in painful emergency, yet degenerated beyond repair needing removal. There may be teeth needing simple fillings or more complex restoration. Some teeth worth saving may need extensive expensive rebuilding, including internal treatment to the root tips. Some teeth may need straightening. Some may need complete surrounding outside, for strength and improved appearance. There may be lost missing teeth needing replacement. All these faults can be corrected.

ALTERNATE PLANS ∽ Differently designed homes can be erected on any residential lot and an individual mouth can often be rebuilt different ways. Some dentists and builders render expected, asked for, satisfactory, simpler, less expensive services. Any of the described dental defects may be the only needed, some minor, some more involved. All dentistry is inter-related, so that often thorough treatment requires combinations of many procedures. Peridental disease of tooth supporting tissues lies deep and the dentist may feel need for such treatment first. It is poor planning to erect a fine home on a swamp or rebuild a mouth before its supporting jaws are restored to good health. Peridental surgery may be necessary.

Some architectural engineering dentists present varied designs for rebuilding a mouth. Remaining defective teeth can be restored different ways. Removable appliances may be made replacing missing teeth, stabilized by existing teeth, needing regular removal daily for cleaning. Fixed bridging appliances may be made, replacing missing teeth, permanently attached to existing teeth rooted in jawbone. These never need being removed and couldn't be. They look, bite, chew, and feel, like the persons own grown. There could be different designs, showing different amounts of gold or other structural metals or showing none, so that even all fixed artificial teeth look perfectly natural. Full dentures may be made replacing all teeth for those who have lost them.

Some mouth reconstruction projects are especially complex. Some problems require trial experimental appliances before the final work is completed. All detailed features take extra time care and cost. Those that are less demanding are less expensive. Any home will provide shelter. Finer homes and dentistry are more expensive and render more satisfaction to those who care about such things.

AN EXAMPLE ∾ An attractive woman came to our office. Numbers of her teeth were missing, several others remained. After examination I described my recommended treatment for full mouth reconstruction including replacement of all missing teeth. They were to be permanently attached in the mouth, covered by natural looking porcelain supported internally by invisible precision metal castings. I explained its benefits. The fee was quoted. She gasped. "Dr. Garfield," she said. "I'll be honest with you. I loved the way you explained things and what you said you'd do. I was going to have another dentist do the work but my husband's partner thinks highly of you and strongly suggested I consult you. You have as I said been recommended highly, but your fees are more than twice those of of the other dentist and I'm sure he's also capable." I felt any dentist the woman whom I will call Mrs. Quandary visited, would be competent, and feeling my fee was fair rechecked calculations. No, there was no mistake. Somehow we continued talking. Suddenly from a few words Mrs. Quandary let slip, it was evident the other dentists plan was for reconstruction which included large appliances needing daily removal for cleaning. Mine were to be permanently attached to the jawbones like natural teeth. I explained the difference and suggested she be sure before deciding.

Mrs. Quandary was intelligent but bewildered by her need, and unexperienced with dental considerations, was lost among the details of dental treatment. Perhaps I was not as thorough as I could have been explaining. As Dr. Hayakawa, the father of semantics would have said, "Oral Reconstruction No. 1, is not Oral Reconstruction No. 2, is not Oral Reconstruction No. 3, is not Oral Reconstruction No. 4."

FEES

"There is hardly anything in the world that someone cannot make a little worse and sell a little cheaper - and the people who consider price alone are this man's lawful prey." - John Ruskin.

Dentistry like everything else must be paid for. Like everything else people feel it costs too much. For those unfamiliar with dentistry, and concerned with its costs, it would be wise to consider the fact that there are few if any endeavors, whose lowest priced products or services, are good practical value. Dentistry is in the position of having some of its most significant features tiny, often invisible. A crude low priced dental appliance is about the same in size as the finest, often bigger. Materials for both cost about the same. There is a great difference in quality.

The basic raw materials, steel and brass, in the small inner works of a watch weigh under one-half ounce. Finer watches usually weigh less. Initial cost for this quantity of such substances may be less than one cent. These raw materials worked and machined for even the cheapest watch could cost a few dollars. Some watch works cost thousands.

A basic unit of modern dentistry is the full jacket or crown which completely surrounds an individual tooth. Least expensive requiring least work is the solid all gold precision crown. Many people think they're too costly. I conducted a personal survey. I cut the natural tooth crown carefully from the root of a tooth I had recently removed, and not saying I was a dentist, visited several jewelers with the following story. "Hello sir. This crown is from the first and only tooth my wife ever had extracted. It meant very much to her. She hated to lose it. I want to surprise her. I secretly asked the dentist to cut the crown off this way. I would like you to mount this tooth crown into a surrounding simple solid gold setting secured to make a ring for her finger." The lowest quoted price was $135.00. It went as high as $275.00 for the simple ring in one shop, that tried to convince me to add diamonds along the sides. I didn't ask how much additional that would have cost. For proper reference to constant rising prices, it is noted that this survey was made in 1965.

Many gold rings made to fit fingers are less expensive. These however, are always from a selection of existing pre-molded designs merely made to fit. The custom made tooth crown mounted ring I described would probably be considered reasonable by many at its lowest price. Both a real dental gold crown and my mythical ring are of gold costing only a small part of their total. The ring needs only to fit its finger comfortably and to hold the cut tooth crown as a setting. A dental gold crown for the mouth must fit precisely, accurately between each tooth on both of its sides, and over the prepared natural tooth it protects perfectly sealing out germs. To make the crown a dentist must cut the tooth scientifically. He often also administers inner tooth treatments. Impressions are taken to make the crown in the dental laboratory more accurately than any ring and a separate appointment is needed to cement it. In the dental laboratory the crowns outer surface is artistically formed to blend with adjacent teeth and its chewing surface is carved to properly interdigitate with teeth of the opposite jaw.

Despite this, dentistry today costs less than ever before. It is not lower in the specific numbers used to measure money paid for particular services, such numbers are unimportant. Dentistry is lower in its real price. The real

TEETH TEETH TEETH

DIAGNOSIS AND TREATMENT PLANNING

cost of anything is not the digits of dollars, francs, marks or pesos paid for purchase, but the amount of labor expended to earn them. The numbers mean little. Standard of living has never been as high and a high standard of living means prices are low. For fewer hours worked today man receives more food, clothing, shelter, entertainment, comfort, medical and dental services. More, better, attractive fillings, inlays and bridges are being put in more people's mouths. Less teeth are lost than ever before in history, and these things are all being paid for with less labor. We complain about having to pay, man always has, and as long as things needed remain needed, man always will. Perhaps someday everything desired will be available. Then what.

Analysis discerns Details of Defect
So Proper Treatment yields Best Effect

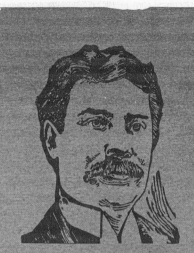

Dr. KING.

Originator of the King
Safe System of Painless
Dentistry and Inventor of
the "Natural Gum" Set
of Teeth.

NO PAIN, NO HIGH PRICES

My $8 sets are the most lifelike and finest fitting plates that dental science can procure. I have the reputation of making the most natural looking, the finest fitting and the best wearing teeth. No set ever leaves my office until our patron is perfectly satisfied as to fit and appearance. I give my personal guarantee for 10 years with each set. No more than $8 charged for the best set at Dr. Kings office unless a special set is desired

DON'T BUY OLD STYLE TEETH. **Full** $**5** **PAINLESS**
Set **EXTRACTION**
FREE

Dr. King's latest invention the "NATURAL GUM" is a wonderful improvement over the old artificial gum. It makes impossible to recognize artificial teeth in the mouth.
This is the only office in LEWISTON where gold crowns and teeth without plates undetectable from natural ones are inserted positively without pain.

CROWN and BRIDGE WORK $5.00   GOLD FILLING, $1.50 up.   OTHERS, 50c up

DR. THOS. JEFFERSON KING.   **TELEPHONE CON.**

38 Lisbon St. (over Doyle Bros.) Off. Hrs. 9 a.m. to 8 p.m. Sundays by appointment. Lewiston. 1891

TEETH TEETH TEETH

110

7

IT NEED NOT HURT ∾ ANESTHESIA

A friend told me of a man who with two others left the state of Washington for fur trapping in severe remote far northern Canada. They expected to be and were snowed in for a long winter. They had a comfortable cabin and ample supplies but couldn't and didn't expect to communicate with others. One suffered a toothache so unbearably painful he shot and killed himself.

The word pain derives from Old French, peine, Middle English, peini, and Latin, poena, all meaning penalty or punishment. These were during times when pain was believed judgment's award for sins performed. Dental neglect is not a sin but will lead to pain.

Pain is discomfort ache and hurt, reaching pangs through to torment, suffered by the body, acting as a biological warning protective mechanism, felt through nerves, calling attention to injury or damaging defects of the body. Most dental treatment like cutting decayed teeth or extracting teeth, involves small professional surgical invasions of the body, which cause controlled local limited body damages. Such professional invasions done by dentists or other surgeons are carefully planned to perform corrective treatment, so that a minimum of body invasion creates maximum curative result. Unfortunately our wonderful automatic pain signal mechanism which helpfully warns of harmful disease and injury, doesn't distinguish between therapeutic invasions that cure and those of damage and disease. Scientific man however, invented anesthetics to eliminate pain sensation permitting comfortable performance of needed therapy.

Pain is conducted by electric like impulse generated by the body, transmitted along nerves to the brain. Nerves contain fat. Most anesthetics are fat solvents. They attract to nerves combining with and affecting them, temporarily altering their ability to conduct electrical impulse, creating anesthesia eliminating pain sensation. None is felt. There is none.

APPREHENSION

Some patients through lack of knowledge, suffer an understandably uncontrollable fear of dentistry and exaggerated pains, ignorance incorrectly anticipates. Mild sedatives available in pharmacies help a relaxed approach to dental appointments. For those especially nervous needing added ease, the dentist may prescribe tranquilizers to be taken before appointments.

TEETH TEETH TEETH

LOCAL ANESTHESIA

Local anesthesia is loss of sensation in a limited part of the body without loss of consciousness. Most dental procedure is performed with local anesthesia at the small operated area, so the patient feels no pain while conscious, comfortable, and cooperative.

TOPICAL SURFACE ANESTHESIA
(close to the surface local anesthesia)

At one time pain of small skin surface operations was considered unpleasant but of short duration and endurable, preferred to the discomfort of deep injection anesthesia. At the moment these surface operation pangs were felt they sometimes seemed unbearable. Modern topical anesthetic solutions applied with a wad of cotton or sprayed on the surface penetrates soft tissues to a shallow depth, permitting simple surgical painless procedures without injections. Close to the surface abscesses can be lanced or opened painlessly. Applied first to the site of an injection the needle is hardly felt going in. Far back in the mouth sprayed on palate and throat topical anesthetics stop annoying gagging. If some pain is ever felt despite topical anesthesia, the treatment went beyond its depth of flesh penetration.

LOCAL INJECTION ANESTHESIA

Most dental procedures, like cutting a tooth cavity for filling or removing a tooth, are beyond the depth penetration of topical anesthetics. Teeth and most mouth parts are enervated by nerves coming from deep within the tissues. To anesthetize such parts the dentist must get to those nerves. To administer anesthesia he is familiar with deep internal head anatomy, so he can reach particular nerves sensing particular teeth. To get to those deep locations with minimum damage to the tissues between, the dentist transmits his anesthetic solutions from outside internally through a fine long thin hollow sharp pointed stainless steel tube called a hypodermic needle. Hypo means under, dermic skin.

Topical anesthesia first applied to the site of penetration prevents pain as the needle enters. Slow emission of solution from the needle tip as it advances along its path may eliminate pain along the way. Awkward pressures sensed during injection, are more of a stretched tissue feeling, as anesthetics enter occupying space like air blowing up a balloon. The surrounding unanesthetized tissues forced to yield around the area feel the stretch. Just as outer appearance varies from person to person so does internal anatomy. The anesthetic is rarely delivered to the exact location desired. A small wait is necessary for the solution to spread and reach affecting the nerve. Sometimes added injections are needed.

TEETH TEETH TEETH

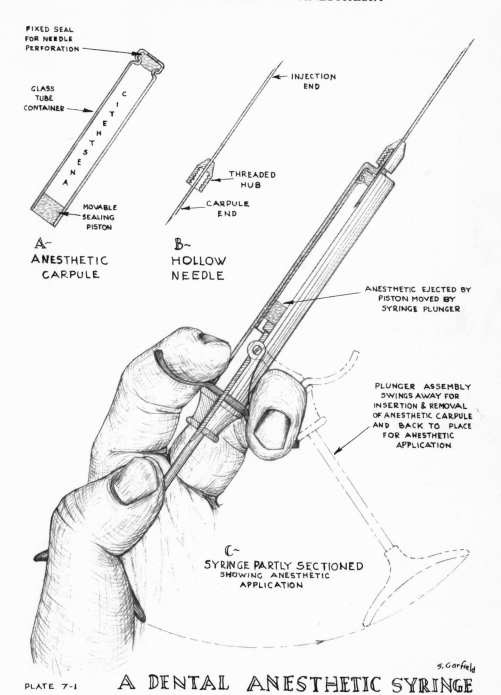

FIXED SEAL
FOR NEEDLE
PERFORATION

GLASS
TUBE
CONTAINER

ANESTHETIC

MOVABLE
SEALING
PISTON

A~
ANESTHETIC
CARPULE

INJECTION
END

THREADED
HUB

CARPULE
END

B~
HOLLOW
NEEDLE

ANESTHETIC EJECTED BY
PISTON MOVED BY
SYRINGE PLUNGER

PLUNGER ASSEMBLY
SWINGS AWAY FOR
INSERTION & REMOVAL
OF ANESTHETIC CARPULE
AND BACK TO PLACE
FOR ANESTHETIC
APPLICATION

C~
SYRINGE PARTLY SECTIONED
SHOWING ANESTHETIC
APPLICATION

S. Garfield

PLATE 7-1

A DENTAL ANESTHETIC SYRINGE

TEETH TEETH TEETH

LOCAL INJECTION EQUIPMENT ∾ Refer to Plate 7-1, A DENTAL ANESTHETIC SYRINGE. Local anesthesia is administered by hypodermic syringe. Injectable anesthetics are conveniently available in individual carpule or cartridge containing about two cubic centimeters of solution. Refer to Plate 7-1, drawing A, The Anesthetic Carpule. The carpule is a short glass tube sealed at one end with a fixed soft rubber or plastic stopper. Its other end seals the solution in with a small internal movable soft rubber or plastic piston. The hypodermic needle is a long thin tube pointed sharp at each end. See drawing B. Closer to one of the ends it is fixed in a female inner screw-threaded hub. The Syringe assembly is usually a metal tube with one end constricted to form a hollow externally screw-threaded male hub. See drawing C. The opposite open end has an attached hingeable saddle like neck, holding within it a movable plunger rod assembly. The neck-rod assembly can be hinged or folded away for insertion of a carpule, and folded back in place for operation.

To use the syringe the needle's female threaded hub is screwed onto the the syringe male threaded end. The neck-rod assembly is folded out of the way so that a carpule may be inserted with its fixed stopper seal end first. As the carpule moves to place, the inner needle point pierces the fixed seal making the solution available to the hollow needle. With carpule in place the neck plunger rod assembly is swung back in line and the syringe is ready for use. The dentist holds the syringe between his index and middle fingers with his thumb on the plunger rod rest. As the plunger is depressed the inner movable piston seal advances into the carpule forcing anesthetic out through the needle.

ANESTHETIC SOLUTIONS ∾ There are different anesthetic solutions. Some people respond better to one than another. Most contain Procaine, a newer name for the drug called novocaine, or similar compounds combined with other refined additives. Most also contain Vasoconstrictors, drugs which tighten narrowing the surrounding blood vessels, so that the anesthetic does not seep away but is kept confined to the local area. Solutions are available with different concentrations of anesthetic and vasoconstrictor, for procedures of different severity and duration. Anesthetics are available without vasoconstrictors for very brief operations, and for the rare patient whose condition favors avoiding such drugs.

UPPER TEETH LOCAL INJECTIONS ∾ Crowns of the upper teeth project down from the upper jaw or maxilla from their roots embedded up inside. The jaw is covered with soft pink gum tissue. Beneath this gum the outer bone surface is thin and porous. Underneath its porous surface the inner bone is spongy and even more porous. Inside the bone fine nerve filaments come from a network above and behind, entering the tip of each root, supplying sensation to each tooth. To anesthetize any tooth of the upper jaw the dentist may first apply topical anesthetic to the local gum surface, painlessly insert his needle through gum towards the bone and deliver the anesthetic. The tissues stretch, ballooning up filling with solution. Gently massaging the area with a finger helps drive the anesthetic Infiltrating to penetrate the porous bone internally, surrounding the nerve fibers altering their physiology, so they can't conduct sensations to the brain. The tooth and surrounding tissues are anesthetized. Dentistry can be performed comfortably. No pain is felt.

LOWER JAW BLOCK ANESTHESIA ∾ Anesthesia for the lower jaw or mandible requires special considerations. The chewing mandible is movable, the largest strongest bone of the face. Like movable beams of machines that exert heavy forces it is dense and tough. Its outer surface is not porous but hard, thick, dense and compact, with few openings. Injection of anesthetic next to particular teeth, expecting the solution to in-filtrate through the dense surface inside to nerves entering the root tips, is usually unsuccessful. Another technique is used.

The lower jawbone is somewhat horseshoe shaped, turning up on each side in the back. Its teeth are embedded along rising from its upper surface. Flesh and gum cover the outside. Beneath the tooth root tips, inside the dense bone, there is a hollow tube-like canal called the Mandibular Canal. The right is called the right mandibular canal, the left is the left mandibular canal. From the front center of the chin, both mandibular canals continue back inside the jawbone, rising with the bone perforating through right and left openings at the bone surface, far back in the throat about one-half inch above the right and left third molars in the average adult. These openings about one-fourth inch diameter in an adult, passing from the inner canals to outside the bone are each called the right and left mandibular foramen. Foramen means opening or passage. Within the flesh, blood vessels and nerve trunks farther in from the head enter the right and left mandibular foramina, run along forward inside each respective canal and divide into fine branches, supplying nutrition and sensation to all the right and left teeth root tips and jaw sides.

The dentist through the mouth directs his needle to perforate the flesh, aiming at the right or left mandibular foramen of the side to be operated. Anesthetic at the site blocks all the internal nerves, anesthetizing all the teeth and the jaw of that side. Many other important body vessels are in the area, the anatomy is complex varying from person to person. Sometimes the patient feels the dentist probing with the needle-point under the flesh,

TEETH TEETH TEETH

for inner familiar bone surface landmarks before depositing his solution. There is no way for any dentist to know exactly where under the flesh his patient's mandibular foramen is. Sometimes several injections are needed for the lower jaw. Some nerve. When anesthesia is obtained any procedure can be performed comfortably without pain.

AFTER THE OPERATION ∞ While any anesthesia remains, until all is gone, there may be some annoying loss of mouth, lip, talking, eating, control. Taste buds are also desensitized and for those who can and care to eat, food isn't fully enjoyed. Within an hour or few the anesthesia slowly dissipates. Sensation gradually returns sometimes with local discomfort. Aspirin is often enough. If necessary the dentist prescribes more powerful drugs to help over the healing period.

NITROUS OXIDE ANALGESIA

Analgesics are drugs that inhibit or abolish pain, through the body's central nervous system, without loss of consciousness. Aspirin is mildly analgesic, codeine more powerful. Some analgesics like codeine could become addictive. Some produce euphoria, a feeling of well being buoyancy that may go on to delightful elation. Nitrous oxide is a colorless gas with pleasant odor and taste. Inhaled it produces a lessening, even complete loss of pain sensation, accompanied by euphoria and even laughter. It's also called Laughing Gas, and in mid 1800's when first popularized was used in entertainments and wild sometimes orgiastic laughing gas parties.

Nitrous oxide taken pure could be dangerous. Nitrous oxide combined with oxygen, inhaled through a nose mask, produces a conscious dreamlike analgesic state making dentistry comfortable even pleasurable for many. Some express regret when treatment is over. A few are annoyed by nitrous. Some patients, especially women, become sexually imaginative under its influence. Unfortunately poor patient, it's only the nitrous. Dentists are cautioned to keep assistants present during nitrous oxide oxygen administration. Some patients refuse dentistry with any other anesthetic. Used as an analgesic while consciousness exists some pain may be felt. I've heard patients say, "It hurts but I don't care. It feels good." Especially successful technique for many, starts with nitrous oxygen analgesia followed by pleasantly accepted local injection anesthesia. Nitrous oxide is more expensive than injectable anesthetics. It produces no unpleasant after effects, in fact its pleasant euphoria often lingers for hours. It is not addictive. Nitrous oxide at high concentration with low oxygen is sometimes used for general anesthesia with loss of consciousness.

TEETH TEETH TEETH

GENERAL ANESTHESIA

General anesthesia affects the entire body with loss of consciousness and all sensation. The patient totally unaware of what happens is essentially asleep, feeling no pain or anything during all procedure. All vital organs, brain, heart, lungs, are under anesthetized control and must be maintained functioning safely while the operation proceeds. Special training is taken by personnel administering such anesthesia. Some dentists limit their practice to Anesthetist as some medical doctors do. Dentistry is performed under general anesthesia in offices and hospitals.

In preparation for general anesthesia the doctor may prescribe premedication drugs to be taken at home. Certain relaxants diminish reflexes, and the patient is cautioned not to drive an automobile to the appointment. Since all organs including the digestive tract are anesthetized, eating and drinking should be avoided for instructed prior hours, and bladder and bowels should be emptied before the operation. The anesthetized disrupted nervous system could unexpectedly cause vomiting, urination, and defecation, an inconvenient stinky mess on the operating table.

The doctor evaluates each patient for choice of anesthetics and means of application. Some patients are afraid of divulging personal secrets while affected. Administration may be of gases breathed into the lungs or solutions injected into the blood vessels, sometimes both are combined. In all cases the anesthetics circulating in blood reach the brain and spinal cord, to desensitize the body's controlling nervous system. The patient unconscious, comfortably safe, is completely unaware of being operated. Within a short time awareness returns. The doctor gives aftercare instructions, and if needed prescribes drugs taken by mouth to relieve a short pain sensed healing period.

INTRAVENOUS ANESTHESIA

Intravenous means into a vein or blood vessel. Intravenous injection is a simple means of general anesthesia for dental surgeries like extracting teeth. After premedication the solution delivered through a thin needle enters a vein of the arm or leg. The patient is told to count slowly while the anesthetic is delivered drop by drop. As anesthesia ensues sleepily, counting slows. Pleasant sleep anesthetic unconsciousness is indicated when counting stops. Operation proceeds painlessly. If the anesthetist sees any sign of returning sensation added drops are injected.

Pentothal sodium, a barbituric acid derivative, is often used. There are others. For longer operations nitrous oxide and oxygen gases may also be

TEETH TEETH TEETH

inhaled. Recovery is pleasant in several minutes and comfortable euphoria may linger for hours. Nausea or headache is rare.

CURARE

Curare, the dried extract of woody vine, was first used as an arrowtip poison by South American jungle Indians. It contains two alkaloid drugs, one paralyzes the heart, one paralyzes muscles. These on the arrow killed the Indians' victims. Pharmacology refined improving this natural extract for use as an additive in general anesthesia. Pharmaceutical curare is a powerful muscle relaxant. In accident cases and for setting bone fractures like broken jaws, curare relaxes patient's complicated muscle systems permitting the surgeon to work unrestrained.

HOSPITAL DENTISTRY

Limited emergency dentistry like tooth extractions and simple denture repairs have been done for medically hospitalized patients for a long time. Dentists and oral surgeons also perform limited dentistry in hospitals for those whose physical condition demands such care. Recently some hospitals have dental divisions with complete modern dental facilities for restorative dentistry of all kinds, from simple fillings to full mouth reconstruction. Similar to medical surgery the patient after prior examination is admitted the night before. The medical staff is available if needed. Major operative procedures are performed by the dentist under general anesthesia controlled by an anesthetist. Impressions are taken for permanent appliances like jackets and bridges to be made in the dental laboratory. Temporary medicated appliances may be inserted. The patient goes home. Simpler finishing phases like cementing bridges and adjustments if needed are usually completed in the dental office.

HYPNOTISM

Hypnotism was probably first unknowingly practiced by primitive man. Animals sometimes seem to hypnotize each other. The Bible's Old and new Testaments indicate hypnotism with phases "laying on of hands" and "calling upon the name of the Lord." Blind have been made to see and lame to walk. Such cures of course were effected where it was the mind that caused physical disfunction. It was mind over body.

In the eighteenth century Franc Anton Mesmer an Austrian medical doctor popularized hypnotism with what he called "animal magnetism." Those were times before chemical anesthesia, and the mind was in greater need searching for a way. To present times hypnotism has experienced fluctuations of acceptance and rejection. Arms and legs have been successfully amputated with hypnotism as sole anesthetic agent, while at many other times the method won't work for minor procedures. Hypnotism works, but not constantly, reliably, unfailingly, dependably. The reasons aren't all known.

Essentially hypnotism is suggestion. The capable therapeutic hypnotist by suggestive technique guides his subjects mind away from pain inducing fears. In some cases hypnotism can create a lethargic dream state, disassociating the mind completely, leaving its body available for painless surgery. I myself have extracted difficult teeth with no anesthesia other than hypnosis, without discomfort shown by the patient. At other times hypnotism failed me completely. It cannot be regularly depended upon day by day for all patients. We don't know why.

In my dental practice I prefer the more dependable liquid and gaseous chemical anesthetics. I rarely use formal hypnotism any longer. However to some extent, everyday, hardly aware of it, probably through personal confidence I emit a form of suggestion dispelling patients fears. You might call this informal hypnotism. It works.

Modern Means Provide Cure
With which we Need No Pain Endure

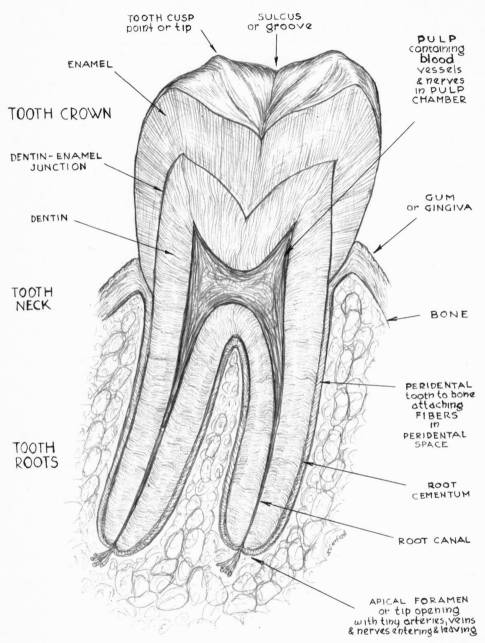

TOOTH CUSP
point or tip

SULCUS
or groove

PULP
containing
blood
vessels
& nerves
in PULP
CHAMBER

ENAMEL

TOOTH CROWN

DENTIN-ENAMEL
JUNCTION

DENTIN

GUM
or GINGIVA

TOOTH
NECK

BONE

PERIDENTAL
tooth to bone
attaching
FIBERS
in
PERIDENTAL
SPACE

TOOTH
ROOTS

ROOT
CEMENTUM

ROOT CANAL

S.Garfield

APICAL FORAMEN
or tip opening
with tiny arteries, veins
& nerves entering & leaving

PLATE 8-1

S.Garfield

SECTION CUT THROUGH AN INDIVIDUAL TOOTH MAGNIFIED

TEETH TEETH TEETH

8

THE INDIVIDUAL TOOTH

This chapter describes the restoration of a tooth at increasing stages of degeneration. It begins with one decayed so slightly it is easily restored with a simple filling. It continues with others more degenerated needing more complex fillings, and inlays, and even further to severely degenerated teeth needing the fully covered protection of surrounding crowns or jackets. Description extends to the repair of a tooth so deteriorated its crown is all rotted away, and root remnants remaining in the jawbone may not even by known of by the person whose mouth they are in. Yet such a tooth if those invisible roots in bone are adequate can often be completely restored with an artificial jacket, stronger than a natural tooth, impervious to decay, looking like a natural tooth undetectable from those mouth grown, often to last for life.

A TOOTH, THE WHOLE TOOTH, NOTHING BUT THE TOOTH

Let's study a tooth thoroughly in detail, child or adult, as a trader examines a slave in the nude. Not for purchase, such teeth can't be bought, but for knowledge, inside and out, for the sake of the health of the tooth that serves us.

Refer to Plate 8-1, SECTION CUT THROUGH AN INDIVIDUAL TOOTH. The erupted visible portion of a tooth is the Crown. Adjacent to the crown's encircling girth which emerges from the gum is the Neck of the tooth. This extends to Roots embedded in supporting bone.

ENAMEL ∾ The tooth's visible exposed outer covering is Enamel, surrounding the crown to the gums at the neck all around. Enamel is the hardest tissue of the body, probably the hardest animal substance known. Like flint it will strike a spark with steel. Enamel is brittle, calcified 97 percent inorganic, plus organic materials. Mature enamel is not considered alive or vital. It contains high mineral content in crystalline arrangement. Tooth crowns are not a single constant color, but vary in shading along their length with enamel thickness and the color of material below. The crown normally ranges in color from yellowish nearer the root to grayish white towards the tip, with tints of blue and slightest evasive hints of pink. These variances are caused by differences in translucency increasing with degree of calcification. Yellowish teeth have thinner enamel through which yellow dentin beneath shows. Grayish teeth are more opaque, less thoroughly calcified, hiding the yellow dentin. An idea of pink can be detected by careful color analysis orginating with the inner blood live pulp and reflections from the gum. Aging enamel may darken and increase resistance to decay. Exact reasons aren't known.

With use, like the soles of shoes, tooth crowns wear away, through their enamel tips and softer substances beneath, shortening in length with age.

DENTIN ∾ Inside under the enamel is Dentin, very similar to ivory. The surface along which dentin meets enamel is called the Dentin-Enamel Junction. The tooth is vulnerable at this junction along which decay that reaches it spreads more rapidly. Dentin is elastic, compressible, has some tensile strength, not brittle like enamel. That's why ivory is good for carving. Dentin contains 72 percent mineral salts and 28 percent organic material. Recent studies under electron-microscope lead some investigators to believe fine nutrient canals and micro-nerves enter dentin from both its inner and outer surfaces. Dentin is considered alive. Dentin is yellow, lighter in youth, not translucent like enamel. It constitutes the inner structural bulk of the tooth, supporting the harder outer enamel surfaced crown from within, extending as roots into supporting bone. Inside the dentin there is a void called the Pulp Chamber. Sometimes later in life along the pulp chamber walls dentin grows again forming an irregular dentin layer called Secondary Dentin, making the pulp chamber smaller. It sometimes occurs as a natural healing attempt against trauma, and adjacent to areas resisting decay. In rare cases secondary dentin fills the entire pulp chamber.

PULP ∾ Within the pulp chamber inside the dentin is the soft organic live Pulp. Pulp is often wrongly called the nerve. It does contain Nerve in addition to other live materials. The nerve supplies sensation to the tooth. Pulp's other tissues nourish the tooth. At the tip end of each root there is a tiny opening to the pulp chamber from the outer bone called the Apical Foramen, apical means tip, foramen means opening or passage, through which all sensory and nutritive vessels enter and leave to service the tooth. There are tiny arteries called arterioles, which supply blood as they enter becoming smaller, forming a network of microscopic looping capillaries which enlarge again into venules which are tiny veins that remove used blood from inside the tooth. There are tiny lymphatic vessels and connective tissue and other specialized tissues and cells. Certain of these when occasion arises act within the pulp chamber helping to defend the tooth from bacterial invasion. THE TOOTH is really quite clever.

TEETH TEETH TEETH

CEMENTUM ∾ Cementum is a thin hard bonelike covering substance, surrounding roots of teeth approaching the enamel towards the tooth's neck. It is perforated at root tips by the apical foramen leading to the inner pulp chamber. Cementum serves to connect short microscopic fibers that attach tooth roots to the bone layer lining, around inside root sockets. Cementum is thicker towards the root tips and may increase in thickness with age, even sometimes moving the root out slightly compensating to some extent for natural wear shortening of the chewing surface. TOOTH CEMENTUM is quite clever too.

THE INDIVIDUAL TOOTH RESTORED

It is a rare mouth family of teeth which hasn't had at least a single member that ever suffered any dental disease. Most mouths have several to many that sicken. In many mouths its most. The most common tooth disease is decay or caries. Caries comes from old Latin karez meaning decay, and old Greek kariez meaning death and destruction. Caries destroys teeth.

FILLINGS ∾ Fillings are the simplest dental restorations. They restore decayed spaces inside teeth by replacement filling of the voids. They're usually made, mixing powder and liquid to a soft mass, placing some into the cavity to harden and then carving off the excess. The simplest filling is the Temporary medicated Filling, called 'temporaries' in dental offices. They satisfy many emergencies. A popular temporary consists of white zinc oxide powder and liquid eugenol. It's an old reliable, helps the aching tooth. A similar preparation is used by physicians in skin ointments. In emergency when help isn't available chewing gum may serve as a temporary filling. It's made with chicle, a gum similar to gutta percha, an old dental material. Chew sugar out of the gum, roll off a tiny piece, place it into the cavity and hope it helps.

To place a Permanent Filling the dentist usually anesthetizes the area, eliminating pain and minimizing discomfort while preparing the cavity. Teeth are cut or prepared with hand instruments and power equipment. Most cutting is power driven. Dentistry demands accuracy. Just as steel parts precisely cut in industry are gripped by vise or chuck for the machining cutter, the operated jaw is securely held while the dentist uses his power drill. Slight slip could cause regretted error.

The dental drill is really misnamed. The tiny cutters inserted into today's ultra-high-speed air rotors and other power driven handpieces are usually diamond coated or carbide burs not used to cut penetrating at the tip like a drill. They cut with hard diamond particles or tiny blades along their sides and ends, revolving like miniature portable precision milling machines. Older slow equipment which turned about five thousand revolutions in a minute, causing vibrations to pound patients teeth and head, as each relatively soft steel blade turning hit to take its cut, has been replaced by ultra speed up to 300,000 R.P.M. Tiny individual cuts, requiring less force taken as each peripheral blade of the whirling cutter another following next so fast smoothly, makes modern toothcutting quite comfortable.

Preparation of the cavity involves removal of decay and other tooth parts, to provide a properly engineered tooth excavation most ideally shaped to support the particular filling material used. Different materials have different structural qualities, considered by the dentist designing cavities, so the remaining healthy tooth part combines with its filling for maximum service. There is no filling material for mouth use that chemically bonds to the tooth. Dental scientists are working on it. Retention or keeping the filling in is accomplished by undercutting some inner cavity locations larger than the opening. See Plate 8-2, RESTORING THE INDIVIDUAL TOOTH, Drawing Series A, Fillings. The soft filling mix put in can't come out after hardening. Where decay leaves only a thin layer of dentin along the inner live pulp the dentist may protect that area with a medicated insulating layer located to permanently stay under the permanent filling.

With passage of time fillings may deteriorate and fall out. Sometimes the securely filled cavity suffers adjacent new surrounding decay enlarging it. Before falling out the patient may feel loosening or it might be dislodged by an examining dentist. Loss of such fillings is lucky. Tooth restorations must be tight to seal out germs. Loose fillings are more dangerous than none. The slight looseness space of surrounding opening is an ideal haven for germs, often causing more damage than annoyance from the open hole.

SILVER AMALGAM FILLINGS ∾ Silver amalgam often called silver for short, sometimes amalgam, is dentistry's most serviceable filling material. In metallurgical language an amalgam is any alloy or mixture of metals one of which is mercury. Throughout the world, dentists probably insert more silver amalgams than any other filling. After the cavity is prepared the amalgam mix is made from two basic metals. One, a finely powdered silver alloy containing small amounts of copper tin and zinc, each added for particular scientific purposes. The other is the liquid metal mercury also called quicksilver, because of its unique quick flowing quality. Mercury, the only metal liquid at ordinary temperatures, freezes into solid metal like any other at 37.96°F. below zero.

The silver alloy powder and liquid mercury mixed, make a soft putty

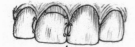

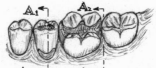

invisible inner undercuts
FRONT FILLINGS~usually plastic
match teeth shades

REAR FILLINGS usually of hard silver alloy & liquid mercury amalgam

section
A₁-A₁

view
A₂-A₂

Fillings are usually compounded of a powder and a liquid to a soft mix. Placed into the prepared tooth cavity they harden in a short time, held by inner regions made wider than outer surface openings. Like concrete most fillings have high compression & low tensile strength

FILLINGS ~ SUPPORTED BY THE TOOTH WHOSE LOST VOIDS THEY FILL & RESTORE
A~

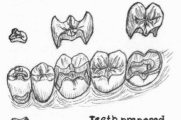
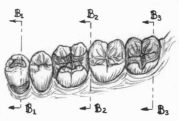

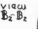

section
B₁~B₁

view
B₂-B₂

section
B₃-B₃

Teeth prepared
tapered for inlays
& inlays tapered to fit them

cemented in use

INLAYS PRECISION CAST OF MOLTEN METAL ALLOYS USUALLY GOLD ARE HIGH IN BOTH COMPRESSION & TENSILE STRENGTH

INLAYS~PARTLY EMBRACE & SUPPORT TEETH THEY RESTORE
B~

front
¾
crown
cast
gold

full
jacket
natural
tooth
shade

rear
¾
crown
cast
gold

full
crown
cast in
gold
could be
natural

thin shell
crown
gold or
stainless steel
~aluminum
for temporary
use

JACKET~CROWN RESTORATIONS CEMENTED IN USE

JACKET~CROWN RESTORATIONS
& TEETH PREPARED FOR THEM

JACKET~CROWNS of HIGH COMPRESSION & TENSILE STRENGTH SURROUND, SUPPORT & PROTECT TEETH
C~

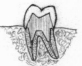

ROOT IN BONE   ENDODONTIA~ROOT SEALED   FOUNDATION PREPARED   POST STRUCTURE   RESTORED

REBUILDING AN ENTIRE TOOTH WHEN ALL BUT ITS ROOTS ARE LOST
D~

PLATE 8-2 RESTORING THE INDIVIDUAL TOOTH S. Gatfield
SOME BASIC PRINCIPLES

TEETH TEETH TEETH

like mass carefully inserted into the prepared tooth. Hardening starts with amalgamation, a process whereby the liquid mercury and alloy powder dissolve into each other, sort of welding strongly together. While this occurs the dentist carves excess amalgam off to proper tooth contour. The patient bites gently down closed on Articulating Paper, a porous paper containing ink. The ink marked higher spots are removed by the dentist making an Occlusal or Bite Adjustment. Chewing should be avoided until the silver amalgam hardens within several hours.

Amalgam is satisfactory for certain fillings but has structural limitations. Like clay brick of building it is strong only in compression. Subjected to tensile or side tearing forces fracture could occur. Silver amalgam is suited to serve surfaces of areas supported by remaining healthy teeth structure and between teeth where support is provided by contacting adjacent teeth. Back in the mouth, compressive chewing forces are high. These are areas that often decay where silver serves well. In time silver fillings may crumble slightly along their edges yet stay safely sealed immediately beneath. This should be checked by a dentist for serviceability or need of replacement.

Silver fillings also have a slight chemical, medical value. Silver compounds are used in some pharmaceutical drugs. Their silver constituent seems to deter some bacterial growth. A disadvantage silver shares with gold and other metals is heat and cold conduction more readily transferred inside to the live pulp than through natural tooth itself. Where indicated, dentists place protective medicated insulators called Bases beneath the metal restoration. Newly filled teeth sensitive to hot and cold temperature slowly adjust as the tooth heals. Silver is rarely placed in front of the mouth since it doesn't match natural tooth shades and sometimes darkens in time.

GOLD FOIL FILLINGS ∾ Pure 24 carat gold, thin foil sheets and other soft gold forms, can be used to make fine dental restorations. Pure gold's soft working quality and inert resistance to corrosion permits especially ideal sealing of cut cavity margins and maintains cleanliness. Pure gold in tiny thin pieces has the quality when absolutely clean of actually welding to itself when forced together under pressure. Bits of the gold are heat annealed to soften and drive off contaminants immediately before placement. Then with high concentrated forces and sometimes unpleasant pounding it is condensed, cold welding to itself, bit by bit gradually filling the cavity. Excess is carved to shape with tiny knives and files. Gold foil fillings are excellent yet not very popular since manipulation of the material is tricky. Such restorations have moderate both compressive and tensile strength limiting them to smaller sizes. Sometimes the condensation pounding forces damage the tooth's inner live pulp.

THE INDIVIDUAL TOOTH

ESTHETIC OR NATURAL LOOKING FILLINGS ⚮ Standards of beauty vary with cultures and customs. At one time people proudly displayed dentistry even adorning their teeth with diamonds set in gold. In modern society most people want natural looking teeth as evidence of youth and perfection. They prefer their dentistry indiscernible. Natural tooth shade filling materials are available making undetectable restorations possible. Two popular types of such substances are synthetic porcelain and acrylic resin. Each has different merits and defects. Neither are strong, their use is limited to front teeth. In most mouths chewing forces in the back could soon wear them down.

Synthetic Porcelain fillings, often called porcelain for short are not really porcelain. The dentist comparing the tooth with a shade selecting guide chooses the closest color. He may combine two or three. Porcelain fillings are made mixing clear phosphoric acid with a silicate powder which determines the shade. In soft plastic state the mix placed into the cavity hardens, and is carved to shape. Perfectly matched fillings may discolor in some mouths sooner than others. Silicate porcelains have good dimensional stability, but sometimes slowly dissolve. They may crumble in time along their edges. Powders are available incorporating fine glass fibers which increase their strength like reinforced concrete with steel rods.

Methyl Methacrylate, an acrylic resin is a more recent dental material. It is also used to make windows of jet aircraft. Powder of selected shades called the polymer is mixed with liquid monomer. Self polymerization causes hardening inside the cavity as both powder and liquid unite and solidify. Acrylic restorations have some tensile strength and are insoluble. They won't crumble at margins. They also may discolor eventually and sometimes warp slightly. Perfectly contoured acrylic restorations sometimes expand from their margins trapping edge stains. Shaved to fit they may expand again.

COMPOSITES are a new family of dental filling materials—the first to match teeth colors and shades, strong enough for use anywhere in the mouth. They seem capable of replacing unsightly silver fillings and of withstanding the heavy chewing grind even of back teeth.

Like the concrete cement of construction that contains rocks, composites are a sort of dental concrete filling for teeth.

Composites incorporate micron-size particles of quartz ceramic or glass, bound by an insoluble resin cement. Mixed of powder and liquid or pastes, they soon solidify to tooth color fillings, close to the hardness of silver and tooth itself. They look like tooth structure in X-ray.

TEETH TEETH TEETH

THE INDIVIDUAL TOOTH

THE GOLD INLAY

Many teeth that support fillings are saved by them. It sometimes happens, a tooth is so neglected not enough remains to hold a filling. To save such a tooth a restoration is needed which will support the tooth. This requires material with high tensile and compressive strength. Gold inlay is the answer. Even where silver amalgam is satisfactory the inlay is often superior, but more expensive. Lacking tensile quality amalgam can crumble and fracture tearing apart. Gold inlays never fail that way and help hold teeth together. Inlays are not better because they're gold, but because they're cast from molten metal. It's the casting that has the strength. Molten silver inlays would also serve though silver is weaker and softer than gold and tarnishes in the mouth. Dental gold castings are not pure gold but alloyed with other metals making them far superior to gold for dentistry. The higher price of inlays is not due to their precious metal cost which is only a small part of the total, but the additional exacting dental office and laboratory procedures needed to make them. For those who prefer whiter inlay color there are lighter gold alloys.

Preparing teeth for cast restorations demands exacting skills. The tooth is cut, usually entered first from the chewing surface, then precisely tapered extending over the sides beyond decayed areas so the gold restoration which replaces missing parts will end sealing on healthy tooth substance. Refer to Plate 8-2, Drawing Series B, Inlays. The rigid inlay made in the laboratory has the identical taper so as to fit exactly to place, restoring all missing parts in gold, sealing closely along all cut margins. The inlays side extensions help hold the tooth together. Making inlays is far more precision demanding than sealing a cavity with a filling, which is squeezed soft into place and forced spreading to fill the void.

LOST WAX CASTING ஒ Dental precision castings are made by the Lost Wax Process. This is an old method of casting originated by early art sculptors and jewelers. The dental profession perfected the technique, so that today some precision parts manufacturers use dental waxes and other materials for making especially accurate small industrial castings. To make a casting an exact model of it must first be made in wax. The cast gold inlay replaces decayed tooth parts plus other parts of the prepared tooth the dentist cuts away. For simple inlays the dentist sometimes carves his wax model on the prepared tooth in his patient's mouth. Most dental castings are carved on accurate models of the prepared tooth in the laboratory. The dentist takes impressions of the prepared teeth from which accurate working models are made. In the laboratory warmed

TEETH TEETH TEETH

soft wax is forced to replace every missing part of the cut tooth. The technician carves the wax, blended to fill all contours and meet adjacent teeth as a full normal tooth would. The model of the opposite jaw is closed as in chewing against the warm soft wax inlay, for forming the chewing surface needed as teeth come together. All cut away tooth parts are restored in wax so the waxed tooth looks complete on the model. The small wax inlay is cooled to harden on the tooth model and carefully removed. The tiny delicate wax model pattern is used to make a precision mold. Fine fire resistant investment powders are mixed with water to a liquid paste, which is carefully painted completely covering every detail of the entire wax inlay model, then placed inside a small steel container. The investment powders harden and dry around the wax model inside. This is put into a burnout oven whose temperature is slowly increased. The investment is heated and as temperature rises high the internal wax melts and completely burns out, leaving a mold void space exactly equal to the wax inlay model.

Dental gold alloy is molten yellow white hot near 2000°F. and under high pressure the liquid gold is forced through a small hole into the mold space of the investment. The gold soon cools hard producing an exact casting of the inlay. The outer investment is easily crumbled away. The casting is cleaned and finish polished. Dentistry's contribution has been the technical perfection of all materials involved, impression and model materials, waxes, investment powders, gold alloys, accurate thermostatic controlled temperature ovens, so that all expansions and contractions involved are calculated and compensated to yield castings that fit teeth precisely.

After trial the inlay is cemented to place. Minor adjustments may be needed. No dental cement has yet been perfected which actually bonds to gold or tooth. Seal and grip are by precise fit. Sensitivity to hot and cold if felt, diminishes and disappears.

JACKETS CAPS CROWNS

Inlays fit or lay largely within the tooth. When more of the tooth is missing, support is needed around the outside. Outer surrounding teeth supports are called Jackets, Caps, or Crowns, all different names for the same thing. A tooth may need restoration of its chewing surface, and around the back and both sides adjacent between its neighbors, yet its visible face looks good and is good. Such a tooth can sometimes be restored with a 3/4 gold crown. Refer to Plate 8-2, Drawing Series C,

Jackets, Crowns. The 3/4 crown leaves a single natural tooth face and completely embraces all other walls plus the chewing surface of the tooth. Such 3/4 crowns show gold along the tooth's natural face edges.

The Full Precision Cast Crown surrounds supporting the entire crown of a tooth. Teeth whose many decayed places, after being cleaned out, leave little more than a spongy network, can often be perfectly restored with a Full Crown. More structurally efficient than strong steel rings holding a wooden barrel together, the full crown like an all metal barrel closed at one end, slipped over the tooth provides maximum protection to the tooth and its contents. Many degenerated teeth whose only alternate was extraction loss, have been preserved for life by full crowns.

Full precision crowns made all of gold are called Gold Crowns. Of course full crowns or jackets all of gold are visibly gold glaring unnatural looking. Natural looking Plastic or Porcelain Jackets can also be precisely made to fully cover and protect teeth. If needed for strength they can be reinforced internally with invisible metal castings.

The Gold Shell Crown is an older approach to full crown protection. They're not completely custom made for the tooth but can be custom adapted. They are hollow thin gold crown shells made available in a large number of tooth shapes and sizes. The dentist selects one closest to the operated tooth, adapts it with scissors and contouring pliers, and may add reinforcing lower melting point gold solder to inside the chewing surface. After checking for fit and bite it is cemented in place. Appearance and marginal adaption are not as ideal as with the precision crown but substantial protection is provided and shell crowns cost less.

Stainless Steel Shell Crowns are sometimes used for children's teeth. Soft Aluminum Shell Crowns are often used for temporary protection to teeth under extensive treatment between dental appointments. Plastic natural looking thin shell Temporary Jackets or crowns are also available.

RESTORING A TOOTH WHOSE CROWN IS ALL GONE

Refer to Plate 8-2, Drawing Series D. Complete rebuilding of a tooth, whose crown is all gone so only roots remain in the jaw, is the most extensive individual tooth restoration possible. Important biological, medical, dental and engineering principles are involved. First roots and bone are examined. They must be capable of supporting the restored crown. Neglected roots are often diseased internally. Endodontic treatment, endo means inside, dontic the tooth, may be needed to seal the roots insuring against inner problems. Endodontic sealing permits cutting inside the roots for internal structural attachment. The roots may be prepared for deep penetrating pins, providing support similar to deep driven piles for tall building foundations and harbor pier construction. The dental engineer may feel it necessary to incorporate an outer embracing band to hold the roots together like a retaining wall. All these tiny features combine in a precise miniature structural foundation casting, which also provides an abutment for a full crown or jacket of choice. This crown restores the individual tooth, and can also sometimes if needed provide support for a bridge replacing other teeth completely missing. All procedures, endodontia, complex root foundation preparation, and crown reconstruction are exacting, may be expensive. Improved living satisfaction is worth the cost.

THE KNOCKED OUT TOOTH

Accidentally and intentionally, teeth are sometimes knocked out of the mouth, crown and root intact. Dental methods exist for restoring and replanting such teeth, even after found on the ground or several days later in grass, brought to the dentist in the bottom of a pocket. Modern dentistry can reinsert such teeth properly treated often to serve for life.

Know Thyself — Says Wisdoms Sage
Knowledge Expands Every Age

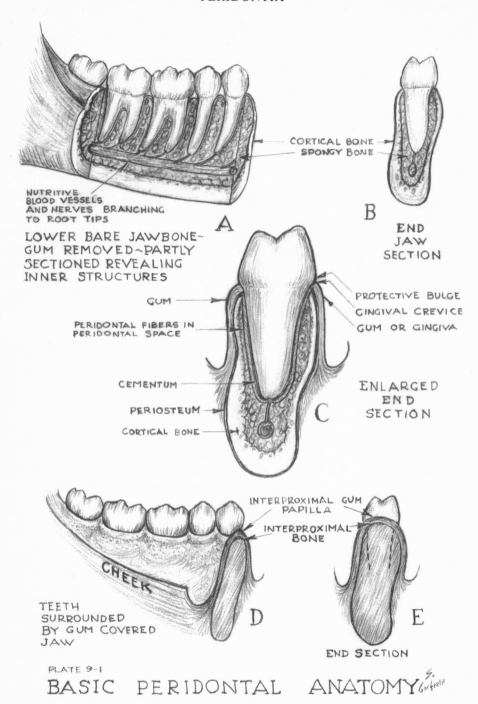

CORTICAL BONE
SPONGY BONE

NUTRITIVE
BLOOD VESSELS
AND NERVES BRANCHING
TO ROOT TIPS

A

B

END
JAW
SECTION

LOWER BARE JAWBONE-
GUM REMOVED~PARTLY
SECTIONED REVEALING
INNER STRUCTURES

GUM

PERIDONTAL FIBERS IN
PERIDONTAL SPACE

PROTECTIVE BULGE
GINGIVAL CREVICE
GUM OR GINGIVA

CEMENTUM

PERIOSTEUM

CORTICAL BONE

C

ENLARGED
END
SECTION

INTERPROXIMAL GUM
PAPILLA

INTERPROXIMAL
BONE

CHEEK

TEETH
SURROUNDED
BY GUM COVERED
JAW

D

E

END SECTION

PLATE 9-1
BASIC PERIDONTAL ANATOMY S. Garfield

TEETH TEETH TEETH

9

PERIDONTIA

Peri means around, dontia the tooth. Peridontia is a branch of dentistry concerned with diseases of tissues that surround, nourish, and support teeth. Dentists with special training who limit their practice to such work are called Peridontists. An older name for common peridontal disease is Pyorrhea.

Human teeth are covered with enamel the hardest animal substance known. Like hard tipped teeth of industrial cutting machines and teeth of earth excavating equipment that scoops through rocks, they must be firmly attached to the structural base that supports them. Peridontal disease destroys attaching gum and jawbone, sometimes causing even undecayed teeth to loosen and fall from the mouth. Many are lost unnecessarily this way. Treatment is available, that will stop, correct and cure such ills. A prevalent attitude that teeth must eventually be lost is wrong. Properly maintained they will serve their host for life.

STRUCTURAL ANATOMY OF TEETH ATTACHMENT

The structural frame of man and other vertebrate animals is the Bone Skeleton. These bones like that of a thumb, legbones of cats and cows, or the jawbone of a mouse or elephant are formed for the functions they serve. We're all alike under the skin and bones. Refer to Plate 9-1, BASIC PERIDONTAL ANATOMY. Under the soft gum the outer hard compact bone surface layer, is called Cortical Bone. Inside under this cortical surface, bone is spongy, and the network of spaces contains marrow fat, blood vessels and nerves. Man's upper and lower jawbones form arches shaping the facial contours, providing walls of bone called Alveolar Ridges, which contain deep sockets or Alveoli that support the roots of teeth.

The outer cortical bone layer extends inside these root sockets where it thins lining the socket walls. Outer surfaces of the alveolar teeth supporting jaw ridges are towards lips and cheeks, while inner surfaces are towards the tongue. Feel this between your fingers if you like. Inside the ridges between the roots of each adjacent tooth the bone is called Interproximal Bone. The interproximal bone narrows rounding towards the teeth necks, forming a tiny curved arch under each tooth crown connecting

TEETH TEETH TEETH

outer and inner jaw surfaces. Tooth roots are dentin, covered with a thin veneer of cement-like bony substance called Cementum. Roots do not completely fill their sockets. There is a thin space usually detectable in X-ray between the root and bone called the Peridontal Space. Within these narrow surrounding confines connecting the cementum covered roots to the root socket bone, there is a mass of fine, short, elastic, radiating microscopic ligaments called Peridontal Fibers. Peridontal also called peridental fibers, suspend teeth in their root sockets or alveoli attaching them to the bone.

This mass of close peridontal fibers forms a layer called the Peridental or Peridontal Membrane, surrounding tooth roots like custom made tiny rugs, also acting as shock absorbers helping protect very hard working teeth, as sometimes experienced when almost imcompressible caramels are finally mastered. Even healthy teeth are not absolutely rigid in jaws. They shouldn't be. They have a minimum of usually undetectable mobility within the confines of their narrow peridental spaces.

Firmly attached to the jaws outer cortical bone surface is a thin fibrous membrance called Periosteum, peri means around, osteum, bone. Periosteum helps nourish bone from outside, and attaches muscles that move bones and supports other soft protective tissues. Periosteum of jawbone attaches a thin layer of Gum tissue or Gingiva. In Caucasian mouths gum is pink. Among darker races gum contains a pigment called melanin and is darker, even brown. Among some the gum is blotched in mixed masses of brown and pink. Normal gum is firm, resilient with a stippled surface. A thin band of attached gum or gingiva extends over the interproximal bone between adjacent teeth under their crowns connecting gum outside the jaw to the gum inside. This is called Interproximal or In-terdental Gum or Papilla.

Around every normal tooth, like a tight collar immediately adjacent to the crown, the attached gingiva becomes a thin knife edged margin like cu-ticle of a fingernail, and for a short distance is not attached to the tooth. The crevice under this unattached gum is called the Gingival Crevice or Sulcus. The gingival crevice is normally closed and clean, as the gum tightly embraces the tooth acting as a sealing gasket to keep dirt out. Around the normal healthy enamel crown of a tooth, the crown portion adjacent to the marginal gum edge protectively bulges. This curving bulge attractively provides shelter to the gingival crevice like eaves of a roof shelter house walls from rain. It deflects food debris from the gingival crevice which is an entry to the underlying peridontal membrane. This crevice must be kept clean. It is the weak point in our peridontal armor. Oral bacteria are insidious and engage in guerrilla like warfare. The patient must use his military toothbrushes, to sweep out the enemy, and toothpicks

TEETH TEETH TEETH

like bayonets and dental floss armamentarium like a well trained soldier fighting back, guarding this vantage point from enemy germ invasion. It's a fight for the life of your teeth.

PREVENTION OF DISEASE

Peridontal treatment starts with regular home care. Unfortunately this usually isn't enough. It's difficult even for dentists to clean their own teeth perfectly. Refer to Plate 9-2, PERIDONTAL DISEASE AND SURGICAL REPAIR. See Drawing Series A which shows the normal condition. Just as dust collects in inactive corners of a room, crevices in surfaces of teeth and between teeth and in fine gum spaces around teeth, all are dirt traps beyond the path of the normal traffic of the mouth. These inaccessible crevices catch and hold debris breeding germs. To avoid dental disease teeth must be kept clean. Patient, "But doctor, I just can't get into every tiny fine space." Dentist, "I agree, you can't. That's why we should visit the dentist or Dental Hygienist for periodic professional Prophylaxis."

PERIDONTAL DISEASE

GINGIVITIS – GUM INFLAMMATION ∞ In a clean healthy mouth tissues can absorb some toxins, effectively combating some germs. When limits are exceeded the germs multiply. The body rushes blood in to counteract fighting infection. Marginal gum edges, bordering the crevices harboring the germs, stretch and swell from thin firm pink to swollen tender red. See Plate 9-2, Drawing C, Gingivitis. This is mild Marginal Gingivitis. Swollen gums increase the crevice providing space for more germs. More bacterial poisons cause more swelling. The tissues stretching become more delicately tender to the touch of the brush, finger, and food. Gingivitis is severe.

IT GETS WORSE – PERIDONTAL POCKETS ∞ Teeth dirt deposits unremoved, harden to become Calculus or Tartar. Calculus is from the same Latin word meaning stone. The invading Siberian Tartars of Mongol, Manchuria and Turkic origin have been described as violent, cruel, unconquerable. Dental calculus is cruel to teeth but can be conquered. Calculus consists of salivary minerals, broken down blood and mouth tissue cells, food debris, various bacteria, fungi and their toxins. Neglected deeper layers become harder and harder, stonelike, as dense as tooth itself, and can often be seen this way on X-ray. It spreads deepening. See Plate 9-2, Drawing D. Visible calculus above gums is called Supragingival calculus. Sub-gingivial calculus is invisible attached to the tooth below inside the gum margin. It spreads deepening unseen causing severe peridontal disease.

The thickening calculus and germs within invade, separating the soft attached gum from tooth and bone spreading, creating Peridontal Pockets. Following germs invading infect and foul the tissues. Mouth odors often become offensive to others who avoid and won't tell the unaware.

The capillaries engorge as blood enters fighting infection. The gums swelling outward become brighter red more painful. Under the gums the rough sub-gingival calculus erodes through the inner tender skin, creating bleeding Ulcers of the lining of gum peridontal pockets, like ulcers of stomachs and intestines. It's a vicious cycle. The red swelling gums trap more dirt, and the germs increase the size of the swollen pockets and infection. Calculus deep within the pockets are beyond home reach and pain makes personal cleaning impossible. See Drawing E.

SCALING AND CURETTAGE – PROPHYLAXIS ∾ Dental treatment consists of carefully removing all hard and soft infectious substances. Scaling removes calculus and softer deposits from around teeth and exposed bone. Curettage is a surgical term for scraping of undesirable material from soft tissue. Just as a gynecologist curets infectious and superfluous growths, or improperly impregnated ovum remnants from uterus walls, the peridontist curets ulcerated epithelium from the inner gum lining. Instruments are tiny scrapers, scalers, files and little spoonlike curets, at the ends of handles delicately applied into and around every recess of every tooth. Electrical ultrasonic instruments are also used. Treatment may be bloody. It's a minor minor operation that must be dextrously thoroughly done. Several successive treatments are sometimes needed in severe cases. Outer tooth surfaces are polished to remove stains. Gums grow back healthy firm and pink. Pockets shrink as swelling recedes and sometimes gums to some extent reattach from below to the teeth and bone.

Miss Aprey Hensive asks, "Won't that hurt doctor." Doctor Perio Dontist, "It needn't hurt at all. In severe cases anesthesia makes procedures completely painless. All the work is close to the surface, so that topical anesthetics simply sprayed or wiped on help." Miss Aprey Hensive, "Do I need anesthetics?" Doctor, "Most people need none. It may hurt a little and bleed, but scaling is quite tolerable. All deposits must be removed. I sometimes tell patients, I'd hurt you more if I didn't hurt you. I've had patients tell me 'It hurts but it feels good.' It's the deeper deposits that do most damage. Those and all others must be removed. In severe cases needing regular periodic treatment, after the first few, the healing tissues hardly hurt at all."

TEETH TEETH TEETH

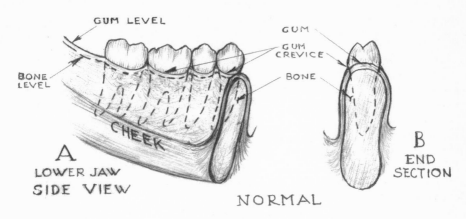

GUM LEVEL

GUM
GUM CREVICE

BONE LEVEL

BONE

CHEEK

A
LOWER JAW SIDE VIEW

B
END SECTION

NORMAL

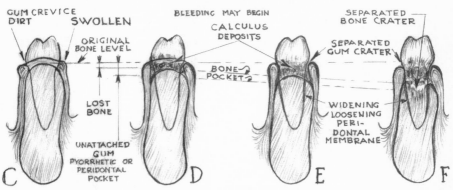

GUM CREVICE
DIRT   SWOLLEN

ORIGINAL BONE LEVEL

LOST BONE

UNATTACHED GUM PYORRHETIC OR PERIODONTAL POCKET

BLEEDING MAY BEGIN
CALCULUS DEPOSITS

BONE POCKET

SEPARATED BONE CRATER

SEPARATED GUM CRATER

WIDENING LOOSENING PERI-DONTAL MEMBRANE

C
GINGIVITIS

D
INCREASING

E
BONE LOSS AND POCKET

F
DEPTH

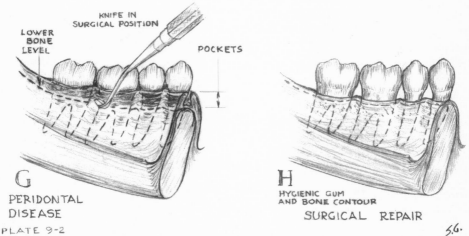

KNIFE IN SURGICAL POSITION

LOWER BONE LEVEL

POCKETS

G
PERIODONTAL DISEASE

H
HYGIENIC GUM AND BONE CONTOUR
SURGICAL REPAIR

PLATE 9-2

S.G.

PERIDONTAL DISEASE AND SURGICAL REPAIR

TEETH TEETH TEETH

AND STILL WORSE ∾ Continued neglect deepens pockets spreading infection further. Just as termites in recesses eat away undermining structures of a house, germs in peridontal pockets destroy supporting bone around teeth roots. Refer to Plate 9-2, Drawing F. The level of pyorrhetic jawbone ridges shrink from the necks of teeth. The total teeth lengths remain unchanged, but bone recession loss shortens the rooted length while the unrooted lengthens correspondingly. This subjects the root attachment to even greater stress. The tooth starts to loosen. In X-ray the peridontal space between root and socket is seen wider permitting greater tooth mobility and bacterial attachment invasion. The NEGLECTED TOOTH may be leaving, on the way out. Its pride hurt. For years THE TOOTH served its master well, yet has been ignored. Like a faithful slave to the end however properly treated anew, it may still serve for life.

Peridontal membrane is organic, subject to bacterial invasion. Anyone finding the skull of a deer, donkey, cow or a human, in forest or desert, can see the strong resistant inorganic teeth in their sockets of inorganic bone. But the teeth are loose may even rattle. The organic peridontal supporting membrane is gone from its space, consumed with the other soft body parts by germs. Germs in pyorrhetic pockets also destroy tooth attachments in live animals. Deep pockets quickly contaminate and can't be scaled, curetted by the dentist every day. Treatment may require surgical correction of the pocket.

PERIDONTAL SURGERY

Anesthesia is applied, usually by local injection. No pain is felt. There's no more discomfort during peridontal surgery than with drilling a tooth. To start, the peridontist tooth by tooth may insert a tiny ruler like instrument called a Peridontal Probe into each pocket measuring its depth. Most surgery is with tiny knives of different shapes. Refer to Plate 9-2, Drawing G. Electro-surgery is also done. Sometimes tissues are ground off with diamond burs. Objective is to remove dirt trapping pockets and reshape surrounding tissues to help maintain cleanliness during normal use. Peridontal surgery is a miniature plastic surgery around teeth. Tissues shaped better hygienically usually look better.

The peridontist uses one or a combination of techniques to achieve his result. Gingivectomy involves cutting away unattached soft pocket tissue from roots and bone. Gingivoplasty is a sort of sculpturing surgery of gums, finely reshaping blending the area for better hygiene and cosmetics. Both are usually combined. In severe peridontal disease the gum doesn't just form pockets as the bone recedes evenly. Under soft tissues, the hidden bone often breaks down irregularly, deeper in some places than others. Between adjacent teeth infection may be so severe the interdental gum papilla often disintegrates completely exposing bone. The outer cortical bone layer, hard as it is, often erodes away. See Plate 9-2, Drawings E & F again. The softer bone beneath disintegrates forming trapping crevices called interproximal bone Craters. All these defects may exist needing correction. When necessary the jawbone itself is reshaped. This is called Osteoplasty, bone shaping. To do this the surgeon may lay a flap.

Laying a Flap, is actually peeling the gum layer as a flap from jawbone surface, like skin lifted from an orange, so the peridontist can see the bone and have better access for reshaping the jaw to a smooth sanitary food deflecting contour. Sometimes Bone Grafts are added. The peridontist recontours the jaw like a landscape architect reshapes a hillside, so its surfaces form an attractive contour that hygienically deflects debris from critical areas for maximum cleanliness. Now the peridontist is also a dental sanitary engineer. After this delicate bone contouring the flap is replaced and if necessary sutured to position.

PERIDONTAL PACK ∾ After most peridontal surgery, a soft claylike dressing called Peridontal Pack, is molded over the area to medicate and protect the wound and promote healing. Sometimes a thin metal foil is first placed under the pack. The pack soon hardens, and helps preserve the healing tissues shape, like a plaster cast applied by orthopedic surgeons. In about a week the pack is removed, stitches if they exist are taken out, and the area is cleaned and medicated. Usually a fresh pack is placed for another week. Sometimes a third pack is used. Occasionally the healed result is not ideal and the peridontist makes minor surgical improvements. It is interesting biologically, that after peridontal surgery when the mouth is restored and maintained, teeth become tighter and can be seen that way in X-ray. Often the soft tissue and bone regrows reattaching to some extent. See Plate 9-2, Drawing H for the healed healthy condition.

Mr. Wade Toolong asks "But doesn't surgical removal of gum pockets expose the roots?" Doctor Perio, "It often does. Of course many people without realizing it have exposed roots from gum and bone recession without going to the dentist." Mr. Toolong, "Won't that look ugly." Doctor Perio, "In cases where a patient's teeth are long, peridontal pocket surgery may make them look longer. Though the improved gum line would look better. In cases where teeth look short the added length improves teeth and gum appearance. In fact gingivoplasty is sometimes used as a plastic surgery of gums just to improve appearance. In any event peridontal treatment preserves teeth that would otherwise be lost."

TEETH TEETH TEETH

OTHER FACTORS

The doctor continues, "I've only explained details of peridontal treatment itself. There are other dental procedures that also help preserve diseased teeth and maintain their peridontal integrity." Patient, "What are they." Doctor, "When teeth are severely degenerated and loose, cosmetic jackets and splinting can be valuable dental treatment. Decay contributes to surrounding disease and that disease hastens tooth decay. The most thorough restoration of a degenerated tooth is a completely outer surrounding jacket. It also provides maximum protection to the tooth within it. Jackets can be made cosmetically natural looking, attractive in appearance. They can cover all the crown and exposed root to the gums and be shaped to more ideally deflect food keeping the area cleaner."

"What is Splinting doctor." "I was just going to tell you. Splinting is the joining of teeth together so that they mutually support each other. Peridontal disease's prime cause of loosening teeth is the loss of supporting bone around them. Just as soil washed from around an erect post driven into it leaves less to hold, so that it can more easily fall, so does the loss of surrounding bone support loosen teeth. Just as fence posts are greatly strengthened, connected above ground by cross-rails, loose teeth are helped tremendously by splinting or joining them together." Patient, "How is that done." Doctor, "There are many types of dental splints. The simplest is wiring teeth together. Wire splinting is considered temporary treatment. If the defect isn't corrected the teeth may loosen again after the wires are removed. Sometimes soft plastics are molded to harden around teeth for temporary splinting. The plastics are also removed after serving their purpose. Plastic holds more rigidly than wires which yield slightly bending." Patient, "I hate the idea of bulky things around my teeth." Dr. Perio, "These are only temporary splints used as part of more extensive treatment. Sometimes removable appliances of different designs serve as splints. They help support weak teeth, distribute the chewing loads and transfer heavy forces from weak teeth to areas more capable of bearing them." Patient, "But doctor I don't like the idea of wearing a removable apparatus, regularly taking it out and replacing it, in and out of my mouth."

Doctor, "The finest splints are permanently fixed splints. Like the tightly nailed cross-rails of fence posts they strengthen teeth most. They are also more expensive." Patient, "But isn't joining teeth as a single rigid unit unattractive." "No, not at all, it need not be. Teeth can be splinted together yet made to appear individual and separate. The finest permanent splints for severely decayed and loose teeth are surrounding jackets. These can be made to join at their point of adjacent contact and yet be sculptured

TEETH TEETH TEETH

to look natural and separate. They can also support and replace missing teeth. They can be shaped to deflect food for maximum hygiene. They can be made to match natural teeth colors and shades, and of materials that keep even cleaner than natural tooth enamel." Patient, "Aren't such appliances expensive doctor." "They may seem to be to some. Though to those that need such work and can afford it, they're worth the price. They involve many modern complex dental techniques." Patient, "Doctor Perio, do you do such work."

Doctor, "That phase of dentistry isn't done by those who limit their practice to peridontal treatment. I can refer you to a doctor that does. Teeth covering fixed splints are usually made by dentists who do mouth reconstruction. In fact any procedure that rebuilds teeth, even a simple filling, also improves conditions of tissues that surround them. All phases of dental treatment are mutually interdependent and help the mouth as a whole." Patient, "Dentistry is more involved that I realized doctor." Doctor, "All practitioners of dental specialities join, using their knowledge to preserve the patient's complete oral health, though some dentists sometimes like to combine different phases of the work themselves just as some medical doctors do."

SOME BIOLOGICAL FACTORS

As bodies from birth reach puberty the outsides of boys and girls show changes, hair on faces and breasts on chests. At the same time inside the body, physiological alterations creating the ability to reproduce their kind leaves teeth and peridontal tissues sensitive and susceptible. The gums sometimes swell bluish red. Sex seems to affect everything, these could be called sexy gums. Hygiene should be thorough. Sensitivity diminishes with maturity.

Women seem to have added problems many ways. For some females, each month with their menstrual cycle, delicate peridontal sensitivities appear in the mouth. Soft tissues inside the mouth, and lining the female genital tract are alike. Some similar drugs are used to treat them. For some women, gum sensitivity and even ulcers occur simultaneously with ulcers in the vulva. Problems often arise during pregnancy. Obstetricians often refer patients for peridontal treatment. Later in women's lives, during menopause, dental difficulties often appear again.

The mouth's soft peridontal tissue surfaces are a special kind of skin. Diseases of other skin, encountered by medical dermatologists sometimes also show symptoms inside the mouth. Various body diseases affect the mouth, diabetes, epilepsy and others. Dentists, peridontists, use medical diagnostic tests and sometimes refer patients to physicians.

TEETH TEETH TEETH

MAINTENANCE CARE

Teeth need regular care to keep them working properly. The Chrysler Corporation guarantees important parts of its man made, non-living automobiles, for five years or 50,000 miles whichever comes first. This guarantee is only effective if the owner shows evidence of proper maintenance every 3 months or 4000 miles, whichever comes first.

After the mouth has been restored to health, keep it clean to keep it healthy. Regular professional prophylaxis is necessary. Mrs. Cara Lotnow asks, "How often should a person have their teeth professionally cleaned doctor." Dr. Wise, "It varies with the person. You can't tell just by looking at the teeth. It's the invisible hidden deposits that do the damage. Some people regularly perform a better job at home, and some mouths form deposits faster than others. Teeth must be cleaned at such frequency that its dirt hasn't a chance to harm. The dentist can tell best. For some people every six months works. Many need prophylaxis every three months. I've had patients with severe peridontal problems who needed their teeth scaled every month. When teeth are really kept clean even deep scaling hardly hurts. The tissues haven't had time to infect becoming sensitive."

Together Mrs. Cara Lotnow and her husband Carey Lotnow ask, "Does that insure doctor, we will never have trouble with our teeth again." Dr. E. N. Formed, Dr. Wise's associate, answers, "No, I'm sorry to say that's one thing we can't promise. That would mean teeth were the only thing guaranteed never to fail. No part of the human body, no machine, however expensive fails to ever fail. Very few are guaranteed for over a year. I will say however, that if teeth are properly maintained they will probably serve their host for life. Neglected, they're lost one by one. Regular care, X-rays and clinical examination, reveals defects while they can be less expensively corrected. Be faithful to your teeth and they'll stay true to you."

Peridontia
Is Teeths Surrounding Situation
Needed for A Firm Foundation

TEETH TEETH TEETH

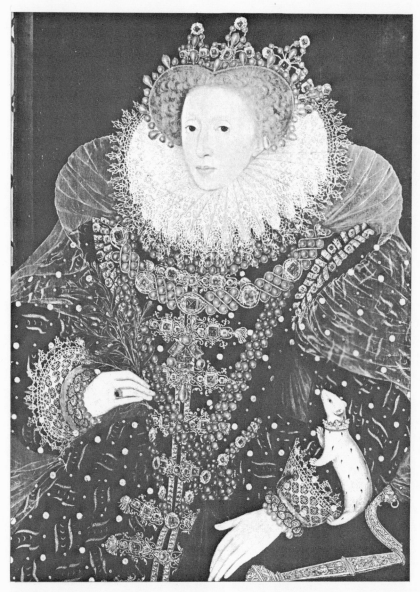

DENTAL DISEASE DOES NOT DISCRIMINATE∾Queen Elizabeth I brilliantly ruled her English Empire from 1558 to 1603. She suffered severe dental disorders as did many of her poor subjects. Decayed teeth and peridontal disease caused pains that cancelled many important conferences. They are said to have influenced international decisions. Some indications are dental infection led to the Queen's death. Animals like her ermine pet also suffer dentally.

TEETH TEETH TEETH

POSTERIOR SUPERIOR ALVEOLAR
BLOOD VESSELS AND NERVES
to & from the Head & Body

ANTERIOR SUPERIOR ALVEOLAR
BLOOD VESSELS AND NERVES
to & from the Head & Body

MAXILLARY SINUS
Air Conditioning Chamber
for breathe from the nose

TEMPORO MANDIBULAR
or JAW-HINGING JOINT

UPPER JAW
or MAXILLA

LOWER JAW
or MANDIBLE

MANDIBULAR FORAMEN
or OPENING
at inner jaw surface

MANDIBULAR BLOOD VESSELS & NERVES
to & from the Head & Body

MENTAL FORAMEN
or OPENING passes
BLOOD VESSELS & NERVES
supplying the lip

S. GARFIELD

ADULT OR SECONDARY TEETH EXPOSED ON THE RIGHT SIDE

BLOOD VESSELS & NERVES SERVICING THE TEETH

FLESH & OUTER BONE REMOVED & SINUS OPENED TO REVEAL INNER DETAILS

TEETH TEETH TEETH

10

SAVE THAT TOOTH ∾ ENDODONTIA

Many endure suffering an abscessed tooth delaying what they fearfully think must result in its eventual extraction loss. Such teeth can be cured, saved, often for life. Tooth abscess is a putrid pus infected region, inside the jawbone around the tooth root tip, where germs have eaten the bone away. The condition can be seen on X-ray as a dark area around the root, surrounded by normal looking lighter bone. Such infections produce poisons absorbed into circulating blood, undermining systemic health.

Jack Melbourne a talented T. V. actor and writer appeared for routine dental examination. He made no special complaint, mentioned no dental discomfort. X-rays of all his teeth revealed a huge abscess surrounding the roots of what had appeared to be a normal looking lower left first molar. It was the largest abscess I had ever encountered. The molar X-ray showed invasion had reached extreme borders of his jaw so that it could easily break in two. I told Jack of my findings and asked if he felt no pain. "My God" he said "That must be it." "What" I asked. Jack replied "My teeth didn't hurt but I've been feeling terrible for quite a while and been thoroughly examined by my medical doctor who could find nothing wrong except that I had a very high white blood count."

White blood corpuscles called leukocytes, normally exist in circulating blood in low numbers. Leukocytes fight germs. When infected, the body increases leukocyte manufacture tremendously to attack the germs. Blood tests revealing high white counts indicate bacterial disease. "Antibiotics," Jack said "only helped temporarily and no source of infection could be found. It must be that abscess." I felt sure it was and called Jack's physician who was delighted to learn of my findings. Endodontic treatment removed the infection, lowered Jack's white count to normal, saved his tooth and restored his health. Bone regrew inside surrounding the tooth roots restoring the strength of Jack's jaw.

Often the pain of an abscessed tooth is severe even excruciating. The magnitude of pain however is not always an indication of the severity of a lesion. Sometimes extreme disease causes no discomfort, so cancers can kill, while even minor dental defects can cause pangs. Our hurt feeling warning mechanism is wonderful but sometimes less than perfect. Westinghouse and General Electric have no better model available.

Endo means inside, dontia the tooth. Endodontia is treatment of

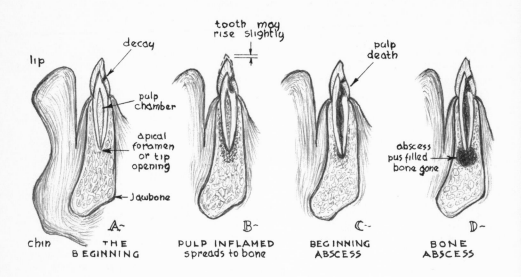

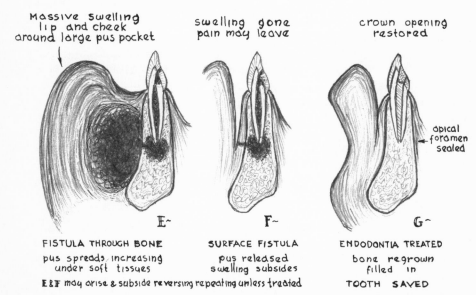

PLATE 10-1

S. Garfield

INCREASING ENDODONTIC DEGENERATION
Shown in section through a lower front jaw

TEETH TEETH TEETH

diseases of the inner tooth pulp and related tissues. Dentists with special training who limit their practice to such work are called Endodontists. An older name for endodontia is root canal work. The soft live inside substances of a tooth is pulp, sometimes wrongly called the nerve. Pulp does contain nerve in addition to blood vessels and other soft tissues. The pulp lies within the pulp chamber which is a space within the tooth crown. The pulp chamber narrows extending into the roots of the teeth as root canals.

INCREASING ENDODONTIC DEGENERATION

Endodontic problems usually start with small decay through the outer enamel which spreads inside to the dentin. Refer to Plate 10-1, INCREASING ENDODONTIC DEGENERATION, Drawing A, The Beginning. Decay continues invading towards the small soft inner pulp which becomes inflammed. Inflammation swelling may spread through the pulp to the surrounding bone and adjacent tissues. Teeth roots and their supporting bone sockets taper. Pressure of the swelling expansion may force the tooth elevated slightly from its socket. See Plate 10-1, Drawing B. Now the tooth is a little higher than its neighbors and is hit more in biting and other mouth movements accentuating the pain. Dental bite adjustment by grinding off the high area gives temporary relief. If decay and inflammation are not eliminated the tooth may rise further hurting again. X-ray shows enamel, dentin, pulp, bone and decay. It cannot show inflammation of pulp or other tissues. Eventually germs enter the pulp, invade the canal causing pulp necrosis or death and perhaps pulp gangrene. See Plate 10-1, Drawing C. X-ray cannot distinguish between normal live pulp and dead pulp. It can show decay through the enamel and dentin, into the pulp.

PULP TEST ∾ Live pulp and its nerve are good electrical conductors. Tooth enamel, dentin and dead pulp are poor conductors. The electrical Pulp Tester instrument sometimes helps. An electrode of the tester is applied to the tooth. The dentist slowly moves a graduated control emitting an increasing electrical current. The patient feels and indicates when a low electric shock is felt at the root tip. Varied sensitivity to conductivity gives the endodontist indication of vitality. Reaction to heat and cold tests applied as a hot instrument or ice chip to the tooth sometimes also helps.

TOOTH DARKENS ∾ Occasionally the dead pulp remains confined inside the canal hardly hurting. The tooth may darken. Germs occupying the dead pulp chamber make it an infection reservoir, a bacterial fortress from which they can attack the body. The body reacts to resist infection. The body's only entry for fighting the germs is through the small apical foramen. This is the tiny root tip opening through which microscopic nerve blood and other vessels, pass from the bone to enter the tooth and service the pulp, entirely inadequate access for fighting infection within.

ABSCESS & CYST ∾ It is ample for germs inside to venture forth attacking, degenerating surrounding bone. They do this successfully forming an Abscess. See Drawing C, Bone Abscess. There probably is pain. The body using other defense mechanisms sometimes tries to limit the abscess growing a fibrous tissue surrounding sac to confine it. Such a lesion is called a Cyst. For some fortunate reason, the roots themselves within abscess and cyst usually resist the infection. The disintegrated bone of abscess or cyst around the root tip is now pus-filled readily discernible in the X-ray as a dark area. The germs multiply. Pus may clog the tiny apical foramen or root tip opening trapping the increasing abscess material. The pressure, caused by increasing poison products against the live surrounding bone, creates severe toothache. At night with days distractions gone, lying down horizontally for sleep increases the head's blood pressure, often making pain unbearable. The tissues are inflammed red, tender, hypersensitive. This can be the most torturous of toothaches.

FISTULA∾The enlarging abscess sometimes reaches the outer bone wall of the jaw, eroding an opening through which the pus escapes, spreading underneath the softer yielding gum flesh. This is a Fistula. The release of pressure from inside the hard bone sometimes relieves the acute pain, while pus spreading infection under the gum increases bodily sickishness. The soft flesh yields stretching filling with more pus. See Plate 10-1, Drawing E. The body resisting rushes additional blood fluids massively swelling the jaw. The surrounding face may be ballooned. Sometimes as pus leaves the fistula bone opening the adjacent flesh is too tough to stretch. The pus may find a path of less resistance, forcing sort of a tissue pus canal for itself, between the gum and bone, traveling to a more distant location where it can and will fill softer flesh or other parts of the body. The patient may become especially sick feverish, yet in misguided ignorance still avoid the dentist. What fools some mortals be. In times before medical control and antibiotics, such infections sometimes spread from abscessed teeth up in towards the brain, and below to the body, even occasionally killing.

Sometimes temporary relief comes as the pus eats an opening through the flesh draining to the mouth. See Plate 10-1, Drawing F. The patient feels better without knowing why. Some even swallow their own pus

TEETH TEETH TEETH

without knowing. Pus does less harm swallowed and digested than spreading inside the body confines infecting vital organs. Sometimes such fistulas drain outside through the face. After drainage inner pus pressures drop and the fistula opening may heal closed. The pus confined inside again, collects again, increasing pressure infection and sickness again. The fistula may open again, close again. Such conditions cannot completely heal themselves.

The delinquent way to relief is extraction of the tooth. After extraction tooth replacement is usually much more expensive than endodontia. I prefer preserving every part of the body, there's little else we really own.

AN INSIDE JOB

Sometimes painless abscessed teeth are discovered in time by X-ray. Sometimes the patient arrives suffering severely. No pain need be felt during any endodontic procedure. X-rays are taken. Anesthesia is applied when necessary. As sensitive as the area is, in cases where pulp and nerve are obviously gone, anesthesia may not even be needed. The immediate object is to release infection pressures from deep within. By scoop or drill the dentist creates an opening to the canal. Pus may gush like a little geyser, green, foul stinking, bloody. Sighs. The patient relieved is enriched as though the flow were oil. He feels the dentist is God. The canal must be cleared. If the chamber contains pulp the dentist inserts a fine barb with tiny hooks like thorns, twisting to engage the pulp, pulling it out dangling like a worm. He uses thin endodontic reamers and files to clear a drainage passage to the abscess.

The final object of endodontia after cleaning and medicating the canal is to fill it and seal the root tip. When this is accomplished infection may still exist in bone around the root outside the tooth. Things however are very different now. The infection reservoir inside the tooth no longer exists. The healthy bone surrounding the abscess area can now control the germs. Within a few months or longer X-ray usually shows the diseased dark area gone, replaced by hard new white regrown bone. See Plate 10-1, Drawing G.

To seal the tooth root canal inside towards its tip, the endodontist must determine its depth, for selection of instrument size. X-rays of a tooth though valuable may show its length distorted. Anatomical natural parts of the mouth often prohibit placing film parallel to the root inside the bone, and no one can tell which direction roots go. They often curve. Measurements of root lengths cannot be taken directly from X-rays to determine the length of root canal instruments. To find the root canal length, the dentist inserts a thin metal instrument of known length, like an

Endodontic Probe or File, into the tooth canal and takes a picture that way. Refer to Plate 10-2, ENDODONTIC DEPTH ANALYSIS.

The X-ray, showing the instrument end related to the root end, helps determine the canal length. Several may be taken. Root canal instruments are long, thin like a pin, tough tapering steel, flexible. Carefully used they will bend and follow curving canals. They are cutting instruments, barbed edged along their length like files. Held between the endodontists skilled fingers, inserted into the canal, moved in and out rotated they cut, cleaning enlarging root canal walls. They are available in a standardized series of increasing diameters. The endodontist starts with thinner files working his way to the measured depth of the root tip. He flushes with medicated solutions occasionally cleaning the canal. X-rays are taken to measure progress along the way. He increases to larger file sizes. When satisfied his path towards the tip is satisfactory for sealing, he cleans dries and sterilizes the canal.

Canals are sealed with Sealing Points cemented permanently to place. Sealing points are small flexible thin tapered points, standardized in sizes exactly equal to canal cutting file and reamer sizes. They come in soft silver and gutta percha. Gutta percha is rubber like. The endodontist selects a sealing point equal in size to the last file used. Root canal medicated cement is mixed to a thin paste and carried into the canal with a file or point. Sometimes a long spiraling wire is dipped into cement, inserted into the canal and rotated between the fingers, screwing pumping the cement towards the tip. Sometimes cement is injected with a syringe. For sealing insurance the endodontist also cement covers his selected sealing point, inserts it to the measured depth spreading the cement into every canal recess. The canal is sealed from invasion at the root tip and outside.

The outer protruding handling length is cut off, the cement hardens, and endodontia is done. Sealing point and cement remain inside the tooth for life. A final check X-ray is usually taken. Sensitivity sometimes felt, gradually disappears. A permanent filling is placed permanently closing the tooth crown's canal access opening.

Endodontia is exacting difficult procedure, especially far back in the mouth where some molars have three canals, each individually needing the same work and all tough to get to. Sometimes an instrument breaks in a canal making sealing more difficult though usually possible. Like with every operation there are failures though most modern endodontia is successful.

Root canal filled teeth sometimes seem to suffer less later decay though we don't know why. If they should suffer they can be restored like any other. If later in life their crown were all lost, a good canal filled root if still

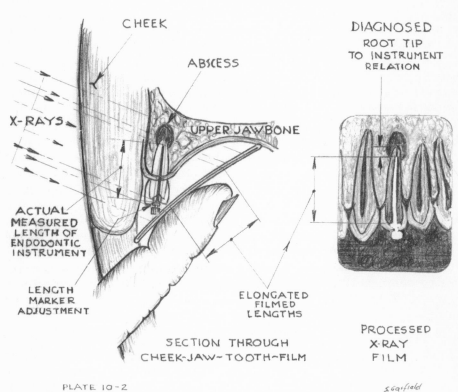

CHEEK

ABSCESS

DIAGNOSED
ROOT TIP
TO INSTRUMENT
RELATION

X-RAYS

UPPER JAWBONE

ACTUAL
MEASURED
LENGTH OF
ENDODONTIC
INSTRUMENT

LENGTH
MARKER
ADJUSTMENT

ELONGATED
FILMED
LENGTHS

PROCESSED
X-RAY
FILM

SECTION THROUGH
CHEEK-JAW-TOOTH-FILM

PLATE 10-2

S.Garfield

ENDODONTIC DEPTH ANALYSIS

TEETH TEETH TEETH

available, could be used to support a new natural looking false crown. Fees may seem expensive though well worth the added life's service. Tibor De Buda, a wonderful gentleman, the father of a friend died in 1962. In 1918 Italy at age 34, he had two upper multi-rooted abscessed molars saved by endodontia. Though several other adjacent teeth had been lost these molars served Mr. De Buda forty-four years until his death in Los Angeles at 78.

AN OUTSIDE JOB

Sometimes the lesion within the bone surrounding the root, is of such nature the endodontist or dentist considers sealing the canal through the crown along the canal to the inside inadequate. He may want to curet or scrape the inner diseased bone around the root, removing all pathological contents. Sometimes the root may curve so severely, the file cannot safely follow the crooked canal, and forcing could perforate the root wall. An endodontic instrument may have broken inside the root blocking the canal, impossible to remove or pass with another instrument. An inner natural obstruction may block the canal. In such case the lesion and root tip are treated from outside, approached from an opening made through the gum covering flesh, and a hole made through the jawbone.

Anesthesia is applied. No pain is felt. X-ray is studied so the endodontist can approach the root tip directly, with least damage to intervening tissues. Inside the mouth he probes the jaw's gum surface with a blunt instrument, feeling for a soft spot where the lesion may be close or even perforating the bone. With a sharp pointed knife he makes a semi-circled cut through the gum to the bone, around the intended bone entry point. The doctor peels the cut gum flap from bone like peel lifted from an orange. He may stitch the flap folded away to adjacent tissues temporarily, or have a surgical assistant hold it retracted for vision and access to the bone. Using a drill the doctor creates a small adequate bone opening to the root tip and surrounding abscess area. He curets the abscess and root scooping the lesion clean of all diseased material. His assistant keeps the field clean.

Where root canal filling sticks beyond the root tip from previous treatment through the crown, he may insure its sealed closure with a hot instrument. The patient anesthetized is awkward but comfortably feels no pain. Since the root tip opening is tiny the doctor may grind a little off to see the canal sealed. He also removes some if he feels the tip is infected. This is called Root Resection or Apicoectomy. Where it was not practical to first fill the canal internally through the crown, he may place a silver or cement sealing filling from outside into the resected root tip canal opening.

TEETH TEETH TEETH

After cleaning and medication the flap is sewed back to its normal position over the bone opening. Within several months or more bone grows refilling the void, completely surrounding the sealed root. There may be a slight semi-circled scar visible if the lip is lifted to look. The tooth is saved often for life.

PULPOTOMY

Pulp is pulp, tomy is from a Greek word tomos meaning surgery, cutting or parting. Pulpotomy is a tiny dental surgery removing only part of a tooth pulp. It sometimes happens a patient visits the dentist and examination discloses decay through enamel and dentin of a tooth crown reaching and infecting some adjacent pulp within the crown. Under painless anesthesia, if removing the decayed pulp and a little more reveals healthy blood vital pulp beneath, sometimes that healthy pulp can be saved. This procedure is called Pulpotomy or Pulp Amputation. It is a smallest amputation of a tiny organ of man. Pulpotomy is quite successful with children, probably because the apical foramen or root tip opening is larger in young teeth, providing more pulp blood circulation. It sometimes succeeds with adults. The pulp's tiny amputated surface is gently cleaned. It is then covered with pulp treatment drugs, sealed in by a protective covering layer of a structural insulator to keep extreme temperature and chewing forces from the pulp. This is called Pulp Capping. Over this a permanent restoration like a filling, inlay or jacket is placed. Pulp treatment drugs encourage growth of a new layer of dentin called Secondary Dentin to form under the pulp cap.

ENDO OUTSIDE THE MOUTH

Endo is an abbreviated term for endodontia or root canal treatment. Endo treatment is occasionally, though not often, performed on natural teeth outside the mouth.

Accidentally and intentionally teeth are sometimes knocked from mouths. Such teeth if available, properly treated, even after several days, can often be reinserted to grow firmly reattached in the bone. An important part of such treatment is the endodontic removal of the tooths inner soft pulp contents and sealing through to the root tips, after which it is replanted in the jawbone, sometimes to serve for life. In certain cases abscessed teeth are extracted by the dentist and through the open root socket the inside surrounding diseased bone is cleaned out. Outside the mouth the tooths inner soft pulp contents are endodontically removed and sealed through to its root tips. It is then replanted to grow reattached in the jawbone.

TEETH TEETH TEETH

OTHER FACTORS

In rare cases even teeth never decayed, without ever having had a filling, suffer death of the pulp and may abscess. Teeth surrounded by dirt deposits and teeth surrounded by peridontal disease, probably from long seepage of toxins through their root walls. Sometimes teeth that are too high in improper bite relations after repeated long time continuous chewing blows suffer death of the pulp. Teeth struck accidental blows may appear unharmed in the X-ray yet eventually the pulp may die. Probably the force tore nutrient vessels entering the root tip. All such teeth can be saved by endodontia.

IF ONLY I HAD PULLED MORT'S TOOTH

I first met Morton and Rhebe Cole during my dental college days at a Saturday night party. They were newly married. I liked them both. Mort and I had mutual scientific interests. We sat together talking most of the evening. Mort was a chemical engineer. He was especially impressed with the fact I had studied professional engineering, had spent several years working as an engineer, loved it, was working part time at it, and yet was leaving the field and studying dentistry as a new profession. Mort had helped develop an entirely new group of technical materials called epoxy resins. Epoxies had remarkable qualities and we discussed the possibility of adapting them for use as an improved dental material. Mort was stimulating, had good ideas. He too was some sort of an unsatiable searcher, had recently started a small plastics business of his own. Perhaps being more creator than business man he abandoned the project and returned to work as a chemical engineer. I liked Mort. I liked the way he talked. I liked the way he thought. He had a wonderful sense of humor. We exchanged names, addresses, and phone numbers, wanting to arrange to get together. That didn't happen for a while but because of mutual friends we did meet by chance occasionally.

Years later I was in dental practice. One day I was flattered, delighted, when Rhebe Cole phoned making an appointment for my professional services. I like Rhebe, she was a good patient. Except for apprehension at the initial moment of injection for anesthesia she was cooperative, pleasant to work with. And the Coles paid their bills promptly too. This helps any dentist like his patient. Rhebe would sometimes bring their infant son Don along to the office. My pretty young assistant Dana with motherly yearning enjoyed cuddling caring for Don while I treated Rhebe. The Coles were parents now establishing a family.

Rhebe mentioned Mort now and then. "Syd," she'd say "I've got to get

Mort to come to see you. His teeth bother him terribly. He needs your help more than I do, but he's so scared of dentists." Eventually Mort did get to the office and he was scared. Taking X-rays was an accomplishment. He squirmed and jerked in fright at every movement. Yet he was warm, so good natured and cleverly funny you couldn't help liking him.

He was far from an ideal patient, but we loved Mort from the first and looked forward to appointments with him. Just as parents should care equally for each of their children, I suppose doctors should have similar feelings towards every patient. Well, this just isn't possible. You treat each individual with best ability but can't help prefer some over others. Occasionally you encounter a patient with traits you detest. Anyway our office always looked forward to Mort Cole's visits.

At this time he was employed at the Von Karman Center of Aerojet General in Azusa California, about twenty five miles from his home in Beverly Hills. He loved the work, spent many hours at it, occasionally objecting to his long daily trips from Beverly Hills, where the Coles enjoyed old friends, to Azusa. The Aerojet company recognized Mort's ability with progressive increases in salary and responsibility. He approached a top position in Aerojet's chemistry section. I recalled early discussion of the epoxy resins back in days we first met. I had since read technical papers concerning epoxies. They have high bonding properties, are strong and inert, all qualities especially valuable for dental restorative materials.

I suggested Mort as a chemical specialist with epoxy background, and I with engineering and dental experience might make a good development team, for adapting and perfecting epoxies for dentistry. They indicated promise as superior cements, fillings, jackets and bridge materials. We discussed this from time to time but Mort had lost interest, absorbed with increasing duties at Aerojet. However he did make and keep dental appointments. His mouth had been neglected for years. We started a major reconstruction project. I explained his dental diagnosis, the procedures needed, and design details of all phases of his treatment. Mort was one of the people who encouraged me to write this book.

In the dental chair he was most unique, especially sensitive and warm, yet funny with his fears all the time. Reacting to any procedure that frightened him of pain, imagined or real, Mort screamed crying out loudly in song, always in tune with music from the sound system of our office. It was funny. He liked listening to the ball game, and when no music was being played he screamed creating tunes of his own. Getting dentistry done wasn't easy and did take longer, but it was fun and was being done.

First, to stop pain and tooth degeneration, all decay was removed. The cavities were filled with medicated strong temporary fillings. We would permanently restore a small part of Mort's mouth and he'd disappear for a few months. Then we'd tackle another area, perhaps do some inlays. Mort might be gone for months again. During one series of appointments we saved a couple of abscessed molars with endodontia. It was much longer before Mort came back after that. But he did, and somehow Mort's mouth was being successfully restored. This apparently was the approach needed and temporary medication care saw that no tooth suffered between work periods.

Sometimes during an appointment scheduled for dentistry we just talked. Some might think we wasted time. If we did, we luxuriously did. As important as teeth are or anything else in life, occasionally it's wonderful to relax and waste time. Such indulgence can be enjoyed by all, without discriminative barrier of monetary means, power, race, color or creed. During harassment of our society's tensioned times, we should all at moments of great need, at least mentally hook our thumbs under our armpits raising our heads proudly back, chest out, and then as really wealthy spendthrifts waste valuable time. And it's the most important time that can be most richly wasted.

Through these years Rhebe came for simpler treatment having her teeth cleaned. The Coles increased to include two boys and a girl. Tooth by tooth Mort's dentistry was getting done, a jacket here, a filling there. With loss of fear his confidence grew. We started missing Mort's musical howling, I'd say "Please Mort, scream a little like in the old days." It wasn't quite the same. He wouldn't scream any more but he did tell good stories.

Eventually all Mort's significant dental needs were satisfied, except for a three tooth bridge replacing a missing upper left second bicuspid being restored and supported by his first bicuspid in front and first molar behind. The bridge was permanently cemented in place Tuesday afternoon October 20, 1964. Our appointment finished early, and rather than have coffee as often served in our office, Mort and I to get away, left for refreshments at the corner coffee shop. As much as I love my work I like leaving for a break with a friend when I can. After some conversation Mort left for home and I returned for my next patient.

The next day October 21, I got home about 7 P.M. As I entered removing my coat the telephone rang. It was my office exchange girl who said I had two messages. One was from a patient in pain waiting on the phone to talk with me. A young man said he suffering severely. I did not know him and he couldn't remember who referred him as a patient. He asked I prescribe a pain killing narcotic by phone. I offered to return, meet him at the office and treat his emergency. He said he was calling from Hollywood, the trip was too far at the time, that he was in great pain and preferred the drug for help over the night. He'd come to the office the following morning. Since he wasn't willing to meet me, I wouldn't prescribe the drugs. He was probably an addict using the technique for a fix.

The next message was to call an unknown Mrs. Schmidt at a given number. I phoned Mrs. Schmidt and heard horribly shocking news. Mort Cole was dead. Mrs. Schmidt was calling for Rhebe who just couldn't call me herself. Mort had been strenuously dieting and exercising. This was a program he created for himself to lose weight. That morning at 8 A.M. he left the house to run a full mile. He ran the mile and back into the house, collapsed. His heart had failed. It was all over. A wonderful person and life were lost. We never know.

I changed scheduled appointments for Friday Oct 23, to attend funeral services at Hillside Cemetary 11 A.M. There were many mourners. Everyone whose life touched Mort's loved him. He was a wonderful person, friend, husband, father. As I left the Chapel walking towards the graveside I saw a group of men I felt were engineers and scientists, probably Mort's Aerojet co-workers. I introduced myself and found they were. In fact some said Mort had spoken of me as his friend and dentist. I told them how Tuesday afternoon I had cemented the bridge in Mort's mouth after which we had coffee. One fellow said, "Knowing Mort, I wish you had pulled his teeth, instead of saving them Tuesday. He wouldn't have run that Wednesday morning mile." Life is unpredictable, unexplainable, and sometimes seems unfair.

From the graveside as we stood sadly, I could see on a far hill two golfers playing.

Difficulties that are Deeply Rooted
Seek Solution Internally Tooth-ed

TEETH TEETH TEETH

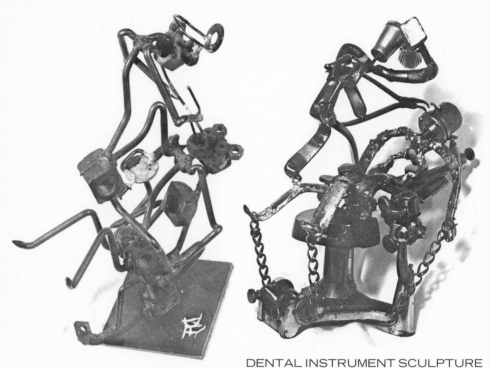

DENTAL INSTRUMENT SCULPTURE
by Dr. John Neufeld Prosth. Dept. Head
Loma Linda U. Dental School

NAIL NUT BOLT SCREW WIRE
Hardware Sculpture by Artist John Duffy
photo by Irving Schapin

SIMILAR IMPRESSIONS OF THE SAME SUBJECT

Professional artist and professional dentist artist, each unknown to the other, created individual versions of the dental surgeon, operating on and over his patient helpless below.

11

ORAL SURGERY

Surgery is that branch of the healing arts and sciences, concerned with correction of deformities and defects, repair of injuries, the cure of disease, relief of suffering, prolongation of life, and the improvement of functional efficiency and appearance, by manual and instrumental operation. Technically speaking almost all dentistry is surgical procedure. Cutting a small tooth cavity and filling it could be called surgery. In England the room in which a dentist treats patients is called the Surgery. In the United States the dentist's treatment room is called an Operatory. The dental degree D.D.S. means Doctor of Dental Surgery. By common practice however, most people think of surgery as technique involving cutting the body with knives and other instruments.

Oral surgery is such procedures performed in regions of the mouth and includes teeth extraction, in performance of which knives are often not used. Many phases of oral surgery involve critical anatomical head structures and the use of general anesthetics. Dentists who take advanced training for such work and limit their practice to oral surgery are called Oral Surgeons.

TEETH EXTRACTION

Teeth are valuable body parts, their loss is to be regretted. They provide more pleasured eating and better health. Only people who've lost many that haven't been replaced can personally appreciate that. Ask one to tell you of dining, limited to cereals and other soft mushy stuff. Teeth are especially important to appearance and provide proper speech. Yet sometimes they degenerate and need extraction.

During early biblical times justice demanded that a man's tooth be removed for knocking out one of another. Today more common causes for taking out teeth are infection, decay, abscess, peridontal disease and their pains. Teeth are also removed to improve bite relations, help neurological problems and for cosmetic purposes. Sometimes extracting teeth is simple. At other times removing even a single tooth is a complicated operation requiring coordinated medical information of the entire body's physical condition, thorough X-ray examination and detailed knowledge of internal anatomy of the parts.

TEETH TEETH TEETH

ORAL SURGERY

Dr. T. W. Brophy both M.D. and D.D.S. a medical doctor and dentist, was an eminent oral surgeon. He wrote an authoritative text 'Oral Surgery' Blakestons, Phil. 1918, still highly respected. In his chapter Extraction of Teeth, a Dr. Fitch tells of a patient who while having an upper right molar extracted by a blacksmith had a large part of his jaw with several other teeth torn away. "The roots of his tooth," said Dr. Fitch, "were greatly bifurcated and dovetailed into the jaw and would not pass out perpendicularly, though a slight lateral movement would have moved them instantly. The jaw proved too weak to support the monstrous pull; it gave way between the first and second molars and with it came the anterior and posterior plates of the antrum. The broken portion extented to the spongy bones of the nose and terminated at the lower edge of the socket of the left front incisor. It contained six sound teeth: the first molar, the bicuspids, cuspid and incisor on the right side. The soft parts were cut away with a knife. A severe hemorrhage ensued and when the patient recovered his face and mouth were excessively deformed."

In ancient time dental knowledge was limited. Instruments were few and crude. There was no thought of germs or antiseptics. There was no anesthesia. Teeth extraction was dangerous, often starting infections which spread into the head and brain causing death. About 300 B. C. a Greek physician Erasistratus invented an instrument he called a "leaden odontogogue" or tooth puller. Erasistratus wrote it was proper to remove teeth only when such a soft instrument could hold gripping them to extract. If the leaden odontogogue yielded bending Erasistratus felt it wiser to let the tooth remain and suffer. This was profound deduction at the time and may merit consideration today. Teeth strongly attached in jawbone have a firm foundation. Some such that are extracted probably could be saved by modern dentistry and should be. However teeth that are firmly fixed and difficult to remove often do need extraction.

SIMPLE EXTRACTIONS ∾ Teeth are usually easiest to remove during early childhood and older age. Such sometimes fall out themselves. The child's first, milk, primary or deciduous teeth, all name variations for the same thing naturally shed unassisted. While the first set erupt to proper place, the secondary or permanent teeth are forming following closely beneath them. The harder permanent enamel crowns impinge against the softer roots of their milk teeth predecessors causing their destruction and disappearance. As the permanent stronger teeth advance closer to the jaw's surface, less and less root of the primary teeth remain holding their visible crowns above the gums. When their root attachments to jawbone are gone the primary teeth crowns left unsupported fall out, lost, making way for their permanent adult successors. Sometimes these first teeth fail to shed naturally and block proper eruption of the permanent teeth. Extraction is usually simple.

Later in life even good permanent teeth may also be lost by themselves, not by natural process but from long neglect leading to disease. Teeth whose roots were amply supported by surrounding jawbone may lose that support. Lack of proper hygiene causes a pyorrhetic or peridontal degeneration of jawbone from around the roots. More and more bone support is lost, leaving the teeth to topple like an erect post in the ground whose surrounding soil is washed away. Such teeth may loosen to the extent people can sometimes pull their own with little pain. Pyorrhetic gorillas and chimpanzees do. It's wiser to have them properly removed by the dentist. Germs are active around infected teeth and can spread invading the body. Extraction again is usually simple and includes medicated prevention against infection.

MOST EXTRACTIONS ∞ Proper preparation for oral surgery includes X-ray, visual examination, and knowledge of the patient's physical condition. In some cases the doctor prescribes premedication like tranquilizers for relaxation, and antibiotics against infection. If general anesthesia is to be used for surgery during sleep, instructions may be given to avoid eating prior to the appointment. The patient who arrives apprehensively may be given relaxants at the office. An attractive woman came to a dental office and said, "Doctor, I'm so scared, I don't want to be too much trouble. I hope you understand, but I almost feel I'd rather have a baby than go through this." A popular jocular reply to such statement occasionally given in dental offices is "Of course Miss or Mrs. Dash, I understand perfectly, I'll help the best I can, please decide soon so that we may know how to best adjust the dental chair."

The patient is seated, properly positioned for the procedure, and draped for cleanliness. Anesthesia is applied so that no pain is felt. Most routine extractions are done under locally injected anesthetics. The doctor thoroughly reviews the X-rays and operation site to best perform his skills. Teeth with longer roots in deeper bone sockets need more effort for removal. X-rays of the root directions are studied, so the tooth may be removed with least resistance along its indicated path. The area is tested seeing anesthesia is profound and the site is cleaned. Extraction difficulties are more apparent to the doctor than patients who feel touch movements but no pain. The dentist may lift the gum separated from around the tooth neck, retracting the soft tissue from bone for better visual access. An assistant keeps these tissues out of the way and the area clean and clear.

Tooth roots are not directly attached to jawbone. They are held within their sockets by fine short radiating microscopic ligaments called

Peridontal Fibers. These fibers must be torn to remove teeth. Peridontal attachments are sometimes very strong making extraction difficult. Most people think teeth are just pulled out with forceps gripping the tooth like ordinary pliers. Sometimes they are, often they're not. Many difficult teeth are efficiently removed without any pulling at all.

Teeth are generally extracted by one or a combination of methods. Refer to Plate 11-1, TEETH EXTRACTION TECHNIQUES. They may be raised or elevated from their sockets in the upper and lower jaws by a variety of strong sharp steel instruments called Elevators. All have handles at one end for control by the surgeon. The Wedge Elevator has a small sharp edged tapered wedge surgical tip, shaped to fit outer curves of tooth roots. Refer to Plate 11-1, Drawing A, Wedge Elevator. Wedge elevators come in a variety of designs for access to teeth in different mouth locations and different size and root shapes. The surgeon inserts the sharp wedge end tip between root and bone and pushes in wiggling, rotating, force driving his wedge instrument. Just as a wedge driven under embedded rock will dislodge raising it, the elevator, as the surgeon skillfully wedges, dislodges the tooth severing its attaching fibers. By skillful use of the wedge elevator alone the dentist may comfortably dislodge the patients tooth completely from its socket. If necessary he will continue or he may have started with a lever elevator.

Lever elevators have their operation end bent as a short arm useful as a lever. Refer to Plate 11-1, Drawing B, Lever Elevator. Levers are also available in many designs. The surgeon places the lever arm of the elevator under a tooth crown bulge. He may insert its tip at a root bifurcation which is a place where the root divides in two. Sometimes he drills a hole in the tooth for engaging his lever tip. Resting the bent base of the lever as a fulcrum against adjacent hard jawbone prominences, the doctor skillfully manipulates the handle, raising the lever elevating the tooth from its socket as a crowbar lifts a rock. He may remove the tooth completely this way. Some elevators are designed to be used for both wedging and lever lifting. Elevators remove many teeth. Sometimes they effectively loosen the tooth for further complete removal with forceps.

Forceps are used to pull teeth. Forceps consist of two handle hinged steel parts with grasping beaks that fold together gripping like pincers, tongs, or mechanical pliers, when their handles are compressed. Refer to Plate 11-1, Drawing C, Forceps. Forceps are also available in varied design for different tooth shapes and sizes at different mouth locations. Many instruments are named according to their use like Universal forceps

TEETH TEETH TEETH

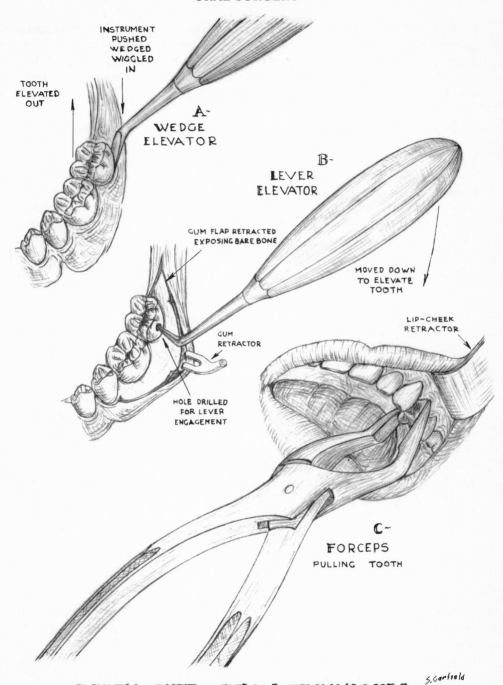

INSTRUMENT
PUSHED
WEDGED
WIGGLED
IN

TOOTH
ELEVATED
OUT

A-
WEDGE
ELEVATOR

B-
LEVER
ELEVATOR

MOVED DOWN
TO ELEVATE
TOOTH

GUM FLAP RETRACTED
EXPOSING BARE BONE

GUM
RETRACTOR

LIP~CHEEK
RETRACTOR

HOLE DRILLED
FOR LEVER
ENGAGEMENT

C~
FORCEPS
PULLING TOOTH

S.Garfield

PLATE 11-1 TEETH EXTRACTION TECHNIQUES

TEETH TEETH TEETH

ORAL SURGERY

that fit many places. Some are named after surgeons who designed them, like Cryer elevators for Dr. Cryer. Other have names taken from similar appearing objects like Cow Horn forceps with little beaks shaped like cows horns.

The surgeon may extract the tooth using only forceps. He selects his instrument and embraces the tooth so its beaks grasp the crown with their tips to the neck. With the tooth securely in his grip the doctor may not yet pull. He firmly forces feeling the root attachment to bone. He may push in slightly, hard, then out, and in, repeating to tear the hold. Some teeth are strongly attached. He may twist, one way, then another, then push again, and in and out. Hard, strong. If musically inclined, since music soothes savage beasts, he may push, pull rhythmically, twist right and left to office melodies. Such surgeons accomplish extractions quicker with jazz than waltzes. If the tooth attachment is especially strong an assistant may help, holding the patient's head for secured resistance against the surgeon's increasing strength. Some teeth are firmly attached to bone and he must pull especially hard. He will never ever grasp the forceps with both hands, and lifting first one leg then the other from the floor, place both shoe soles flat against the patient's chest pushing, driving with his thighs, thrusting with his back, pulling with both arms to get the tooth out.

When the peridontal attaching fibers are felt separating, he cautiously, as in the diagnosed X-ray, removes the tooth along its root direction, sometimes a curved path, causing least damage to the patient. These procedures require tense control within the surgeon, yet are often performed so smoothly the patient is surprised when shown his extracted tooth. The wound is inspected, tiny scooplike curettes like little spoons if needed, are used to deeply scrape out any infectious abscess or cystic materials. The surgeon may use small files to shape the bone socket edges smooth for more ideal healing. If doubt exists an after operation X-ray will be taken before the patient is released. Medicants may be applied inside the socket. As blood starts clotting healing has already started. The surgeon may suture or sew the gums stretched over the vacated opening closing the wound. Just as a seamstress has a variety of needles, threads and stitches, for different sewing needs, so does the surgeon. Don't ask him to patch a pocket or shorten a hem, he charges too much. The area is cleansed. No pain has been felt through all procedure. The anesthetic is still effective.

Aspirin products may be taken to prevent pain as anesthesia leaves. Even beneficial operations cause certain temporary damage to an area. If the doctor feels need he may prescribe stronger pain prevention drugs, sleep inducers, and antibiotics against infection. Home care instructions are given.

TEETH TEETH TEETH

MULTIPLE EXTRACTIONS ∾ Prolonged dental neglect sometimes leads to extensive degeneration with many or all teeth beyond possibility of salvage. When this has been established early removal is best. Though pain may not be constant and the disease seems to be tolerated, germ toxins are being absorbed, circulating in the blood, affecting general health. Toxins around the teeth cause continuing jawbone loss, so that prolonged delay may leave insufficient bone to satisfactorily support a denture.

The dental treatment plan and patient's health determine the numbers of teeth removed at one time. In rare cases all teeth, even many, may be extracted in a single appointment. More conservative procedure schedules several appointments, during which usually back teeth are removed first and front teeth last.

For multiple extractions the surgeon often starts cutting the narrow gum strips between adjacent teeth, then separating the inner and outer gum, peels it away from the teeth like the skin from an orange to expose the bone. With X-ray referral, teeth are removed in planned sequence considering their root lengths and directions, so that bone around already emptied sockets yields, permitting least damages as following teeth are taken out. Infectious abscess and cystic substances are also removed. When many adjacent teeth have been neglected, the degenerating bone around them often is rather irregular. If only teeth extraction is done the resulting healed toothless jaw's shape in many cases will not provide the best possible form for supporting dentures.

When necessary Alveoplasty is performed. This is a plastic surgical reshaping of the jaw to supply a better base foundation for the dental appliance to follow. Sharp bone spicules that could painfully pinch under a denture through the gums, are smoothed. Where bone is flat or shallow, extensions may be deepened for better removable denture grip and mouth form hygiene. The soft tissues are trimmed to provide a better stitched healing seam. Medications are applied. Gum flaps that had been peeled away are replaced and stitched or sutured to cover protecting the wound. Still under anesthesia no pain was felt.

HOME CARE

Proper home care hastens recovery and healing, helps prevent complications and suffering. Many unexpected variations, that are not apparent occur in oral surgery. The specific instructions given by the surgeon should be followed with precedence over any other. Some general principles for after oral surgery care are explained.

Do not disturb the wound. Maintenance of the original blood clot helps healing. Even rinsing during the first few hours could cause trouble.

Cleansing mouthwashes help, though certain contained drugs could rupture the fresh blood clot, and delay early delicate healing. Keep quiet, relax, rest with the head raised. Excitement and loud talking elevates the blood pressure and moves muscles of the area which could tear the wound. When the operation is far back towards the throat, avoid opening the mouth wide for examination in a mirror or showing a friend. The stretching muscles easily rupture the healing wound inviting infection. Avoid sucking the site or tongue probing. Resting seated in a chair keeps the head's blood pressure lower which is less disturbing to head wounds than lying flat in bed. If bed rest is needed elevating the head on a high pillow helps. A small amount of blood seepage is to be expected. Biting on a soft wad of clean cotton gauze, held firmly gently at the site between the jaws, helps pressure control the hemorrhage. Sometimes a moistened tea bag within the wad helps. Tea contains tannic acid, a hemostat, or blood stopping drug. If excessive bleeding persistently continues call the doctor. Do not toothbrush the area until healing is substantial.

Sometimes upper teeth have root tips reaching to the nasal sinuses. When such teeth are removed nose blowing should be avoided for a week or more. The extraction site is a potential passageway, and the nose blowing inner pressure could disturb early delicate healing tissues, causing serious infection.

Some swelling is expected as a natural body response delivering healing fluids to the area. The doctor will prescribe drugs if needed, which help reduce swelling yet stimulate beneficial body fluid circulation. Ice packs help reduce swelling and may be advised. They're sometimes recommended as often as 30 minutes of each awake hour the first day or two. They may also lessen pain.

Pain is usually controlled with one or two aspirin tablets taken about every three hours. If needed, stronger drugs, sleeping aids, and drugs against infection, will be prescribed.

Eating and drinking should be avoided for the first few hours. If hungry sip liquids keeping away from the operated area. Softer foods are safer. Heavy chewing over the site could tear the wound, driving food in, creating infections. Chew at other places.

HEALING

Post operative, or after the operation appointments are sometimes needed. Within the wound, tiny bits of bone shed after surgery, food particles may collect, infect, causing pain, disturbing healing. Treatment is cleansing and medication. The patient should help keep the area clean. Newly forming soft granulation tissues with fine branching blood

TEETH TEETH TEETH

capillaries, soon grows in filling the void as healing progresses shrinking the wound. Sutures if placed are removed usually in about a week or more. They may come out themselves yet the dentist should be visited for assurance. Healing time varies, progressing as the soft granulation tissue is replaced by new bone growth, filling in from the bottom moving up along the socket walls, while the soft gum tissues close. Usually the gums unite closing the opening within three weeks.

DRY SOCKET

An infrequent complication causing severe pain is "dry socket" or Alveolar Osteitis, an inflammation infection of the newly exposed bone walls surrounding the inner extracted socket itself. This may occur despite excellent surgery. Often because of patient negligence, or despite home care by conditions not completely understood, probably related to poor general health or started by loss of the initial healing blood clot. Pus is absent, the bone is bare, a foul odor and severe radiating pains persist. It sometimes begins as early as the second day after extraction, in rare cases lasting a month and more. Daily office treatment may be needed, consisting of cleansing irrigations and medical dressing. Antibiotics help. Drains may be inserted to delay surface closure promoting healing from the bottom up. The patient must be careful to keep food debris from the socket and may be instructed to use a syringe for regular home flushing. Modern drugs and methods have reduced this problem substantially.

EXTRACTION COMPLICATIONS

Various factors may complicate tooth removal. Some more common are described. Ankylosis is the consolidated attachment of two separate parts growing to unite fixed as one. In arthritis, ankylosis of finger and other bone joints limits use of the parts requiring skilled orthopedic surgery for repair. In rare cases ankylosis occurs within jaw hinge joints also needing specialized procedure. Teeth sometimes ankylose to their jawbone sockets, especially difficult to remove. If treatment were limited to mere increase of pulling power the attaching bone might tear away. The surgeon uses any and all means, power cutting drills and burrs, tiny chisels at angles he feels best for removing the tooth, if necessary piece by piece, for least body damage. He may consider it wiser to leave some parts in.

Tooth roots normally taper thinner towards their tips to the advantage of most extractions. Exostosis of a tooth root is an abnormal increase of the root bulk towards the tip, so that it is thicker there than other parts towards the outer bone surface. Bone will yield and stretch. If the root exostosis is

TEETH TEETH TEETH

not excessive, removal may be possible by careful manipulation. If root exostosis is too big the tooth usually cannot be completely removed as one piece through the smaller opening. Sometimes it is cut in pieces. Sometimes the roots bone path is enlarged. Sometimes paths are made from other directions through the bone, to remove the parts. New bone grows in filling those voids as with normal root sockets of extracted teeth.

More often teeth are restricted from direct simple removal by irregularities of their root shape. They may have rather straight roots, turning hooked sharply at the tip, extending beyond range of the straight part. When the tooth is withdrawn, this hooked tip often breaks, left at the bottom. The surgeon sometimes can tease it out with fine root tip instruments. Sometimes it's best to leave such pieces in place. Removal could require major surgery to surrounding parts. Sometimes root tips of upper teeth are close to the lower floor of the nose sinuses. Probing could drive them beyond, through into the sinus cavity causing further complications. Small root pieces are often well tolerated left deep in bone. Sometimes after long periods they make their own way to the surface. If necessary the surgeon removes the tip through other created access.

Some teeth with multiple roots have roots which diverge, or spread forking apart wider than the opening range of their crown neck coming through the bone. Some teeth with multiple roots spread out from the neck invisibly under the bone, then turn their tips in towards each other encircling bone, like a bow legged cowboy around the body of his mounted horse. If X-ray examination were not used and increasing pulling forces applied, either the tooth would break at the neck or tear away with attached jawbone. Such accidents have happened. The oral surgeon plans procedure to best suit the situation. He may prefer to section the tooth cutting off the crown separately, then separate the roots, delivering each with least damage along its individual path. He may split the crown so its parts remain attached to each root section for withdrawal. He uses chisels, drills, any other instruments, and imaginative ingenuity, to complete his small technical surgery.

IMPACTED TEETH ∾ Impacted teeth are those which cannot erupt into normal position, being blocked by obstruction. They may be completely embedded invisible within bone, blocked unseen just below the surface with only a tough fibrous gum layer covering, or have only part of their crown seen coming through. If the obstruction is removed, impacted teeth often erupt themselves, making their way to proper position. THE IMPACTED TOOTH seems to have a brain of its own. Any tooth may impact, most common are third molars, wisdom teeth. Third molar impactions are more usual in the lower jaw where their malpositions cause many difficulties.

TEETH TEETH TEETH

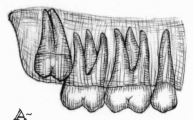

A~
VERTICAL IMPACTION

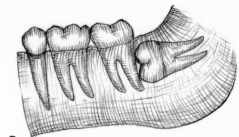

B~
HORIZONTAL IMPACTION

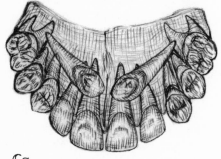

C~
LATERAL IMPACTION
OF BOTH UPPER CUSPIDS CROSSING
ROOTS OF ADJACENT TEETH

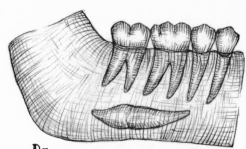

D~
A LOWER CUSPID IMPACTED UNDER
ROOTS OF OTHER TEETH

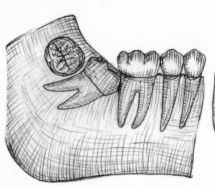

E~
CROSS IMPACTION
OF THIRD MOLAR

ANGLED IMPACTION
OF SECOND MOLAR

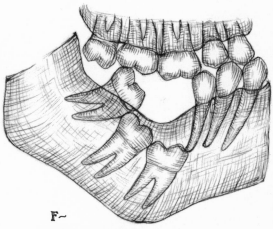

F~
A COMPLEX COLLECTION OF IMPACTED MOLARS
CONTRIBUTING TO THE PROBLEM OF
A MALFORMED JAW

PLATE 11-2 **VARIETY OF TEETH IMPACTION** S. Garfield

TEETH TEETH TEETH

Towards the mouth front, cuspids or eye teeth also often block.

The prime reason for failure of eruption impaction, is jaw under-development. Soft food, consumed increasingly by recent generations is good for lazy eaters, the business of food processors and those that make meat grinders, but results in less force used chewing and less time spent chewing. Today machines chew for us. This decrease in muscular skeletal jaw function results in decreased jaw development. Jaws are becoming smaller than they used to be.

In man's changing evolutionary biology all things did not coordinate ideally. By heredity man's chromosomes and genes continue delivering to embryos the full number of tooth germs, that go on forming tooth buds becoming all our teeth of the same full size. There just isn't enough space in smaller jaws for all these teeth to get through. Impaction results. Third molar impaction is most common, since they're the last teeth to erupt, having to take whatever space is left at the end of the less developed jaw. Lower wisdom teeth impaction gets especially involved squeezing in, because the mandible bone surface is harder and changes its direction, turning up at the third molar location. Front canines impact getting involved at the right and left turning points of the jaw. THE TOOTH is frustrated by modern times much like his living host.

Our progressing biological development though not coordinated perfectly is trying to catch up, striving steadily ahead. With increasing frequency teeth of new generations especially third molars occasionally fail to appear. This does not indicate man is becoming less wise but his WISDOM TEETH, all wise and considerate, prefer not to intrude when not needed. Impacted teeth removal is one dentistry's contributions for correction of imperfection in natural development.

Impacted teeth are found in many irregular anatomical positions. Refer to Plate 11-2, VARIETY OF TEETH IMPACTION. Surgical classification groups these positions into categories such as Horizontal impactions, Vertical impactions, Angular impactions, others. These are descriptive names used for convenience by man as a surgical aid. THE INDEPENDENT IMPACTED TOOTH with a strong will of its own, though often found in the standard postures described, may locate itself in almost any imaginable position or complicated combination.

It's not always necessary to remove impacted teeth. If they cause no trouble though they often do, and are regularly observed to see no problems arise, it may be safe to leave the tooth in place and avoid what is sometimes a rather uncomfortable operation. The dentist can best decide. Problems do arise however with patients unexpectedly alarmed by pain, or more fortunately detected earlier, during routine dental examination.

The impacted wisdom tooth, last to erupt, may assume position such

ORAL SURGERY

that its hard enamel cusp pointed crown, which forms first as with all teeth, is directed against the softer fully rooted properly erupted second molar. While the impacted third molar roots are forming and after completion, their misdirected eruption pressures against the second molar roots can cause great pain and sometimes destroy the more valuable second. Also the forward directed pressure against that second molar, often transfers along through all teeth forward by tooth to tooth contact, sometimes forcing unattractive crowding irregularities of the smaller rooted, less firmly fixed front teeth.

The third molar may be partially erupted through, blocked by a small encircling ring of overlying flap of tough fibrous tissue called Operculum. Operculum is from an Old Latin word meaning cover or lid. It names many biological objects. The horny plate used to close the foot opening of the shells of certain snails is called operculum. The plug of mucous which forms closing a woman's cervix opening to the uterus after impregnation is also called operculum. In the mouth the operculum partially covers the slightly erupted tooth, leaving a gum tissue opening vulnerable to food entrapment, infection and decay of the submerged molar. They also cause Pericoronal, peri means around, coronal crown, infections of soft tissues surrounding the tooth. These are often painful and may spread into severely swelling the cheek and throat. If tough operculum is the sole impacting agent, after surgical removal infection subsides and the tooth erupts to place. Often in addition to operculum the tooth is also blocked by surrounding bone and the adjacent second molar.

Often an impacted tooth is blocked by another tooth and bone. If the impacted tooth is valued its obstacles are removed permitting eruption. When a sound third molar is kept back by a severely decayed second, sometimes good planning is removing the decayed second molar whereby the third often goes forward erupting into the more useful second molar position. It's usually better keeping the second molar which is more ideal for the position it holds and removing the impacted third. Generally the impacted tooth is taken out. Sometimes this is complex procedure.

Surgical intention is to cause minimum trauma. If the tooth is completely embedded in bone, passage is made from the least damaging direction. If the molar is partially through a restricted bone opening, the opening may be enlarged. The tooth may be split into smaller parts individually removable through the limited passage. Often some surrounding bone is removed and the tooth is also split. Access to impacted third molars is difficult. Closely coordinated surgical assistance is valuable. Judgement and dexterity are very important, space is limited. This a time oral surgeons always prefer women with big mouths and are glad to be able to use them.

TEETH TEETH TEETH

ORAL SURGERY

The doctor knows the intimate anatomy of all involved parts. Through the wide open mouth of his tightly closed or wide eyed patient he may use a power drill to cut and section bone or tooth as needed. He may place a chisel edge between cleavage lines of the almost inaccessible part of the tooth. Chisel handle in one hand, surgical mallet in the other or an assistant's hand, the end is struck one or more blows splitting the tooth. The bewildered patient shocked through head structures, confused, wonders what's done and perplexed praying hopes the doctor knows what he's doing. He does. The patient asleep under general anesthesia is comfortably unaware throughout.

Sometimes pounding, especially the upper jaw of people with fragile facial tissues shows a day or so later as dark bruises under eyes as though punched. I'm glad to make this available as an excuse if desired, for those who have been punched. This soon disappears. Just as teeth may be irregularly positioned, branching nerves of the area are sometimes intimately involved with deeper parts, difficult or impossible to avoid. Removing such a tooth could on rare occasions damage such a nerve causing Paresthesia, a local numb loss of tactile sensation or touch, sometimes accompanied by a prickling burning feeling. This slowly disappears as sensation usually returns.

NEOPLASMS

From Latin, neo means new, plasm means form. Neoplasms are new formations of tissue, or tumors that arise without definitely known cause from cells of normal tissue. They serve no useful function growing at expense of the healthy part or organism. They are independently identifiable in character. Some enclosed within sacs often including fluids are called Cysts or Cystic Tumors. Many tumors of different appearance starting from different soft and hard tissues affect teeth jaws mouth and the face. There are soft tissue tumors originating in lips, cheeks, gums and tongue that sometimes also contain hard tissues like bone or teeth. They may remain attached, limited to the place they grow from, or spread expanding invading deforming surrounding regions. There are tumors that originate within jawbone containing soft tissue, mixed soft and hard, or hard tissue, growing confined within the bone boundaries damaging their immediate area. They also sometimes spread, stretch, perforate the bone, invade and deform adjacent parts. There are tumors of teethy tooth parts and jaw parts, that appear away from the mouth and head at distant apparently unrelated parts of the body.

Some are Benign meaning gentle or mild, remaining rather limited and confined, considered aside from the disfigurement they cause relatively harmless. Others like Cancers are malignant, evil or dangerous, yet if treated in time frequently curable. If neglected they may spread killing within the head. Sometimes they grow leaving the mouth and head through the neck, to cause impairment of function in other places again causing death.

Dentists are in an especially advantageous position to see these growths in regions of the mouth. Dental university and post graduate instruction include training in benign and malignant tumors of head, face, mouth and neck, and ways to recognize them. A valuable tool for diagnosis and detection of neoplasms is biopsy.

BIOPSY

Biopsy is removal of tissue from the living body for diagnostic examination by microscope. Sometimes when the lesion is small the specimen may include its complete removal for examination. With larger tumors the surgeon removes a representative section containing the doubtful plus adjacent normal tissue. To prevent deterioration the specimen is immediately placed in preservative like 10 percent formalin. In the pathology laboratory the sample is prepared. If it contains hard tissues like bone or teeth these are chemically decalcified so the entire specimen is soft. Standardized stains are applied, giving different color values to the varied cell constituents and other structures. The sample is then placed in a liquid transparent paraffin that fills all voids, hardens and supports the specimen. Sometimes it is frozen. With a machine called a microtome the specimen is cut into slices 5 to 7 microns in thickness. One micron is 1/1000 of a millimeter or .00004 of an inch. Under a high power microscope an Oral Pathologist studies the specimen. Tissue cells of malignant or deadly neoplasms demonstrate particular characteristics that distinguish them from benign or harmless tumors and normal tissues.

SOME TUMORS

Thorough description of mouth tumors is far beyond scope of this book. Several of popular dental significance are described.

Papilloma is a generally harmless or benign soft tissue tumor found on the epithelium or skin or the delicate surface lining or mucosa of lip, cheek, gum, palate, tongue and under the tongue. It is a small wartlike cauliflower looking mass, slightly paler or greyer than surrounding flesh. They sometimes cover larger areas or patches. They may appear at any age more usually during fifties and sixties. Treatment of simple classic benign papilloma is surgical excision or removal. With neglect or trauma from poor fitting dental appliances or rough infected teeth, they could become ulcerated, infected and bleed. They sometimes degenerate to malignancy. When possibility is suspected the surgeon takes a biopsy.

Tori is plural for a tumor called Torus, just as cacti is plural for cactus. Tori are benign or harmless osteogenic tumors. Osteo means bone, genic means originating from. They are also called Osteomas, they're bone tumors. Oma is a word ending meaning tumor. Tori are usually bi-lateral, meaning similiar and oppsite on both sides of the body center line. Tori are tumors of bone covered with gingiva or gum, extending into the mouth from the jaw surface as bump lumps, sometimes large as walnuts, generally smoothly formed with a walnut like surface. They are adherent to the natural anatomic bone contour, intimately connected with a pedicle or stemlike attachment. Tori are fairly common. They increase slowly in size. Many people are unaware of tori existence in their mouth until called to their attention when discovered during routine dental examination. Thoma's 'Oral Surgery' describes the case of a physician whose mouth tori were given little attention until they grew to such size interference with tongue and speech occurred. Tori of the upper jaw grow along each side of the palate center line, from the top extending down into the mouth lessening oral cavity volume. They are called Torus Palatinus. Tori of the lower jaw are called Torus Mandibularis. These generally grow on right and left inner sides of the mandible below the teeth more usually towards the front. Tori generally cause little trouble, unless teeth are lost, at which time they interfere with proper construction of dentures and should be removed. Surgery when indicated is rarely serious. After anesthesia the doctor slits the soft gum covering tissue through to the tumor bone, deflects it from the surface for visual exposure and access. Tori are generally removed with chisels and the resultant surface smoothed to contour with bone files. Since the separated soft covering tissue flap is now larger than the new properly shaped surface, the excess is cut to size and sutured together in place. Healing follows.

Odontogenic tumors are tumors originating generated from tooth tissues. There are many kinds of odontogenic tumors. Some are specialized, like harmless Enamelomas which are miniature tumors like droplets of tiny pearls, consisting solely of enamel. They are often called Enamel Pearls and Enamel Drops. Enamelomas are found as isolated structures between roots of individual teeth but more usually attached to the bifurcation or forked separation of bicuspid and molar roots. They are rare.

The Compound Composite Odontoma is an especially unique benign odontogenic tumor. These growths are composed largely of teeth. Sometimes several hundred. Some of its teeth may be full sized, well formed. Most are small, even tiny, deformed. Many are only rudimentary parts of teeth. This odontoma occurs in both upper and lower jaws, sometimes blocking eruption of normal teeth. They have been found in other body parts. The tumor usually forms when the patient is young, and may be present unknown for years, confined within normal jaw boundaries. Sometimes it grows erupting as a mass, extending far beyond the bone causing great facial asymmetry. When a small tumor is removed bone quickly refills. When the neoplasm is large there is danger of jaw fracture after removal. Bordering bone surrounding the tumor location may be very thin, patients should be especially careful. Such jaws have fractured even from yawning and rolling in bed. Correction may require jaw wiring, splinting, and adding bone grafts. Again bone regrows filling into the healing spaces.

Other types of tumors in other body parts sometimes contain teeth or parts of teeth. The Dermoid Cyst or Teratoma seems sex related. It is found in male testicles, and female ovaries. More common in the ovary, this tumor sometimes reaches the size of a coconut. They often contain well formed teeth in jawbone sections, skin, hair and other tissues. Dentists individually and as a professional group are primarily concerned with their patients and society's welfare. No dentist or oral surgeon ever engaged in agitation, picketing with signs, or other organized strike activities, in jurisdictional dispute with urological, obstetric, genital or gynecological surgeons, concerning determination of rights for treatment or removal of these teeth and related parts from testicles or ovaries.

AN INTERESTING CASE ∾ Tumors are completely nondiscriminating, properly irritated they arise from any cause whatsoever. I had been treating for some time a young man I will call Jack. At one of Jack's visits I saw a small growth beneath his tongue. The underside of the tongue has along its center, running from the tip back, a thin webbed flesh attaching to the floor of the mouth. It is called frenulum linquae or Tongue Frenum. The frenum's forward free edge thickens into a tough tissue cord that stretches, tightening when the tongue is lifted or extended. The cordlike ligament limits tongue extension from the mouth. If the frenum is especially short the tongue extension may be so limited as to impair speech and the person usually a child, is said to be Tongue Tied. Surgery of such lingual frenum usually releases the tongue for proper speech. Frenums are also cut to relieve certain peridontal tissue problems and eliminate interference with dentures. At the frenum base where it attaches to the mouth floor, adjacent to each side, there are tiny exits of salivary ducts which deliver saliva to the mouth from the sublingual salivary glands under the tongue. In the normal mouth tiny bumps the size of pin heads may be seen at these salivary duct exits.

In Jack's mouth they were three or four times as large. I called this to Jack's attention mentioning I did not remember seeing them that way before. "Yes doctor," Jack said, "I know, I get them once in a while, they come and go. I don't know why. They never bother me." I palpated feeling the area gently with my fingertips in search of hard lumps. Sometimes salivary ducts fill with calcified mineral deposits of little stones, blocking saliva flow, causing inflammation and pain. These require removal, like gall stones which form blocking bile in their ducts. I checked with X-ray. There was no evidence of salivary stones. I could find no cause for the lesion.

I explained tumors and biopsy to Jack, asked that he watch the area and report any rapid growth irregularities promptly to me. During several following appointments I saw the nodules apparently harmlessly come and go. One day the tumor was massive, almost one-half inch in diameter almost as big as a marble, bumpy, soft, pink, pendulously attached around the base of the frenum. The surrounding area was severely inflammed. I showed this to Jack with a mirror, who said he once saw it almost half the size, but it had never been as large or painful before. I again explained tumor significance and the value of biopsy. The growth was totally, generously excised, and sent to a pathology laboratory. The pathologists's biopsy report arrived saying the tumor consisted of two basic materials, both benign or harmless. One a small amount of normal salivary duct tissue. The other consisted of cellular material comprising a superficial mucocele. No malignancy was observed. Mucoceles are small cystic tumors that sometimes appear on the delicate mouth surface from trauma like stretch tears and other irritations. We were both relieved.

Jack's surgical wound healed rapidly. Soon after, another small mucocele appeared as before. Jack could think of no irritation cause.

A following appointment Jack arrived excited. "Doctor," he said, "I know just what causes these tumors. I should have known before. It's when I make love to my girl friend." He told me passionate, intimate detail. "I stretch my tongue very much tightly and it tears underneath. I've watched it. I know. Look." There was another moderate size mucocele, a tumor of love or love making, under Jack's tongue. Perhaps it was worth it.

An excellent companionate story to this one concerning my male dental patient is another I discovered involving a medical doctor's female patient. This also concerns a lesion of the mouth, though it was not a tumor. See Plate 11-3, A STRANGE CASE OF PALATITIS.

TEETH TEETH TEETH

A STRANGE CASE OF PALATITIS

HERBERT RATTNER, M.D.
CHICAGO

A NEW clinical experience is always stimulating and as such should be shared with one's colleagues. It is in that spirit that I record the following case.

For quite some time I had been observing a comely young woman for soreness of the roof of the mouth. Although never severe, it was at all times bothersome, particularly so during the menstrual periods when invariably the symptoms were aggravated. Examination showed that her complaint was due to an inflammatory patch on the hard palate—a rather well circumscribed patch about 3 cm. in diameter, slightly edematous, and studded with punctate hemorrhages. It was only slightly tender to touch.

I had never before observed a lesion quite like it, nor could I fit it into any definite dermatologic category—except to suspect that it was due to irritation of some sort. The history, however—and a rather exhaustive history, I thought—failed to reveal any clews. Then, too, the clinical exacerbations coincided each time with the onset of menses. Throughout this period she was also in frequent consultation with her internist for a train of symptoms which he considered were due to psychosomatic rather than to organic disease, for complete and repeated laboratory studies, roentgenologic and clinical examinations had failed to reveal anything abnormal other than the inflammatory patch on the palate.

Treatment with a soothing preparation for use as a mouthwash, a diet of bland and soft foods and sedation afforded only slight relief. Hormonal therapy, instituted on an empiric basis, was also without benefit. A clinical test ruled out the possibility of a fixed drug eruption, and, finally because the case had taxed whatever ingenuity I could muster, it was suggested that a biopsy be performed with the hope that a histologic study would be of some help. The young woman overheard the suggestion to her physician and heard me repeat that I still held the opinion that the lesion was a simple inflammatory reaction such as might result from trauma. It was then—when the term "trauma" was used instead of irritation—that she asked whether the lesion might not be due to fellatio, only she spoke in the vernacular. The menstrual exacerbations? She had practiced the art only during the menstrual periods.

The biopsy, of course, was deferred and subsequent events proved how right she was. The lesion healed in due course, and then, possessed of a highly developed sense of curiosity—she actually reproduced the lesion.

I have since wondered on many occasions whether to be proud of or chagrined at my naivete and failure to solve the case until I encountered a zestful report in the French literature of another case which had similarly puzzled the physician. It is quoted in Ronchese's interesting monograph, "Occupational Marks."[1] In my patient, however, the lesion was avocational—I believe.

104 South Michigan Avenue.

1. Ronchese, F.: Occupational Marks and Other Physical Signs: A Guide to Personal Identification, New York, Grune & Stratton, Inc., 1948, p. 167.

Reprinted from the Archives of Dermatology Oct.1949, Vol.60 p.624
Copyright 1949 by American Medical Association
PLATE 11-3

TEETH TEETH TEETH

PRE-CANCEROUS LESIONS

Exact causes of cancer or carcinoma are still unknown. Accelerated research would hasten disclosure and eradication of its diseases. We do know, physical and chemical irritation to tissues, over prolonged periods, often create lesions called pre-cancerous, which if neglected and subjected to further abuse can become cancerous. On the other hand cancer also occurs without precedence by anything we recognize as precancerous. We don't know why. In the mouth ill fitting dentures, jagged edges of infected teeth, irritating, abusing soft cheek lining gums and tongue for long times, and even shorter periods, have caused specific lesions, not yet deadly themselves which upon continued mistreatment degenerate to cancer. Tobacco has proven a contributing factor.

Leukoplakia is a precancerous lesion commonly found in the mouth. Leuko means white, plakia means flat or plate. It appears as a white area on lining of cheeks, gums, lips and tongue. Some of these white patches come and go harmlessly. The pre-malignant lesion forms Hyperkeratosis, or thickening of the outer layer of skin. In its area the soft pink lining denses, lessening in transparency becoming whitish pearly gray, in more advanced stages fissured with tiny crackled crevices. Leukoplakia is aggravated by trauma such as jagged tooth edges and intensified by tobacco. It sometimes seems to start from heavy smoking alone, appearing at the site where inhaled smoke impinges on the lining of the mouth, on lips where cigarettes cigars and pipe stems are constantly held. A common location is cheek lining, adjacent to the biting surfaces of upper and lower back teeth especially when these teeth need repair. Cheek biting is a factor. In the back of the mouth jagged chewing edges sometimes nip adjacent cheek tissues. Their bruised ulcerated surface becomes more susceptible.

Often where these white patches are seen in mouths of smokers the tissues become normal when the teeth are repaired and smoking stops. If smoking resumes the white patches often return. I have seen leukoplakia return in mouths of heavy smokers who said they had stopped, but whom I saw from the corner of my eye smile and wink slyly at the dental assistant. Some patients say they've stopped without winking. For those who prefer fooling the doctor "Good Luck!" This is fine, and will always work for people who can arrange agreements with mouth linings not to be affected by smoke. Or they may prefer to bribe cancer. Neither will be successful. Patients who delight at deceiving their doctor, are sadly foolishly, making unfortunate fools of themselves. Leukoplakia seems more frequent among men than women, though occurrence among women seems to be increasing. It has also been associated with lack of vitamins, especially A. Leukoplakia can be cured, if neglected it sometimes turns cancerous,

TEETH TEETH TEETH

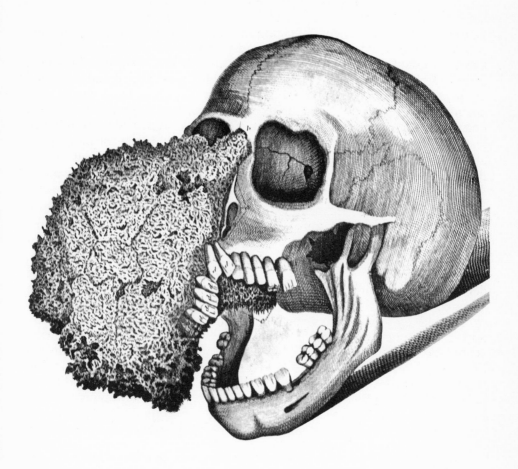

A Rare Extreme Example CANCEROUS HARD BONE or OSSEOUS TUMOR
Grown From And Destroying The Skull Face of A Woman

This death dealing monstrous tumor, containing teeth it displaced, could have been caused by disease of the teeth. Such tumors of bone, bulging from the face, completely or partly flesh covered in life, are horribly disfiguring. Unfortunates who suffer their repulsive appearance live ashamed reclused, avoid being seen by others. Never very common, such tumors are rare in modern society, curable if treated in time with modern methods.

Reproduction of an etching from "The History and Treatment of the Diseases of The Teeth", a highly esteemed treatise of its time, by Joseph Fox, Member of The Royal College of Surgeons, London, England, 1806.

TEETH TEETH TEETH

spreading back to the throat and beyond into the body. Biopsy is advised.

AN INTERESTING CASE ∾ Fred Duhearny was a fine actor. Middle aged, good looking, intelligent, he had performed in theater and for the screen. He starred as a famous detective in a small successful motion picture series. He was my friend, a heavy smoker and avoided dental affiliations.

One day Fred came to the office with a toothache. His cheek linings, right and left, were leukoplakic adjacent to jagged seriously decayed teeth. I suggested thorough examination, and treatment of his entire mouth, but Fred insisted only his one aching bicuspid be filled. I corrected that problem, explained leukoplakia, smoking, dental health and biopsy. He said he would stop smoking. At strong insistence he returned in two weeks. Leukoplakia had substantially subsided. We met socially now and then. Fred was smoking again.

Over a year later he returned with another toothache. He was still smoking heavily. Comparing with detailed descriptions written in his earlier records I showed Fred in a mirror how his cheek leukoplakia had enlarged. Again I asked he stop smoking, suggested further restorative dentistry and advised biopsy. Pain gone, he wouldn't make another appointment. He continued smoking.

Perhaps six months later he came for another filling. Leukoplakia was even larger, spreading and changing in character. It was heavily fissured with cracks surrounding higher ulcerous malignant looking lumps. There were small leukoplakic spots towards the throat. I showed Fred with a mirror, strongly insisted on biopsy and referral to an oral surgeon, explaining that if necessary conservative surgery would probably eliminate the condition, providing he stopped smoking and corrected other oral defects. He refused to follow my advice, never returned as a patient. However Fred continued as my friend, we met at gatherings. He was always smoking. I remember once at a party in his own apartment Fred told me he was in care of a gastro-intestinal specialist and could eat little but bland spaghetti.

A few months later, a girl Nina he had referred to my office as a new patient told me Fred was in the hospital. I visited him. He was suffering intestinal problems. A few months later Nina told me Fred died of cancer spread throughout his body.

ACCIDENTS

Minor dental accidents are treated in most dental offices, broken teeth and teeth knocked out. Blows that knock out teeth sometimes originate

TEETH TEETH TEETH

from a fist that also breaks the jaw. Blows that knock out teeth and break jaws sometimes originate from automobile collisions that also smash surrounding parts of the face and skull.

Faces are created by outer visible skin covered flesh, supported inside by their particular forms of bones of the lower and upper jaws and higher bones of the skull. Those who are beautiful or handsome happen to possess especially attractive combined arrangements of all these things. It's just good luck. Skull bones act as a structural container protecting their valuable inner contents. They also serve as a base for attachment of various nerve controlled muscles which terminate in facial flesh of lips, cheeks, eyes and lids, nose and other parts. They also coordinate with a complex series of masticatory muscles that drop and raise the lower jaw to open and close the mouth. When nerves of human emotion cause these muscles to contract, coordinated with others that automatically relax, they pull different soft parts of the face towards inner bones creating facial expressions like laughter, snicker, cry, hate, horror, alarm. When these muscles and others activate the lower jaw and tongue, speech and chewing are accomplished. Some people can wiggle their ears.

When accident occurs like a face hitting a steering wheel, flesh may crush, a tooth or many may loosen or be lost, a jaw may break. When structural bones are broken drastic changes occur. Coordination is out of control. The same muscles that create expressions, guiding soft face parts to bones, now pull broken bone and the flesh attached to it, away from proper places. The structural form of the face may seriously deform. It's just bad luck. One side, or part of a side, may pull up or down, right or left, inwards one place, out another, to any possible position. The seen outer soft face soon swells hiding the details of damage.

Restoration of the structurally damaged face is intimately involved with articulation and geometry of teeth and jaw actions. Usually dental accidents limited to jaw fractures are treated by oral surgeons. Sometimes fractured and displaced broken jawbone fragments are only part of a smashed face and head. Such reconstruction is usually done by Maxillofacial Surgeons, men who often have both D.D.S. and M.D. training.

BROKEN JAW ∾ Luckily dental accident damage often limits to jaws. Because of their forward prominence like automobile bumpers, lower jaws are hit first. Not being as strong as bumpers when hit hard they break. The surgeon's basic structural objectives are to restore the broken jawbone sections to proper position, and to insure that teeth of both jaws relate properly to each other with the jaws in proper position. Since jaw muscles exert high forces the surgeon must join all disrupted parts together strongly, exactly securely in place, until the broken parts heal rigidly

TEETH TEETH TEETH

together. Broken jawbone sections usually contain adjacent teeth, used by the surgeon to help establish proper relations and secure fixation. He wraps turns of short soft thin wires, around each tooth neck, joining their endings towards lip and cheek, with a tightly twisted excess needed for further use. Heavier steel arch wires or special bracket arch strips with little lugs along their length, are formed to fit around the jaw's outer tooth surfaces shaped to the normal jaw contour.

With assistance the broken jaw segments are held related properly, while the stronger contoured arch wire or bracket strip is fastened around the teeth, with each tooth excess twisted wire tab. Now the broken sections are held wired together properly. On the opposite even if unbroken jaw, wire tabs are also turned and twisted around each tooth. An arch wire or bracket arch strip is also made to fit that jaw and secured attached with the wire tabs. Both jaws are now brought together properly related with their teeth properly interdigitated. The surgeon applies intermaxillary or between-jaw wires tying upper and lower jaws together in properly closed position. The patient feeds taking liquid, high fat protein vitamin fortified diet, sipped between the teeth, often from a hand tilted, long beaked, narrow necked, small teapot. Some manage nips of gin, bourbon and scotch. Healing is usually within one to two months during later parts of which some even manage to love.

MORE SEVERE DAMAGE ∞ Sometimes an accident is disastrous and treatment for facial injury though extreme is subordinated to maintenance of life itself. When time for facial restoration arrives detailed examination is made. X-rays are taken from different directions. Stereoscopic X-rays may be made to help visualize damage in third depth dimension. These help locate displaced bones and contaminating foreign objects. Anatomical identity and location of every bone fragment must be determined. Heavy facial swelling often makes thorough examination possible only under general anesthesia. Restoration of such a face is a challenge. The surgeon must be a skilled anatomist, sculptor and engineer. He may plot with drawings on a sample skull specimen and paper, the patient's fractures and displaced bones for his reconstruction plan. Vital decisions must be made.

Some loose teeth and tiny bone fragments are discarded, most are precious beyond price. All significant displaced jaw and other bones must be relocated and held positioned until healed.

The patient is anesthetized, no pain is felt. Often curare derivatives are administered as muscle relaxants. The surgeon, anatomical sculptor, remolds the facial parts. Sometimes bones can be manipulated to place by hand, fixed to position by surgical steel wires, screws or brackets. After healed these may or may not be removed.

TEETH TEETH TEETH

ORAL SURGERY

The geometric mechanical key to facial reconstruction, is the relation of upper and lower teeth and jaws to each other, correlated with the right and left temporo-mandibular hinging joints of the lower jaw to the skull. The surgeon often starts reuniting bigger broken jaw parts, then continues rejoining teeth to teeth and jaw to jaw to skull relations. Like an engineer he checks the united fit of static or non-movable related structures, and motion paths of those that move. After all local parts are properly jig-saw-puzzle fit together, they must be rigidly held that way until healed.

Sometimes from outside through perforated flesh, long rods threaded at one end are screwed into jaw and other bone parts. Sometimes parts are too small or fragile so that a screw could cause surgical fracture. Sometimes, under the flesh, small embracing clamps are used to hold the bones. These metal clamps may have female threaded holes, into which from outside through facial flesh, long rods male threaded at one end may be screwed. Such patients have rods temporarily fixed to each bone needing control, going through holes radiating outside their face. Now on the outside, double grip adjustable clamps are placed, along each steel rod. These clamps also serve to secure added outer connecting rods, by which the surgeon establishes an outside the head rigid structural network. By means of the outer framework all bones can be adjusted, and held accurately rigidly positioned until healed. Sometimes the patient's head is shaved and a plaster cast molded around the skull to serve as a base for stabilization. After inner bone structures are related the surgeon manipulates outer facial flesh for cosmetic restoration.

All this is done with the patient anesthetized unaware. Sometimes severe accidents unfortunately leave cosmetic reconstruction to be done without need of any anesthesia by a mortician.

During treatment of more complicated cases, the patient looks rather strange with a large high plaster skull projection, wires, radiating pins, adjustable clamps and connecting rods. He is not a man from planet Mars. He is usually a man from a serious automobile accident perhaps wishing he were on Mars. After the bones heal positioned the network is removed, never completely forgotten. If satisfactory teeth to teeth occlusion was not attainable in the hospital, or if teeth were lost, necessary corrections are done by the dentist. More ideal facial affects if needed may also be accomplished by soft tissue plastic surgery. Results are remarkable.

A CHANGE OF FACE

The face is the prime individual, physical, identifying characteristic of a person. Faces are available in great variety of sizes, shapes, types, colors and surface finishes. Younger are more desirable than older faces. Antique

TEETH TEETH TEETH

faces have very little commercial value at all. When a face first appears it is soft, smooth, tender to touch. As growth occurs reaching sexual maturity half of the faces develop hair on their lower surfaces. This apparently is considered undesirable by many, since every day and even more often, the small accrued increment is removed with a sharp steel blade or electric clipper. Despite this repeated shaving, these hairs keep coming back, while later in life in many cases higher up on the head, hair greatly desired falls fading away. Upon maturity and earlier the other half of faces undergo other behavior patterns. They become dissatisfied with their lip shades and regularly cover such surfaces with a reddish grease. Sometimes they use other colors. Applications are also made around the eyes. These faces later in life do not lose hair from the head top. All faces have teeth which if neglected fail.

MAL FORMATIONS ∽ From birth inherited through the embryo, or from improper development or misfortunately acquired disease, some suffer severe facial disfigurement from malformations of the jaws. Certain bones like chins which should provide normal contour, may fail to grow to proper prominence, leaving that part missing. Those or other facial parts may overgrow, creating ugly mammoth features. These disfigurements small or large are usually symmetrical, the same on both right and left sides. Sometimes they're asymmetrical, limited to one side, from which they converge blending towards the center, meeting the other relatively normal half of the face. People with such disfigurement suffer emotionally, socially and financially. Their number is greater than realized since many self-consciously recluse, avoiding contact with others. Means are available for improving such faces and the lives of the people they face. Face-jaw reconstruction is usually performed by maxillofacial surgeons. Since teeth relations are often critically involved dentists are consulted when needed.

FACIAL DEFECT DETAILS ∽ Agnathia is absence of an upper or lower jaw or both. Hemignathia is absence of one side of a jaw. Retrognathia is a lack of jaw development. Retrognathia of the mandible or lower jaw could exist to such extent no jaw is apparent at all. The nose and upper lip jut pointed forward, leading cruel society to describe the condition as Bird Face. Prognathia is excess forward projection of a jaw. More common in the lower jaw it is called Mandibular Prognathism. To some extent mild prognathism can be helped by orthodontic application of forces with tooth brackets and wires. Prognathic deformity may be associated with excess pituitary gland growth hormone production. If hormone secretion is especially high in early life, the person grows to a well proportioned giant. If after normal size and proportions have been

TEETH TEETH TEETH

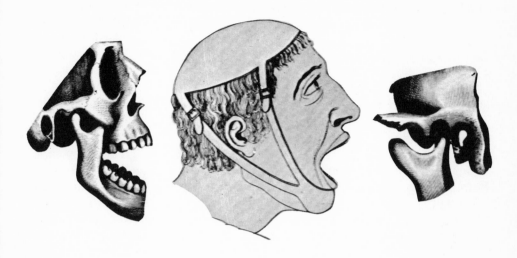

DISLOCATED JAW ∾ From an etching in "The History and Treatment of the Diseases of The Teeth" an esteemed treatise of its time, by Joseph Fox, Surgeon, London 1806.

The head's Jaw-Hinging Joint, also called Temporomandibular Joint and Mandibular Joint, is not as firmly held as that of a door hinge. The human jaw even in ordinary opening-closing action, in addition to turning, changes its location within the normal anatomical range of its socket. Sometimes it dislocates, slipping from place, locking so the jaw cannot close. If alarmed the person should relax, and may manage proper relocation themselves. It can be corrected by a dentist.

In early times, before Xrays showing teeth root size and direction, and modern surgical instruments, lower jaws would often dislocate when teeth were pulled from them.

Center Drawing is of a Head Apparatus Assembly, suggested by Dr. Fox in 1806 to prevent jaw dislocation while extracting lower teeth. Left Drawing shows a dislocated jaw, slipped forward from its rear socket so that the jaw cannot close. Right Drawing is an enlarged view of the jaw joint in its normal rear socket position.

In todays world, jaws still dislocate, less while teeth are being extracted, sometimes in fist fights and accidents, and even at times from wide yawning. Appliances similar to above are sometimes used to help.

TEETH TEETH TEETH

reached, the pituitary later becomes overactive, a condition called Acromegaly results. This creates gigantic enlargement of the tongue and lower jaw. Over the eyes bony ridges may become excessively prominent. Hands and feet sometimes also enlarge. Such ugly enlargement disfiguration misrepresents the personality of its unfortunate victim. They're often gentle people.

Excessively large jaw is also inherited characteristic. The Hapsburgs were a famous royal family founded about year 1100. Eighteen generations of its members ruled Austria, Spain, Italy and other parts of Europe. They inherited and popularized the then desired jutting Hapsburg jaw and lips. Standards of beauty change with cultures and time. Uganda women of African Congo stretched their lips increasingly, by insertion in cut holes of wooden discs up to six inch diameter and more, for greater appeal to Ugandanese men. Japanese infant girls had their feet tied and deformed from infancy, for tiny sized appeal to Japanese men. During Hitler's height of power his mustache was emulated by many German men. If during Hapsburg days present techniques were available, plastic surgeons may have been engaged to enlarge lips and jaws of envying neighbors.

TREATMENT TECHNIQUE ∽ Procedures for changing these deformed faces have been perfected. They apply surgical ingenuity and skill. Photographs, X-rays and accurate models are made and studied. The surgeon as artist engineer, may superimpose experimental new face proposal drawings over photos and X-rays, to plan and predict the operative result. Steel templates may be plotted and made for surgical guides, to help cut the anesthetized patient's bones. Access to inside the head is difficult. As much procedure as possible is done through the mouth, avoiding outer scars. When openings through facial flesh must be made, entries are located at head sites and angles almost indiscernible when healed. The surgeon avoids damage to vital muscles, blood vessels and nerves. Parts are added by bone graft, modern inert plastics and metals. Excess bone parts are removed carefully according to plan.

An especially clever simple instrument for sawing bone from outside the face is the Gigli saw. The saw consists of two fine twisted, very strong, very flexible steel alloy wires with serrated sharp sawlike edges. The saw is fastened to the end of a sharp straight or curved thick large needle. The needle is inserted through from outside the flesh, accurately located and angulated close around the bone to be cut. It pulls the flexible saw around the site, emerging at two small protected face flesh points for surgical manipulation. The doctor grasps one wire end in each of his hands, and with the patient held by assistants, strokes the saw around through the bone

TEETH TEETH TEETH

like a strip of cloth over the toe of a shoe being shined. Facial damage is minimum. Cut inner ends are connected by wires, screws, brackets or any other means. Some inner fastenings are left permanently after healing. These and other imaginative surgical methods have improved jaws, faces, and lives of many people, and will for many more.

Direct Approach — When Neediest
Delivers Relief Demanded Speediest

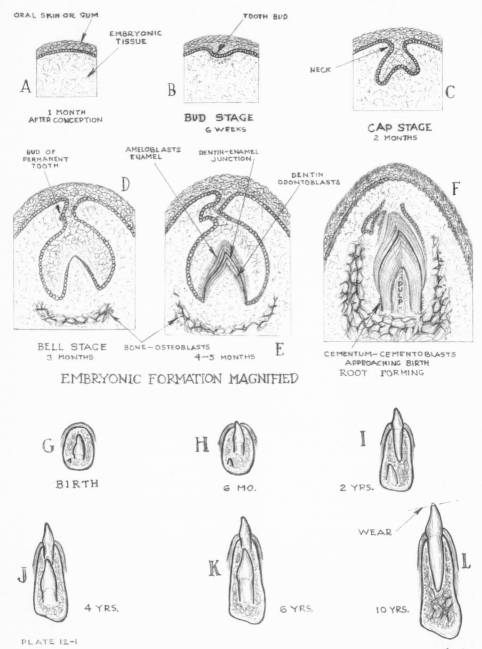

ORAL SKIN OR GUM
EMBRYONIC TISSUE
A
1 MONTH AFTER CONCEPTION

TOOTH BUD
B
BUD STAGE
6 WEEKS

NECK
C
CAP STAGE
2 MONTHS

BUD OF PERMANENT TOOTH
D

AMELOBLASTS ENAMEL
DENTIN~ENAMEL JUNCTION
DENTIN ODONTOBLASTS

BELL STAGE
3 MONTHS

BONE~OSTEOBLASTS
4~5 MONTHS
E

F
PULP
CEMENTUM~CEMENTOBLASTS
APPROACHING BIRTH
ROOT FORMING

EMBRYONIC FORMATION MAGNIFIED

G
BIRTH

H
6 MO.

I
2 YRS.

J
4 YRS.

K
6 YRS.

WEAR
L
10 YRS.

PLATE 12-1

TOOTH FORMATION~ERUPTION~RESORPTION
SHOWN IN SECTIONS THROUGH A TOOTH IN THE JAW   TIMES & SIZES APPROXIMATE

TEETH TEETH TEETH

12

DENTISTRY FOR CHILDREN ∾ PEDODONTIA

An excellent time to start treating an infant's teeth is when the child is only about one eighth of an inch long. You would need a special instrument to see him and hardly recognize him if you did. He looks much like an elephant, tiger, skunk, baboon, or dolphin, in the same condition. He has a small tail. It is about 250 days before his birthdate. He is an embryo developing in his mother's uterus, and it is only three weeks since her ovum was fertilized by his father's spermatozoon. She probably does not even know she is pregnant and he may be greatly concerned. At this time a depression called the Oral Groove is already forming what will later be the mouth connecting to the gut. Treatment consists of nourishing balanced diet food including vitamins, calcium, phosphorous and flourides for the mother. Her body factory is in process of reorganization for production of her new product. Her hormones are in delicate balance and her gums are susceptible to infection. She should be extra careful to keep her teeth clean.

When the embryo child is about six weeks old, less than one half of an inch long, certain cells of the oral epithelium or skin, start gathering into several up to ten little round thickenings at different points along each primitive jaw. This is the first sign or beginning or Primordia of the teeth, also called the Tooth Germs or Buds. At about four and a half months after conception the fetus has grown to 7 1/2 inches long. The mother may feel it moving inside. The heart can be heard beating. Its sex has developed one way or the other we hope, to become a he or she. The Enamel Organs of some of the primary teeth have established crown tips. Primordia of the first permanent molar adult teeth often already are appearing. The lips, tongue and jaws are fairly well organized. The tail is gone. The being doesn't look much like an elephant, tiger, skunk, baboon or dolphin any longer. It may grow up to behave like one.

The mother manufacturing her baby within herself should be supplying good dietary food materials for his teeth and body. When the creature is finally delivered through the automatic life conveying apparatus from inside its producer, first becoming a helpless member of society, crowns of all twenty primary or baby teeth are establishing within the jaws. Several may be forming roots. Some permanent teeth are on their way. The child is born. Occasionally an aggressive infant appears at birth with central incisors already erupting through.

TEETH TEETH TEETH

THE RISE AND FALL OF THE TOOTH

Teeth do not grow increasing in size like eyes, or a nose or toes, or peaches on trees, which after budding arise as a small organic entirety, then grow expanding bigger and bigger until mature fully formed. Beginning under the flesh each part of a tooth as it appears stays the same size it is. Starting at the top of the crown, teeth form and deposit layer by layer, elongating incrementally, increasing in length adding towards the root, until its root tip is reached as the tooth forms full. Teeth only seem to grow as they move erupting through flesh, exposing more and more of themselves, merely changing location, from inside to out seen rising above the surface. After maturity teeth get shorter with use, again layer by layer, being worn away like the cutting edge of a knife from the outside.

The beginnings of tooth formation start in the embryo about the sixth week, even before the jawbone itself. Bone appears later to surround support and join the teeth providing structure for the jaw. EMBRYONIC YOUNG TEETH are independent little things, involving in adventures more dramatic than most people realize, all under their own noses.

FORMATION OR BIRTH OF THE TOOTH ∾ We will accompany teeth on a trip of development aided by Plate 12-1, TEETH FORMATION-ERUPTION-RESORPTION, Drawing Series, Embryonic Formation Magnified.

Drawing A at about one month after conception, shows a greatly magnified sectional view through the surface of primitive embryonic oral or mouth opening covered by a layer of oral epithelium or skin. Drawing B at six conceived weeks shows one of ten little round thickened skin swellings which are the primordia or beginning tooth buds of the primary or first set of teeth of each primitive jaw to be. The skin here depresses as an indentation into underlying soft embryonic flesh. The depression continues deepening, entering the tissue a short distance, as a tube of skin like rubber around a finger poked into a blown balloon. Then the skin tube end flattens spreading out like a mushroom, and its borders curve reaching ahead embracing adjacent tissues like a bowl or cap as in Drawing C. Embryologists call this the Cap Stage of the tooth. It is sort of a double walled skin cap connected by its necked tube to the outer skin.

The next stage, Drawing D, called the Bell Stage is especially dramatic. The drama starts very tiny, in a space smaller than occupied by all angels dancing on a pinhead, though this tooth drama is real and does take place. It has had repeated performances through all past centuries in all of mankind's mouths, and has many many billions of productions ahead to go. Exciting things happen during the bell stage. The skin neck thins

TEETH TEETH TEETH

bending to a side and extending even further. See Drawing D again. The outer wall of the cap spreads out now more, like a bell rounding spherically, providing a crypt for the tooth to form in. The inner lining of skin starts moving back pointed towards the neck, cleverly assuming the form of the tip of the crown of the tooth it will be. The Creator has bestowed its soul as THE TOOTH is being born. Later, in the bell stage, Drawing E, the thin neck bends projecting even further forming an accentuated side extension. Here within that nook starts the beginning or primordia of the secondary or permanent tooth bud of the later adult tooth to be. These things all take place, forming all of our teeth.

Inside the bell, drama intensifies as the tissues reorganize. Like exciting characters in a Chinese play, varied specialized cells appear to perform special tasks. Between the walls of the doubled skin bell, cells called Ameloblasts arise, and start depositing a material later to calcify becoming enamel, around on the outer layer of the inner skin of the tooth crown form. God is the greatest playwriter director of them all. Outside this inner skin tooth contour, inside the bell chamber, other microscopic cells called Odontoblasts appear. These create, depositing material that will become dentin. The contact surface of enamel and dentin along the tooth crown's shape is the Dentin-Enamel Junction of the future tooth. Within the mouth of the bell chamber the tissues are organizing into Tooth Pulp containing nerve and blood vessels. See drawings D, E, F. The director of the play is an expert coordinator. At the same time the Creator's stagehands appear as other cells called Osteoblasts. These deposit increasing spicules or bits of bone around the scene to support and attach the tooth, forming the structural jawbone to be.

Drawing F shows the primary tooth crown established rather independently approaching maturation. Its skin connecting neck, from the former outer skin nourishing surface, like the umbilical cord of a born child is needed no longer. The crown is moving to erupt towards the surface. Enamel and dentin are calcifying, being increasingly deposited layer by layer, as ameloblasts within the enamel crown area of the bell and odontoblasts on the root side continue activity. Adding dentin is lining part of the pulp chamber and forming the lengthening root. The primary tooth is on its way. As the root establishes diverging from the crown a new character cell appears on the scene. These called Cementoblasts, Drawing F, manufacture and deposit a thin bonelike layer of material called cementum around the outer root surface. Cementum helps attach teeth to bone. The secondary or permanent tooth bud is also finding its independence. It seeks a vantage point to continue its formation and development behind the primary crown. The bone is increasing as needed, in size and strength for the jaws.

TEETH TEETH TEETH

This knowledge has all been gathered by scientific investigators, using material from lower animals and human unborn cadavers of all ages, either aborted by accident, medical necessity, or lost other ways of life's misfortunes. All such research helps advance modern dentistry.

In the human animal the six anterior primary child's teeth are succeeded by six similar larger secondary permanent adult teeth. The child has no primary premolars or bicuspids. Behind each anterior cuspid in the child's jaws upper and lower, there are first and second primary molars. These primary or baby molars are succeeded by first and second adult bicuspids that follow erupting beneath them. Behind the second bicuspid, each side of each jaw, adult first second and third molars arise, as the growing jaw increases providing space for them. These molars have no predecessors. They originate and develop directly from tooth buds of jaw epithelium just as the primary teeth did.

RESORPTION ∾ Up to the third month in the womb the unborn is called an Embryo. From then till birth the Being is called Fetus. Through embryonic and fetal stages internal toothbirth is part of the preparation process for external childbirth and continues after. The following series Plate 12-1, of drawings G through L starting with birth, shows development, growth, eruption, maturity and death or resorption loss, of a primary child tooth replaced by its succeeding permanent adult tooth. These drawings are of a lower front jawbone section, growing evolving with its primary and secondary teeth within. Sizes and ages are only approximate yet give good representation of the changing situation.

At birth, Drawing G, no teeth have yet erupted. The jawbone cross section isn't much larger than the primary tooth crown that almost fills it. The secondary tooth crown tip is tiny, hardly started behind, below its predecessor. Little jawbone exists or is needed for nursing. Chewing muscles are undeveloped. As muscles grow chewing starts, as can be told by mothers whose tender nursing nipples are sometimes nipped. As the primary tooth crown grows lengthening, muscles and bone accommodate to meet the increasing need. Six months after birth, Drawing H, the front tooth tip can be seen erupting through. Its root is lengthening. At two years, Drawing I, the jaw has grown to provide for the matured baby tooth, crown totally erupted, structurally fully rooted. The developing larger adult tooth crown is following behind below, separated by a bone layer.

Now another exciting change takes place. As the secondary tooth crown enlarges it strengthens. It becomes ambitious assuming the role of conquering invader. THE PERMANENT CROWN takes advantage of organic tissue cellular behavior tactics. Like a wise military leader it calls to arms as ally troops another microscopic cell. The Osteoclast. The osteoclast is a cell of the human body devoted to destruction of bone. As the permanent tooth lengthens from beneath, its tip advances towards the primary tooth root. Like advancing soldiers osteoclasts before its path attack resorbing the bone clearing the way. As careful obedient militia they forge ahead cleverly, never damaging the permanent tooth following. When the permanent crown reaches the primary root, see Drawing J, the osteoclasts continue attack resorbing through cementum and root dentin. The adult tooth grows increasing its rooted length, advancing its crown destroying its predecessor. See Drawing K.

Ambitious permanent teeth have always engaged in such underground activity. They are ruthless. Yet no evidence is known revealing them or osteoclasts to conduct organized undercover actions undermining any governmental society. The permanent advance continues until the impotent primary root attachment is lost so that it falls, shed naturally from the mouth. Sometimes it weakly wobbles, and mother or dad jerks tearing it away. Some lower animals like monkeys pull their own primary teeth. Some primary teeth have later interesting experiences outside the mouth. Placed under the pillow supporting the head of the sleeping child from whose mouth they were lost, they reappear as coins of different denominations in the morning.

Plate 12-1, Drawing L, shows the permanent tooth fully erupted and formed. Its tip is already being worn away. Permanent teeth are harder, stronger, longer than primary teeth they oust. They also start erupting before fully formed. They too wear away with use and suffer from neglect.

TEETHING

Adam and Eve were the only people to appear on Earth fully grown teethed without teething. Since their time human born, like kittens puppies calves and other animals, expected to feed at the breast from birth, arrive with toothless gums. While inside its maker mother the child feeds through an umbilical cord of arteries and veins, like the assembled collection of cables and tubes which first nurtured space men as they ventured from their mother missile. All is coordinated. At birth teeth aren't needed. Babies mouth parts are ideally adapted for nature's earlier outer environment feeding from mothers breasts. Infants soft tender lips are designed to fit, grasping around the darker areolar ring of the teat, sealing clinging to suction suck its food between bare soft gums from deep within the mammary protuberance. This fulfills more than needed nourishment. It has been found children who are breast fed are less inclined towards thumb sucking and other habits which lead later in life to irregular unattractive teeth arrangements. They suffer less orthodontic deformity. The child has

TEETH TEETH TEETH

good greedy taste. He may switch from one breast to the other, both are nice. Psychiatrists say some fathers, even good ones, sometimes feel jealous of their own nursing children, others may be envious too.

Milk is extracted, by lactiferous glands from mother's blood deep within her breast. It is biologically manufacture controlled to ideally fill infant needs. Milk mothers bodies make, contains needed baby body building materials including calcium, fluorides and other substances for forming teeth and bones. Mother feeding herself and child should also consume the milk of other animals plus other balanced foods for both.

Breast feeding includes self giving love from mother to child, as also seen in lower animals. Modern woman increasingly feels this feature of nature old fashioned. It doesn't go well with sports cars, cocktails and cigarettes, casually held between fingers in long holders while noses tilt and eyes raise. And why should women nurse children, men don't. Some husbands are adapting, learning to nurse though only with bottles till now; they wash dishes, diapers and floors. Some do well ironing clothes. Some women of course fix cords on vacuum cleaners and plugs in walls. More and more mates are rebelling these changes in roles of the sexes, increasing the frequency of divorce. This social conflict is not in the best interest of teeth, or children in whose mouths they grow, or fathers and mothers in whose mouths they exist or are lost. It is not the responsibility of THE TOOTH.

TEETHING DETAILS ∽ Teething is the process of baby teeth erupting from their inner jaw forming location, through the flesh surface to outside for use. Infants react differently to teething. One grows comfortably, family loved though sometimes inconvenienced, working with enjoying its baby ways, until an early thrill of parenthood suddenly discovers the white emerging tip of a tooth. And teething continues that way. Other children suffer pain, crying, wailing, biting in objection at the hurt in their mouth, drooling saliva screaming, while their teeth come through. Both behaviors are considered normal. Some children are luckier than others. The child gets its twenty primary teeth between one half to two and one half years of age during a rather continuous two years of teething procedure.

Teeth have been blamed for many childhood diseases, colds, diarrheas, fevers. Their eruption may lower resistance, but does not cause sickness. Germs are to blame as in later life. Infants are delicate. It is just as possible the baby's sickness sensitivity created the dental difficulty. If the infant does sicken or fever when teething, a physician should be consulted. At this early age teeth problems are so involved with other health factors, treatment is more usually within realm of the medical doctor who will recommend dental care if needed.

TEETH TEETH TEETH

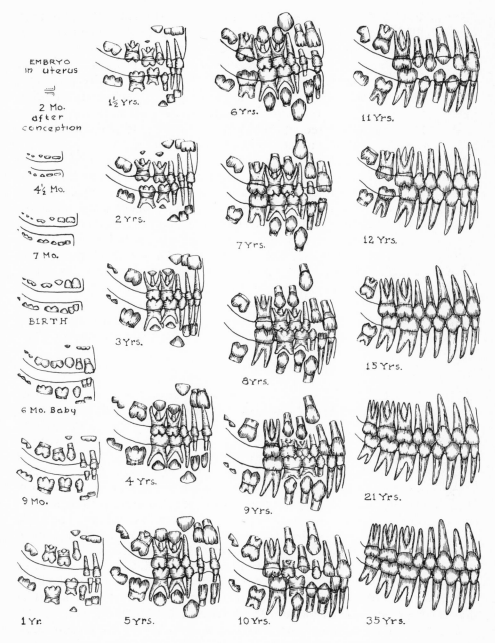

EMBRYO in uterus

2 Mo. after conception

4½ Mo.

7 Mo.

BIRTH

6 Mo. Baby

9 Mo.

1 Yr.

1½ Yrs.

2 Yrs.

3 Yrs.

4 Yrs.

5 Yrs.

6 Yrs.

7 Yrs.

8 Yrs.

9 Yrs.

10 Yrs.

11 Yrs.

12 Yrs.

15 Yrs.

21 Yrs.

35 Yrs.

CODE~ ◐ Primary or baby teeth ◑ secondary or adult teeth Representations all approximate

SUCCESSIVE DEVELOPMENT OF HUMAN TEETH S. Corfield

PLATE 12-2

TEETH TEETH TEETH

TEETHING AIDS ∞ As tooth tips approach forcefully, cutting through tender gums, they hurt some children to crankiness, they can't eat or sleep. This sometimes starts at six months with the first erupting teeth, though more often at a year and a half when the broad surface molars with their many pointed cusps force their way through. Babies are especially active putting all sorts of things in baby mouths, biting, chewing, like kittens and puppies. This is normal, the child like other animals is helping cut its own teeth from outside. Some misinformed mothers try to stop such gnawing, they can't and shouldn't, though they may drive themselves and the baby frantic trying.

Avoid ash trays, ant poison bottles, knife, fork and lip stick container chewing. Rubber teething rings and other soft toys help prevent accidents. Falling with hard objects in the mouth can cause severe dental damage. Though natural at these times for children to chew do not give babies tobacco plug. Chewing tobacco stains rugs, is disgusting and old fashioned. It's even being seen less in movies of the Old West.

The teething child may frequently wake, crying, time after time through the night. Parents loyally at first volunteer eagerly, then after a while disgusted resentfully take turns. Milk in a cup or bottle pacifies infants but should not be overdone. Children learn to use the crying wake, enjoying what for them is middle of the night parental attention parties. They generally stop when teeth are erupted, unless parents permit them to extend such technique for other personal purposes.

GENERATIONS OF TEETH

Formation of children's primary teeth, their eruption loss and replacement with permanent adult teeth, contribute to what may be considered a series of two successive teeth generations experienced within mouths during the life of each person they inhabit. Just as lifetime generations of man vary so do times of each tooth's appearance and loss.

Plate 12-2, SUCCESSIVE DEVELOPMENT OF HUMAN TEETH, portrays development of primary and permanent teeth from life's beginning to maturity. This series was drawn by the author with help from a similar series created by I. Schour D.D.S. and M. Massler D.D.S. University of Illinois, College of Dentistry. All teeth sizes, ages of formation eruption and loss are approximate. Variations are considered normal. Each drawing has an upper and lower single line representing the visible edge of upper and lower jaw surfaces. Teeth are shown forming within these jaw lines, invisible, growing approaching the surface. The time each tooth is shown to meet the jaw line and cross it to outside approximates the time of normal eruption. Each drawing representing the

TEETH TEETH TEETH

condition at its age, shows the state of teeth forming invisible inside the jaws and those crossing the jaw line surface seen erupted above.

The drawings show upper and lower right teeth in jaws from that side. Conditions are similarly opposite on the left side. In the mouth side teeth lie in a rather straight line parallel with the cheeks, while the front teeth turn in towards the front center of the head. These drawings show the entire side of teeth with the front teeth turned out, all teeth of the side shown in a flat plane for clarity.

Drawing 2 Months after conception of the embryo in the uterus which is 7 months before birth, shows beginnings of what might be called the first forming generation of teeth. The tooth buds appear as tiniest dots within the primitive jaw lines in the enlarged view. The next drawing of the 4 1/2 Month old fetus in the uterus, 4 1/2 months before birth, shows the incisal edges of all ten primary teeth taking distinctive shape. Drawing 7 Months after conception, 2 months before birth shows the growing jaws with larger primary teeth tips and the beginning appearance of permanent teeth. The next drawing at Birth shows well formed tips of all primary teeth, continuing permanent teeth development, all still unerupted invisible inside the jaws. Drawing 6 Months after birth shows beginning of what could be called the generation of erupting primary or baby teeth. The front incisors are crossing the jaw line drawn seen coming through. Lower teeth usually precede uppers, girls often before boys.

MAMELONS ∾ At this time an interesting characteristic of newly erupted front teeth may be noticed. Close observation of a child or the drawing discloses that the teeth's cutting edges rather than being a continuous smooth line has three little scalloped curves projecting from its biting edge border, like little round saw teeth. These are called Mamelons. They appear on both primary and secondary front incisors, most prominently on permanent central and lateral incisors. Parents sometimes worry thinking they're malformations. Mamelons are normal and wear away in time with use. They probably help incisal edges cut erupting through gums. Drawings 9 Months through 3 Years show the primary teeth growing incrementally, roots lengthening, crowns erupting, until all twenty appear fulfilling the primary erupted generation of teeth. The secondary permanent teeth unseen beneath, are simultaneously enlarging approaching. Drawing 4 Years shows the crowns of permanent front teeth formed already advancing to destroy into the primary root tips. It is interesting that first and second permanent bicuspid crowns which are narrower, approach into and enter between the wider spread roots of the primary molars which they later destroy and succeed.

At 6 Years of age the primary teeth are accompanied by erupting crowns of the first permanent molars also called the six year molars. This starts

TEETH TEETH TEETH

what might be considered a mixed generation of primary and secondary dentition. Within a year at 7 Years of age some primary front teeth are gone, seen replaced by permanent successors. The generation of mixed dentition increasing, replaces primary with permanent successors until at about 11 Years the permanent teeth have completely taken over, though all are not yet fully formed and properly placed. At 12 Years second permanent molars are seen erupting. At fifteen they're full and positioned. At 21 Years of age all thirty two teeth including the third molars of wisdom have ususally completed the generation of permanent teeth. Drawing 35 Years shows the erupted tooth crowns somewhat worn from use. There may be some thickening of the roots as sometimes normally occurs from an increasing deposition of cementum around their sides.

This generation of natural permanent teeth if given proper care can be expected to last for life. Neglected they're lost leaving occupants toothless for a barren generation of no teeth. Dentistry can help such people with succeeding generations of artificial denture teeth.

CHILD GUIDANCE

Every person has an individual personality affected by heredity and environment. Even growing plants respond to better gardening with better buds, blossoms and fruit. Parental behavior molds the growing child. Some older people themselves have not had proper care, being little more than children just grown older, larger in size, with more happenings that happened during the more numerous days they've lived. When parents around a child display inadequate feelings, expressing a dread of dentistry, it is unreasonable to expect a sudden brief apparent change of attitude to convince the child, who is wiser than they think. Such a child would be a fool. "Don't do as I do, do as I say" won't work.

To properly guide children parents themselves must be informed. Just as progressive doctors continue study of newer findings, fathers and mothers should reach forward with society's progress for new information guiding their selves and children towards right directions. This includes awareness of modern dentistry's values.

Mother should start early showing her watching child the way, playfully brushing her own teeth over the washbowl. Then she can help her baby brush, as both together watch playfully in the mirror. It can be fun for mother and son and little girls too. When a parental medical or dental appointment approaches, all should look forward to the experience with the child anticipating the trip as a treat. The dental waiting room, office, powerful lights, and automatic moving chairs that go up and down, can be a young adventure. Meeting assistants and dentists as friends, all

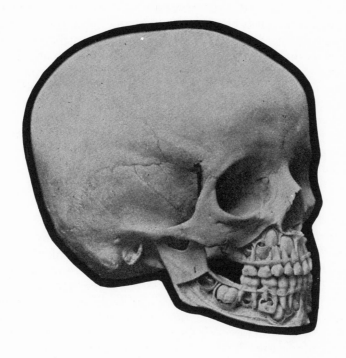

SKULL OF FOUR YR. OLD CHILD
front jawbone layer removed revealing
primary, baby or child teeth succeeded by
secondary, adult or permanent teeth

TEETH TEETH TEETH

contribute to the child's education, guided towards later treatment of their own.

DENTISTRY FOR CHILDREN

Principles of treatment for children is similar to those for adults. Some doctors of dentistry treat both children and adults as some medical doctors do. In medicine, increasing knowledge of complex conditions and changes of children's bodies as they grow from birth, led to the specialty of pediatrics. Similarly in dentistry, complications of treatment involving formation and eruption of primary teeth as jaws grow, then loss of these early teeth replaced by permanent dentition, led some doctors to devote themselves to dentistry for children.

Pedo means foot or beginning. Dontia refers to the tooth. Pedodontists are dentists who undertake special studies in children's dental problems and limit their practice to such work. They treat children from birth usually until the adult dentition of twenty eight teeth including second molars erupt at about age fifteen.

Some pedodontists serve their youthful patients even longer. Adolescents may develop an attachment of confidence towards the pedodontist, preferring to continue with him. Doctors sometimes treat such patients into early adulthood, perhaps to eighteen. Then the new grown-up feels awkwardly misplaced among children in the office, and prefers going to another dentist as a young man or woman among men and women.

AT THE OFFICE ∽ Sometimes an ambitious, even under a year old infant, crawling or learning to walk stumbles alarmed, falls on its face, fractures front teeth, and is rushed by distressed mother for emergency treatment. Dental visits are best planned by an appointment, after all twenty primary teeth are erupted at about two or two and a half years of age.

The pedodontist is an understanding friend of young people. His waiting room is often a musical playroom, with child sized chairs and tables, toys, pictures and books, where little patients feel comfortable among other boys and girls. I know a pedodontist who dresses like a cowboy in his office, which looks like a Western ranch house. Children love coming to their cowboy doctor. They don't need being lasso'd or tied to the chair. It's the parents who come along to this dental office. Feelings of ease extend into treatment rooms where children are seated in smaller dental chairs. Drills and other instruments are also smaller, for the smaller mouths of smaller bodies of younger people. The first visit as a tour guided by dentist and helpers discovers all the newness. X-rays are taken for an easy start.

TEETH TEETH TEETH

Confidence grows as the child is gently introduced to treatment, first having teeth cleaned with the same little turning parts used later to drill and fix cavities.

AROUND CHILDREN'S TEETH

Disease of the tissues around teeth are more common in later life. Children have not yet lived the accumulated years of neglect leading to peridontal degeneration. Yet such disease does occur in children, more frequent among primitive people, low socio-economic groups, and in war suffered areas where probable cause is lack of oral hygiene and proper nutrition. Teeth irregularities which trap dirt, and diseases of the body like diabetes, also cause trouble to tooth supporting tissues. Children's most common peridontal disorder is gingivitis or gum inflammation. Primary cause is dirt. Neglect leads to more severe problems which can be avoided by cleanliness.

Teeth are best cleaned after every meal. Until about age six or seven, parental help brushing is advised, with examples of parents seen cleaning their own teeth. Some children like Disclosing Tablets. These are little colored pills containing harmless chemical stains, usually red, which when chewed and swished around the mouth brightly color the dirt on teeth surfaces. They help as a test for cleanliness. The child brushes until all disclosing stains disappear. The tablets do not stain teeth. In addition to home care, children like parents, need regular more thorough professional office cleaning treatments of unaccessible areas hard to reach.

Like adults, children's teeth accumulate deposits from many sources. Food, salivary minerals, mucous, mouth tissue cells, and germs and molds that grow within them. Some young teeth stain dark brown and green. A pedodontist told me a story of little Fred, whose older sister Agnes asked that the dentist be sure to clean his teeth before school started. "Yes Fred," the doctor said, "Your teeth do look terrible all covered with that green stain." Little Fred said, "Oh, I don't mind the stains doctor, it's Agnes who wants them cleaned. Green is my favorite color."

Fluorides professionally applied to tooth surfaces, and in toothpaste and drinking water is valuable. Proper balanced diet and avoidance of sugars and refined starches helps.

PRESERVING CHILDRENS TEETH AND JAWS

Some misinformed people have the old incorrect belief, that since primary or baby teeth are lost early, if they are decayed restoring them is waste of money and time. Parents say "Yes, why fill teeth that aren't even supposed to last long and naturally fall out anyway." Doctor P. E. Dow, "Defective baby teeth should be restored for several reasons. Tooth decay is actual germ infection inside the tooth, within a short time they can sometimes cause long lasting damage. A child whose teeth hurt can't eat, its general health may be affected. Decay in and around a primary tooth may spread, infecting adjacent permanent teeth following close beneath to erupt. Children are delicate. Germs of tooth infection may enter the throat and beyond inside the body, even seriously undermining general health. Decayed baby teeth often cause disfiguring improper positions of permanent teeth, far more expensive to correct later."

"Teeth, first primary babys, and then succeeding permanents, are both normally arranged in a smooth curve around the jaw arches, next to each other. Adjacent teeth touch at their broadest extremities called contact points. Each baby tooth occupies keeping its space, to act as a passageway when the tooth is lost, for entrance into position of its following erupting permanent successor which should replace it for life. Primary teeth not only maintain space for their successors, their healthy hard contact with each other also provides a mechanical fixity encouraging the jaw to grow. It is probable that if forming tooth buds were experimentally removed from growing jaws, those jaws developing without teeth would never attain full normal size."

"As jaws grow a natural force exists moving teeth forward along the jaw arch towards the front. All are kept in place aligned by their healthy hard contacts. Between these contacts, dirt accumulates most, needing most cleaning. It is here teeth frequently decay as hard contacting tooth surfaces rot soft. The continuing forward forces move the teeth forward, closing into each other's soft decayed yielding areas. Teeth decay irregularly, so that hard remaining parts cause deflections from normal tooth arch form. Some irregularities lock primary teeth into each other, so that those ready to shed are held in place. Beneath these decayed irregular teeth, the succeeding permanent teeth continue growing, moving to erupt. If strong enough they will force through."

"Often their proper path isn't available any longer. The primary decayed teeth closed together and locked, block passage, so that their permanent successors forcing erupt displaced irregularly, through one side or another wherever weaker tissues yield. The child may grow with permanent crooked teeth and jaws irregularly out of line." Parents, "Oh."

YOUNG TEETH DENTAL DETAILS

Nerves inside children's primary teeth have low pain sensitivity. Anesthesia is rarely required for removing decay, cavity cutting and

TEETH TEETH TEETH

filling. As with adults anesthetics are usually used for permanent teeth.

Most common restorations for cavities in children's teeth especially back in the mouth is silver filling. Gold inlays aren't popular since baby tooth life is rather limited. A popular idea that children's teeth are easily filled in less time is wrong. They are smaller yet require careful technical consideration. Often small restorations are more difficult to do than large.

If tooth degeneration extends deep into nerve pulp, the pedodontist first uses endodontic treatment for those conditions. When a primary tooth too badly broken down to support a filling is needed to keep its neighbors in line and maintain space for its successor, it can often be saved until permanent tooth eruption with a shell crown. Children's shell crowns are of thin hollow stainless steel made to match children's teeth crown forms. They fit around over supporting the tooth from outside. They are available in varied tooth crown shapes and sizes. The pedodontist selects one closest to the treated tooth, adapts it with trimming scissors and contouring pliers. After decay is removed and medication applied, the cemented shell crown provides chewing for the child and also helps support the adjacent teeth as long as necessary.

In front of the mouth where appearance is important, children's teeth like adult can be restored with natural color fillings. More active than adults children play, chase, fight, fall, fracture teeth. Full jackets will restore those badly broken and bridges any lost. Teeth knocked out of the mouth can often be reinserted into the jaw for lifetime service. They should be picked up, even from dirty streets, if found even a day or more after loss, brought to the dentist who with modern methods may be able to replant them in the jaw for perpetual use.

FIRST MOLARS ∽ Especially important back teeth which are often neglected and suffer seriously, are the first permanent molars, right and left, above and below. They deserve this cautious description. They erupt at about six years. They are permanent teeth intended to last for life. They have broad cusped chewing surfaces, held by strong widespread supporting roots capable of heavy chewing. They hold strategic position to mouth welfare, in fact the first molars are called the Keys of the Dental Arch. They are the first permanent teeth to erupt in the rear, behind first and second baby molars, and are often mistaken for baby teeth expected to be lost. Some parents neglectful towards primary teeth have equal unconcern for these, so that they are often allowed to degenerate needing extraction. This is serious. Their space vacancy causes even harder to care for second molars further back, to drop tilting forward misaligned, causing food trapping infection and their following later loss if unattended.

There are modern methods of removing unerupted incompletely formed less needed third molars or wisdom teeth, transplanting them into sites of first molar extraction where they sometimes take hold, continue to grow and erupt useful for life. Even YOUNG WISDOM TEETH are wise and serve man when they can.

PREVENTIVE ORTHODONTICS

In addition to treating teeth and their supporting tissues, pedodontists are sort of control engineers of children's changing teeth. While maintaining the health of teeth along their change from primary to secondary dentition, they prevent conditions causing orthodontic malformations and eliminate those they can that create them.

SPACE MAINTAINERS ∞ Through neglect or other cause, sometimes primary teeth are lost before they should be, leaving a space in the jaw, before their permanents beneath have developed enough to erupt filling into the void. Left abandoned such spaces often grow deformed, closed smaller or completely, by surrounding growth forces. This blocks eruption of the permanent tooth causing later problems. When loss of such primary teeth cannot be avoided pedodontists preserve the space with space maintainers. Refer to Plate 12-3, SPACE MAINTENANCE. Drawing A shows mixed primary and secondary teeth with their normal ideal space maintainer. This is the normal second primary molar crown preserving the distance, filling it, between the erupted permanent first molar behind and first bicuspid in front. The second permanent bicuspid is forming following beneath.

Drawing C shows the result of neglect. In this child's mouth the second primary molar was lost early, yet no provision made to keep its space. Before the bicuspid could erupt from below, the permanent first molar and even the following second tilted far forward improperly. The second permanent bicuspid was kept down blocked trapped, invisible inside the jaw. This can only be seen with X-ray. It may make its way out cramped through a side, crooked towards the cheek or tongue. Drawing B shows a space maintainer in use. Bands are cemented around the crowns of first permanent molar and first bicuspid. These are held apart by two attached thin rigid wire bars, maintaining space necessary for eruption of the second bicuspid between them. When the bicuspid erupts properly the pedodontist removes the space maintainer. So give three cheers and three cheers more for space maintainers and pedodontists and the Captain of the Pinafore.

To prevent orthodontic or crooked teeth problems, pedodontists use varied techniques. They correct bad personal habits like thumbsucking

TEETH TEETH TEETH

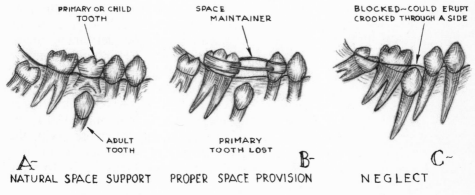

PRIMARY OR CHILD
TOOTH

SPACE
MAINTAINER

BLOCKED~COULD ERUPT
CROOKED THROUGH A SIDE

ADULT
TOOTH

PRIMARY
TOOTH LOST

A~

B~

C~

NATURAL SPACE SUPPORT   PROPER SPACE PROVISION   NEGLECT

PLATE 12-3 SPACE MAINTENANCE   S. Garfield

TEETH TEETH TEETH

which cause tooth irregularity. They may perform minor orthodontic treatment to early irregularities which if neglected become more serious. When such problems are beyond their realm pedodontists refer patients to orthodontic specialists.

Early Care for Young People
Make Mans Future Rewards More Reapful

13

ORTHODONTIA

Lifes path is pleasant walked lightly free, fortune found along the way. For some its sometimes wonderful. Others less lucky find roads rough, stumble fall and bruise. A few strong fortunates strive and survive even bearing burdens. Emotional burden is sometimes severe, may make life a struggle. Dental disfigurement can create such burdens. It need not. Many malformations of teeth and jaws,accepted in the past as misfortunes of fate, causing anquish to some sensitive, can now be corrected by orthodontia.

Ortho is part of a word, meaning straight, correct or upright. Dontia is the tooth. Orthodontia is a branch of dentistry concerned with correction of improper positioned teeth and jaws, for improvement of appearance, emotional and physical health. Dentists who undertake special studies and limit their practice to such work are called Orthodontists.

Natural things in nature, and natural things in people, and people things in people, sometimes imperfect cause trouble. Unexpected tidal waves, earthquakes, mountain slides, floods, damage and kill. Like abnormal faults of our physical Earth, defects also trouble its living beings. Incorrect teeth and jaw positions are found among fish and lower land animals, and are increasing among races of man. Irregular teeth-jaw relations are not limited to unattractive appearance and psychological disadvantage. Crowded crevices between misaligned teeth are hard to clean cause decay, infection, peridontal disease and tooth loss.

CROOKED TEETH CAUSE AND CURE

Some children at birth inherit the dental defects of irregular ugly teeth. Some grow with jaws too small, so their teeth crowd crooked erupting through. Young growing bone is soft pliable, when subjected to even light constant force will yield to its direction. Some infants tender toothed jaws deform sucking around bottles poorly designed artificial nursing nipples. Some children's jawbones and teeth deform around their own sucked thumb. A young child sleeping for long, on the same side, in the same single position, head weight pressing the same sided jaw upon its supporting arm rest, could cause the soft jaw to grow deformed from that side. A nervous child's tongue muscles thrusting forward against its teeth could force them to grow bucked out. Tight lip muscles might pull them back, properly or too far in. When teeth of a jaw erupt from ideal position, as both jaws are brought together, mismating teeth of the opposite jaw could cause either soft boned jaw to grow deflected forward or back, yielding to the stronger tooth position. Parental neglect to treat a child's baby or primary teeth can cause its following permanent adult teeth to come through incorrectly.

Fortunately the same plastic quality of bone that permits misdirected forces to deform teeth and faces can be used by orthodontists to correct them. They combine biological knowledge of teeth and bone with orthodontic engineering principles, to design individual corrective appliances for each patient's problem. With this apparatus in the mouth, they can apply forces of magnitude they desire, to teeth and bone they desire, in directions they desire. They move malformed parts of the patient to normal attractive places. Where extent of deformation is beyond orthodontic treatment oral and maxillofacial surgery can help.

Modern orthodontia is constantly progressing, becoming more available to more children whose growing elastic bones readily respond. Adults are also being helped. Mature patients ask, "Can adults actually be helped by orthodontia." Doctor, "Of course, with latest orthodontic technique more and more men and women are treated successfully. People are increasingly appreciative of personal appearance value. With older patients orthodontia is usually part of other extensive restorative procedure. In long neglected mouths, where some teeth are lost, the contact support formerly provided by the lost teeth to remaining teeth is gone. These often drift and are forced by chewing into poor positions. If such teeth are first straightened by orthodontia, better bridges and other appliances can be made. Results look better, are healthier and feel better." Patient, "Doesn't that take extra time." "Yes, it does, and extra cost. It is not always indicated, but when advisable is worth it. The dentist can best decide."

NORMAL DEVELOPMENT

In growing children's mouths, tooth arrangements and numbers are complicated by changing combinations of primary teeth not yet lost, and secondary or permanent teeth erupting to place. The orthodontists result is directed towards the permanent adult dentition. As teeth develop and grow to erupt, they experience a natural orthodontia of their own. Each tooth individually approaches only approximately its final proper place. As all successively follow each other, each is guided by contacting adjacent neighbors, and by opposing angulated contacts of their opposite jaw opponents, directing them all to place. As crowns reach full final eruption they normally appear in attractive, intricately coordinated, clever pattern.

TEETH TEETH TEETH

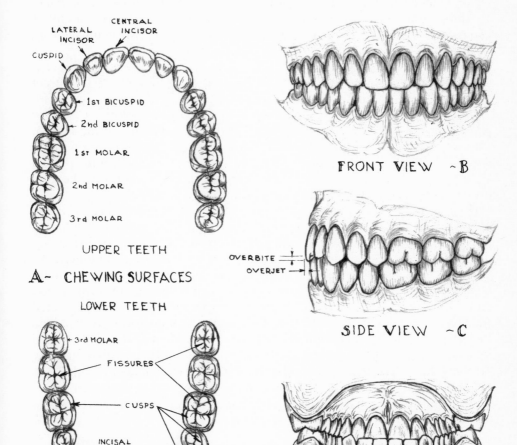

LATERAL
INCISOR
CENTRAL
INCISOR
CUSPID

1st BICUSPID

2nd BICUSPID

1st MOLAR

2nd MOLAR

3rd MOLAR

UPPER TEETH

A- CHEWING SURFACES

LOWER TEETH

3rd MOLAR

FISSURES

CUSPS

INCISAL
EDGES

CENTRAL INCISOR

FRONT VIEW ~B

OVERBITE
OVERJET

SIDE VIEW ~C

BACK VIEW ~D
FROM INSIDE THE MOUTH
LOOKING FORWARD~TONGUE OMITTED

PLATE 13-1 NORMAL TEETH RELATIONS S.Garfield
PERMANENT OR ADULT

TEETH TEETH TEETH

This arrangement is the goal of the orthodontist. A full set of adult teeth number thirty two. The last four molars called wisdom teeth are fully formed erupting between age 18 and 25 years.

NORMAL TEETH RELATIONS ∽Refer to Plate 13-1, NORMAL TEETH RELATIONS, which shows several normally related views of upper and lower permanent adult teeth. Upper and lower, right and left teeth are symmetrical, opposite on each side of the body's center. The upper teeth arch is larger all around than the lower. When teeth are in Occlusion or closed together faces of the upper teeth crowns normally extend beyond the lowers all around. Feel this with your finger with teeth closed. Above and below, from the vertical center of the head outward towards both sides right and left, front teeth or anteriors are Central Incisors, Lateral Incisors, and Cuspids also called eye teeth or canines. They all have single roots. They all have single Incisal, cutting or biting edges, for biting and tearing through foods. The cuspid tooth crown is somewhat thicker with a single spearlike point or cusp. Upper cuspids have the longest roots in the mouth. Front teeth have hereditary vestiges of function as weapons of defense and offense, more in the female than male of our species. They are also sometimes used in tender love bites, sometimes not so tender.

Following behind cuspids are the back teeth. First and second Bicuspids also called Pre-molars, then first, second and third Molars. These usually have two or more roots. They have broad, chewing, grinding surfaces called their occlusal surface. Occlusal means to close or meet. When back teeth are closed together meeting in occlusion, they act as vertical stops for the jaws and determine the height of the head and face. Back teeth perform the heavy work of chewing, crushing food for digestion.

While front teeth have single narrow bite edges, occlusal or chewing surfaces of back teeth divide into two ranges, like little mountains of narrow pointed projecting prominences. One is outward along towards the cheeks, one inside towards the tongue. The pointed projections of these prominences are called Cusps. They are like tiny mountain peaks. Between outer cusps towards the cheek and inner cusps towards the tongue, along the occlusal surface center, there are tiny gorge or ravine like crevices or Fissures. When jaws normally close together tips of the outer or cheek side cusps of lower teeth, cleverly fit up into or interdigitate with the central fissures of the upper teeth. Tips of the inner or tongue side cusps of the upper back teeth fit down into the central fissures of the lower back teeth.

Man does not chew directly up and down. Normal chewing includes sideways grinding somewhat like cows, as the tiny slanting walls of opposing cusps slide along against each other, as tooth cusp peaks fit into opposing teeth fissures. I'ts quite a clever arrangement, try it. Ideal

TEETH TEETH TEETH

occlusion throughout the mouth rarely exists and isn't necessary. The orthodontist strives for an attractive, satisfactory functional result approximating the ideal.

Plate 13-1, Drawing Series A shows an upper jaw turned up opened wide above its mated lower. Details of the teeth chewing or occlusal surfaces are presented. Drawing B is a front closed view. Drawing C is a side closed view. Overjet is distance the front surface of upper teeth project ahead of their mating lowers. Overbite is distance the incisal edge of upper front teeth extend down below hiding that much of their mating lowers. These are both normal relations and obvious in all views showing the teeth closed. Drawing D is a view from back inside the closed mouth looking forward. The tongue is omitted from the drawing to reveal the teeth relations.

THINGS LOOK BAD

Probably no other part of human anatomy varies as much as teeth. Orthodontic irregularity occurs in great variety. Teeth may crowd or spread, tilt in, out, any direction, to one side or any others. Sometimes they erupt not normally from the jaw's top edge but from the jawbone side, inside or outside. They may twist or turn. Either jaw upper or lower could be receded, retruded back or Retrognathic. All mean the same. Retro means back, gnathic jaw. Either jaw could jut forward as an excess overjet, protruded or Prognathic. Pro means forward. Either of these, or normal related jaws, could have teeth receded back in retruded position, or protruded bucked far out forward.

Crossbite is a condition, such that lower teeth of a side instead of being under their uppers properly partly inward, cross over extending outside beyond. This could be minor hardly discernible, or so severe the jaw deforms the whole face to a side. Double Crossbite is a symmetrical condition in which lower teeth of both sides extend out beyond their uppers. It exists with especially wide lower jaw or extremely narrow upper. Closed bite, or excessive overbite, can be so extreme either arch is far too small or big for its opposite.

When such jaws come together, teeth of one arch instead of contact stopping closed, pass completely inside outside, each beyond the other. The jaws stop by biting hurting into mouth flesh. Eating is awkward uncomfortable, mouths tender sore. In Open Bite, a few over erupted teeth of opposite jaws hit first, preventing further jaw closure, so most teeth remain separated open apart, as though biting on a stone back in the mouth. Such mouths can never completely close.

All these things may exist individually as described, or combined in

TEETH TEETH TEETH

minor or major degree. Some so slight treatment is not recommended. Sometimes so severe treatment is mandatory for the patient's appearance, mental and physical health. Orthodontia can be of great value, improving bones of such jaws and positions of such teeth. Mother, "My misunderstood child is ugly as sin. She's selfish, cruel and crosseyed. Her teeth are crooked and her nose too long. When light isn't bright she's sometime mistaken for a werewolf. Yet doctor, she always stops scratching people when they bleed profusely. I would like her to become a famous leading lady screen and television star. Can orthodontia make her gorgeous, gentle, beautiful, tender, kind, talented and charming." "No."

INSIDE INFORMATION ∾ It was once believed teeth moved through bone as a result of bones fluid resiliency. Like a stick forced through thick mud flowing around it. As early as 1911 Dr. Albin Oppenheim of Vienna used orthodontic appliances on monkeys, studying the histological and physiological behavior of teeth and bone. Histology is microscopic study of biological tissues. Physiology is study of the function or behavior of cells, tissues,and organs, of the living body. These and other researches revealed living bone tissue is constantly being rebuilt and replaced through life.

When forces are applied inside the mouth, above the gum to the crown of a tooth, they transfer through the tooth root to the inside bone around it. Inside the bone along the pressured side of the root, microscopic living body cells called osteoclasts appear. They consume the bone ahead on the pressure side. The tooth loosens, as force continues, moves. On the side the root moves away from, other microscopic cells called osteoblasts create and deposit new bone filling the void. Osteoclasts on the root pressured side resorb bone. Osteoblasts on the following side fill in new bone. Osteoclasts and osteoblasts are the same cells intimately involved in normal continual bone replacement during life. It could be said the orthodontist uses them both to grow teeth and jaws to better positions.

While moving, the tooth is always slightly loose. When it reaches final destination, the orthodontist ends force application, osteoclasts stop destroying the bone. Osteoblasts grow new bone all around the root tightening the tooth in final position. The bone itself similarly responds to the force, also growing to some extent with the teeth towards the guided direction.

While teeth move through bone, a natural thin root covering layer of bonelike material called cementum, protects the roots from damage. If applied pressures are too high cementum damage may result, and the tooth root also resorbs being destroyed. The orthodontist treats his patient so teeth and bone will move to position in the least time without damage. He

TEETH TEETH TEETH

adjusts his forces to suit the conditions. Tooth movement speed varies greatly. A rough average might be an eighth of an inch a year. Movement is usually slower in adults. Extensive orthodontic changes sometimes take a long time, even two or three years. It takes time to do a difficult job. Good things are worth waiting for.

OUTSIDE INSIDE INFORMATION ∾ The orthodontist engineer reshapes his patient, applying forces in the mouth to push and pull between tooth and bone parts of the head. If a controlled force is exerted between teeth or jaw parts of equal size and strength, each moves equally in opposite directions. Pushing separates them, pulling brings them together. Sometimes this is done.

More often different mislocated parts must each be moved by themselves in particular directions. Knowing the intimate nature of bone and teeth, the orthodontist uses mouth segments of greater strength which move less, as force is applied, for resistant anchorage to move weaker parts further. When a firm tooth needs moving, several other teeth together may be used as united resistance, to move the single stronger. Forces may be applied between different parts of a single jaw or from one jaw to the other. Sometimes even this is not enough, even greater resistance is needed. To grow changes in especially rigid segments or entire jaws, the orthodontist may feel no structures within the mouth strong enough. He uses the patient's skull as anchorage. Apparatus is designed for attaching to teeth and jaws inside the mouth, passing between the lips, exerting forces and attaching to the head outside the mouth. Such treatment is performed more usually with children. It seems awkward, but yields valuable results sometimes otherwise unobtainable.

MEASURING UP ∾ Orthodontic patients should be in good physical condition. Teeth and supporting tissues manipulated for movement must be healthy. Needed general dentistry is finished first. Examination of cases limited to simple tooth position improvements only requires dental X-rays and models of the teeth and jaws. More significant orthodontia demands more detailed examination. Outside visual observation of the head and face though valuable is limited. Facial flesh is soft and kind, blending to minimize defects of hidden teeth and bone irregularities beneath. To treat most cases properly the orthodontist needs knowledge of inner structures. Full side and front Cephalometric X-rays of the head are taken. Cephalo means head, metric measurements. Front and side face photos are often valuable. These give the doctor more accurate measurements of the inner skull, jawbone, and teeth related to each other, and to the outer flesh of the face.

TEETH TEETH TEETH

THE ORTHODONTIC SURVEY ∾ Patient photos X-rays and mouth models are studied. Each tooth posture is evaluated. Some may be too far in or out, some tilt back or forward, some are crowded, or spaced far apart, some twist one way or another, some suffer combined faults. Each tooth is evaluated for relative position along its jaw, and to the teeth of the opposite jaw. Upper and lower jaws are judged for relation to each other, and as a combined working assembly related to the head. The orthodontist determines which parts need moving, in which directions how far. He may be able to sketch and predict approximately the face's final improved appearance. Using his specialized orthodontic form of non-surgical facial plastic surgery, the orthodontist performs a life moving sculpture of teeth, jaws, and face.

EXTRACTION FOR ORTHODONTIA ∾ When teeth are too crowded for straightening into jaws too small to fit them all, the orthodontist may remove an unnecessary few. In the back if erupted, or even unerupted if necessary, wisdom teeth are taken out. Towards the front first bicuspids are often most practical. They usually supply the amount of space needed If other teeth are severely decayed they may be removed instead.

Mother, "But doctor, if bones will grow following teeth as they orthodontically move, why extract any at all. Won't Johns jaws increase in size providing space for the teeth being straightened." Orthodontist, "Yes it would grow larger. If John's jaw were too small for his face we would encourage its growth. I could avoid extraction, but it would not be practical for John. His jaw size is good as it is. Also enlarging a jaw takes much more treatment time and trouble, and costs more. It is done when advisable. Johnnie's final more ideal, less crowded condition with those unneeded bicupids gone, will stay cleaner keeping his teeth healthier longer. Removing his two bicuspids will give us an attractive better arrangement faster. One is decayed anyway."

GETTING STRAIGHTENED OUT

Irregulary erupted teeth are like juvenile delinquents strayed from their proper path. In rare cases, if not too seriously involved, they may straighten out by themselves. Left alone, shifting without help, they usually become even more seriously involved. They degenerate and suffer. They may even be lost beyond salavation. Delinquencies originate from heredity, neglect, or poor environment, or as is often the case combinations. They can always be helped. They need understanding to be treated properly. They must cooperate. They must be taken strongly in hand, yet gently and firmly slowly guided towards their proper direction. This all requires effort, time,

TEETH TEETH TEETH

and money. It's worth it. Returned to normal, they are healthier, happier, look better, and lead longer more useful lives.

APPROACHING THE PROBLEM ∾ Orthodontic appliances are custom designed for each individual patients problem. They fit only the mouth they're made for. Both fixed and removable apparatus are used. Fixed apparatus are cemented, attached to the teeth. They cannot be removed by the patient. Day and night, in the mouth contantly, they work guiding teeth and surrounding tissues. Patients talk, eat, sleep, with their orthodontic apparatus. Properly controlled, it works all the time, bringing mouth parts to place. Fixed appliances tend more to trap food, need extra cleaning care. Both fixed and removable sometimes affect speech a little during treatment. Always less than patients imagine. Speech is better than ever when treatment is over.

Removable apparatus are patient inserted and removed daily for cleaning. If annoyed, patients can take them out to eat or talk. They may if desired only be worn while sleeping. You can even sleep without them. Patients are treated only while they're worn. Out of action, the resisting tissues tend to relapse back to improper places. Patients sometimes try to fool the doctor, saying they wore appliances they didn't. They can't fool their teeth.

Patient, "Which are better doctor, fixed or removable." Orthodontist, "They're both good and have their place. Generally finer results can be accomplished with fixed apparatus. They firmly grip each tooth. Forces can be more accurately controlled and delivered, to every tooth and their supporting following bone. They can be moved to more precise positions. Being constantly worn, treatment is continually applied. Most orthodontia in this country, especially with children, is with fixed apparatus. In Europe more removable appliances are used, though fixed technique is increasing."

Patient, "Why use removable appliances." Doctor, "Fine orthodontic results can be accomplished with removable equipment in many cases. They are often more convenient, especially for actors, or those with special dates or conferences. The president of the mortgage and loan company doesn't want being seen with braces on his teeth. More luscious kisses can be delivered without hardware in a mouth. Adults we hope, can be better depended on to intelligently replace mouth appliances. I did however have a mother patient, whose seven year old daughter constantly had to remind and coax her to wear her removable orthodontic equipment. I don't know anything about the woman's kisses."

TEETH TEETH TEETH

FIXED ORTHODONTIA

Refer to Plate 13-2, ORTHODONTIC APPLIANCES. See Drawing A, Fixed Orthodontic Apparatus. Fixed orthodontic appliances also called Braces, are attached in the mouth by metal Bands, cemented to firmly embrace individual teeth. The orthodontist studies the case and designs corrective appliances on models of his patient's misaligned teeth and jaws. He decides which teeth need banding, sometimes all. Each band is a small encircling narrow ring of thin stainless steel, individually formed to fit tightly around and hold its particular tooth. Attached to the outer face of the band is a tiny metal bracket. The bracket is used to control the tooth. Brackets are available in great variety with tiny hooks, holes, and slots, of different sizes and shapes, for appying forces to the tooth. Forces are applied by means of rubber band elastics, springs, and wires, to move the tooth. Resistance for these forces are supplied by arch wires. Arch wires are formed to fit outside the teeth around the entire jaw arch. The arch wire serves as a basic foundation, for attachment at points along its length, of individual elastics and springs to the teeth brackets. These forces guide each tooth to its proper place in the arch, and assemble all the teeth as a functional unit, to their proper form around the arch.

There are many types of arch wires. Some are heavy rigid hard, acting as an immovable foundation around the jaw teeth, from which at places along its length forces are applied to each tooth, pushing, pulling, turning as needed. Some are light thin resilient wires, also serving as springs themselves. These are bent adjacent to particular teeth needing corrections of different amounts, away from the teeth at different angles. At each tooth location, the wire is later forced into and attached to its particular slot of each tooth band bracket. The very force needed to bring the wire into the bracket is calculated to act restoring the tooth to its desired position.

Sometimes two arch wires, called twin arch wires, are so bent related to each other, such that when each is forced into its separate, short distance apart slot, on the same tooth bracket, their differentiated exerted forces correct the tooth's position. Rather than being round, some arch wires are flat in cross section, or rectangular, or square. Such wires are twisted in addition to being bent. The combined bend and twist is so calculated, that when the wire is forced attached into its precise bracket slot receptacle, bend and twist join exerting the needed correction forces.

Mrs. Wanda Knowe asks, "Which method is best doctor." Dr. Arthur Dauntest, "They're all good. Some better for correcting certain deformities than others. Some orthodontists prefer using one way over another. Some change methods as the case proceeds and needs change. Many use combined techniques. There are many ways to skin cats and straighten

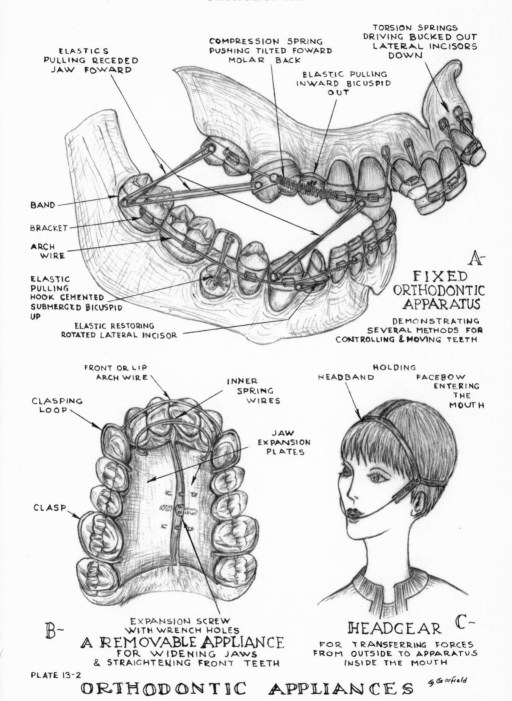

ELASTICS
PULLING RECEDED
JAW FOWARD

COMPRESSION SPRING
PUSHING TILTED FOWARD
MOLAR BACK

TORSION SPRINGS
DRIVING BUCKED OUT
LATERAL INCISORS
DOWN

ELASTIC PULLING
INWARD BICUSPID
OUT

BAND

BRACKET

ARCH
WIRE

ELASTIC
PULLING
HOOK CEMENTED
SUBMERGED BICUSPID
UP

ELASTIC RESTORING
ROTATED LATERAL INCISOR

A-
FIXED
ORTHODONTIC
APPARATUS

DEMONSTRATING
SEVERAL METHODS FOR
CONTROLLING & MOVING TEETH

FRONT OR LIP
ARCH WIRE

INNER
SPRING
WIRES

CLASPING
LOOP

JAW
EXPANSION
PLATES

CLASP

HOLDING
HEADBAND

FACEBOW
ENTERING
THE
MOUTH

B-
A REMOVABLE APPLIANCE
FOR WIDENING JAWS
& STRAIGHTENING FRONT TEETH

EXPANSION SCREW
WITH WRENCH HOLES

HEADGEAR C-
FOR TRANSFERRING FORCES
FROM OUTSIDE TO APPARATUS
INSIDE THE MOUTH

PLATE 13-2
ORTHODONTIC APPLIANCES

G. Garfield

TEETH TEETH TEETH

teeth. Orthodontia is a complex field involving intricate detail. Advancements are constantly being made. These are only basic descriptions of some popular techniques illustrating general orthodontic principles."

INSTALLATION OF FIXED ORTHODONTIC EQUIPMENT ∾ In the mouth crowded irregular teeth usually touch tight. Space must be provided between such adjacent teeth, so the thin metal bands only thousands of an inch thick, can be placed around between them. In the laboratory, on the rigid model, as bands are made to fit each tooth model, space is provided by cutting separation with a thin saw allowing for later fiι. The orthodontist must create separation space between each adjacent tooth for its band thickness. There are several separation methods. One stretches a small strip of rubber thin, forcing it between the teeth. The stretched rubber pulling back thickens, starting minor local orthodontic movement, providing enough space within hours.

The teeth are cleaned and dried. One by one each bracketed band is removed from its model tooth, and cemented to its corresponding mouth tooth. After cement hardens in several minutes the excess is removed. The banded teeth are ready for their controlling forces, applied by means of the arch wire. The orthodontist positions the arch wire, so each part is aligned with its related bracketed tooth. If uncertain he refers to the patient's model. He attaches particular parts of the arch wire, to their particular bracket receptacles. Along the arch wires length, he forces particular bent portions into their particular tooth bracket slots. The restorative forces are already acting. The patient feels them through roots and bone. If uncertain of any tooth's applied force magnitude, the orthodontist can measure it with a sensitive Stress Gage in ounces. If too high so tissues might damage, he lessens the load, too low it is raised. One by another tooth the orthodontic hardware is assembled in the patient's mouth.

To insure every activating arch wire segment stays properly related working in its bracket, they are locked in. Each bracket in addition to spring arch wire receptacle slots, has tiny tying wire slots. The orthodontist uses short lengths of soft ligature wire, to tie the arch wire to each bracket. With ligature tying pliers he twists each tying wire tight. Often all wires are twisted one by one all around, and the patient has a unique appearance, with the thin stainless wires like long wiry whiskers spreading gleaming from the mouth. With cutters the orthodontist snips each close, then bends the excess away, avoiding bruising lip and cheek lining. There are also other ways of locking wires to brackets. Refer to Plate 13-2, Drawing A again.

TEETH TEETH TEETH

Additional springs or elastics may be applied for special needs between particular teeth. The orthodontic forces are already acting moving the patient's parts. Crowded teeth are being spread, separated brought together. Twisted teeth returned. Bucked out teeth brought back in, in teeth straightened out. Each to its proper place, all to an attractive functional arch form.

For changing relations of opposite jaws, elastics or springs are applied between them. Crossbites slowly though surely move, uncrossing to right or left. Jaws attractively changing, improving back or forward. Treatment progresses constructively. The ugly duckling is being beautified, soon to see herself mirrored that way and admired by others.

HEADGEAR ∾ In most cases orthodontic treatment and appliances are confined inside the mouth. Sometimes the problem cannot be corrected by forces applied only inside, and it is necessary to transfer activating energy, from inside to outside the mouth. Headgear is used. Refer to Plate 13-2, Drawing C, Headgear. Headgear consist of two basic parts. A Headband assembly of soft cloth or plastic, adjustable comfortably tight, fitting around using the patient's head as resistant anchorage. Near the ears on each side of the head, the headband has receptacle slots, for attaching and receiving forces from the facebow.

The Facebow is a light compact rigid wire assembly, that transfers force to orthodontic hardware inside the mouth, from the head held outside band assembly. From each headband side receptacle slot, the facebow wire comes forward close to the face, turning in forward in front of the mouth like a bow. There from the center two smaller wires go back on each side, entering the mouth between the lips, fitting into receptacle slots of the teeths fixed orthodontic hardware. Headgear hardware is removable and replaceable for eating, kissing and other conveniences. It can comfortably be talked and slept with. It only works while in place. Headgear hardware is awkward but accomplishes valuable corrections otherwise uncorrectable.

FINISHING TOUCHES ∾ Treatment progresses improving improper teeth and jaw relations. The orthodontist makes needed adjustments at intervals. So that working forces keep actively fresh, patients are supplied with elastics and instructions for home replacement. As mouth parts each move to their place, their hardware parts whose jobs are done are removed. Defects lessen and disappear. Active treatment is over at the appointment of relief, when all bands and wires are removed, as the patient delights, feeling with cheeks, probing tongue and fingers, all newly free tooth

TEETH TEETH TEETH

surfaces. What seemed like a long time is a short investment for the new better faced life.

Mrs. T. H. Inker asks, "What about the spaces between adjacent teeth doctor. The thin space where bands were removed." Doctor, "Thats an intelligent question. Those spaces usually close themselves. If they don't simpler orthodontic devices close them in a short time."

In rare cases despite every orthodontic effort a tooth will not move. It is Ankylosed or fixed rigid to the bone like an arthritic joint. We don't know all causes of tooth ankyloses. It's unpredictable and rare. When important such teeth are removed and properly replaced by other dental methods.

A DOUBTFUL APPROPRIATE STORY

A man was with a friend in a hotel lobby when he noticed an apparent stranger staring at him. The person approaching said, "Joseph Brown, it's years since I've seen you. I hope you remember me. You look so different, I've never seen anyone change so much. You were tall and stout Joe, you seem to have shrunk short and thin. It's incredible, especially the changes in your face. Your hair was black and full, now its baldish blonde. And your complexion has changed. And your teeth Joe. I remember how crooked ugly they were. I saw you talking They're beautiful. My! How you've changed." The man replied, "I'm not Joseph Brown, I'm Frank Smith." "My God," he cried, "Even your name has changed."

REMOVABLE ORTHODONTIA

Removable orthodontic appliances can be inserted in the mouth and removed by the patient whenever desired. They're generally a single assembly of several parts for moving teeth of an individual jaw. Their basic structural bulk like the base of removable dentures for eating, is usually a piece of pink or clear rigid plastic. Orthodontic denture bases are hardly noticeable. They often fit inside the jaw arches, within the teeth's inner surfaces, extending over adjacent gum covered jawbone. Bases are thin for minimum tongue interference. Upper appliance bases cover those inner tooth surfaces and the palate. Lower appliances fit behind the teeth, under the tongue, and back on both sides.

Embedded in the plastic bases are thin stainless spring steel wires, extending as clasps for attaching to teeth, holding the appliance in the mouth. Other wires extend as activating springs, exerting forces against misplaced teeth for moving them to proper place.

Removable appliances are used most for correcting front teeth faults. Refer to Plate 13-2, Drawing B, A Removable Appliance. It often happens that within the range of the six anterior teeth from cuspid to cuspid, right to left, the tooth arch form rather than being smoothly curved, teeth attractively in line, jags irregularly, teeth in, out, twisted. The appliance is made with a visible wire in front of the teeth called the Labial or Lip Wire. This wire forms the shape of an attractive arch. It covers the six front teeth, contacting the most forward projections of those deflected out. The labial wire acts as a controlling barrier rail, to which the teeth are brought, establishing a proper front form. On each side of the cuspids, right and left, the wire bends towards their bite edge corner space, between the cuspids and following bicuspids. There the wire turns in behind the teeth, being embedded fixed in the hidden plastic denture base.

Behind the backs of the same front teeth other springlike wires unseen, are also attached to the plastic base and contact the inside teeth back bulked projections. Other parts of the denture have wire Clasps for holding the appliance in place. Refer again to Plate 13-2 Drawing B which shows an appliance for straightening front teeth and also spreading a narrow jaw wider.

The orthodontist adjusts the labial wire to push forward projections back, and the inner wire Springs to move backward irregularities forward. Treatment proceeds as the front and back spring wires, approaching each other, straighten the teeth between them. Treatment ends with teeth brought attractively aligned to the smoothly formed arch lip wire, by the wire springs behind them. With treatment completed the appliance is no longer needed.

Removable apparatus can also be designed for irregular teeth of other parts of the mouth. At special locations in the plastic base, springs or hooks for holding elastics, are used to pull particular teeth to proper places.

Removable appliances can move jaws right and left and back and forward. Separate apparatus are made for each jaw, each is held in place by clasps, each is insertable and removable by the patient whenever desired. In both orthodontic dentures, hooks are located at appropriate places, so that elastics stretched between them daily, by the patient, pulls the jaws growing to their proper place. Jaw relocation is more difficult with removable equipment. As mouths open for talking and other purposes, the very elastics used for jaw pulling may pull the clasped devices from their teeth.

ACTIVATORS

Orthodontic Activators are especially interesting removable apparatus for improving improper jaw relations. They use force to guide jaws growing to

TEETH TEETH TEETH

place like other appliances, and also use help of the patient's personal normal neuropsychological response pattern.

Activators are made on patients models, mounted related to each other as the jaws are improperly related in the head. An upper plastic base is made to fit inside the upper model teeth and jaw clearing the tongue. A lower plastic base is made fitting inside the lower model teeth and jaw clearing the tongue. The models with their bases within them are separated and remounted by the orthodontist to the improved jaw relationship desired. In this normal jaw related position, upper and lower bases are joined together as a single unit. Clasps are attached to hold the both-jaw joined together activator assembly, to the teeth of only one jaw, upper or lower.

When the activator is placed clasped in the mouth it's quite a mouthful. Adjustments are made. The tongue fits within it, and the device, filling relatively nonfunctional space, is far more readily accepted than inexperienced observers realize. It either hangs down from the upper jaw or rises from the lower, as sort of a bouncing mouthful as the jaws open and close. When they close together the correctly related activator base causes hitting conflict with its misrelated jaw. Patients seem to tease the position subconsciously, opening closing, delivering forces moving their jaws to place. At the same time amazingly, the neuro-psychological responses help move the jaw even further from interference, to its proper position, as both reactions combine growing the jaw right or left, back or forth to their new improved place.

JAW SPREADING AND NARROWING

When forces are applied to a rigid material surface resting on teeth and their adjacent gum covered bone, the entire area moves as a unit growing in the directed direction. This helps spread narrow jaws wider. Refer to Plate 13-2 Drawing B. On a model of the jaw needing treatment, upper or lower, a plastic base is made fitting inside its jaw and teeth. The base is split along its center, separated in two base plate sections right and left. Each plate section half has wire clasps for attaching to teeth of its side. Along the separation center incorporated in each section half, is a thin tiny expansion screw assembly, acting as the sole agent joining the plate halves together. Half the screw housing assembly is embedded in the right plastic plate, half in the left.

At the center separation there is a tiny screw, which if turned spreads the two plate halves, moving them wider apart. With the halves closed held together by the expansion screw assembly, as made on the model of the narrow jaw, the appliance is placed in the mouth. With a tiny wrench as instructed by the orthodontist, the patient turns the screw a prescribed amount each or each number of days told. As the screw turns day by day, by week by month, the halves separate spreading the jaws, moving, growing them wider apart.

If the section halves movements were limited to this action, as the jaws grew apart in the front of the mouth, an increasing equal space would develop at the jaw center, between the right and left halves of teeth, and it does. Usually in narrow jaws the front teeth are crowded irregularly crooked. Usually in the same appliance towards the front, additional orthodontic attachments are incorporated, to move the front teeth correcting for the central spread, distributing them attractively along the new widening arch. See Plate 13-2 Drawing B again. Sometimes the problem is so involved the jaw is first widened. Later another appliance is used for front teeth manipulation.

Similar screw appliances can contract over wide jaws narrowing them to normal. The expansion screw assembly itself is first turned with the wrench, opened widest apart. Turned in the opposite direction, it will now close, and can be used as a contraction screw. On a model of the wide jaw needing narrowing, a plastic base is made, incorporating along its center the wide opened screw attached to right and left sections. Along the center, between the sections continuous front to back, a space is provided equal to the screw assembly widened opening. Each section half rather than having only sufficient clasps to hold to the teeth of its side, has from inside clasping extensions around to the outside, embracing both inside and outside of the teeth of its side.

Placed in the mouth the patient is instructed to turn the screw so that it contracts. The halves are brought together, pulling the teeth and jaw sides closer. Treatment ends when the jaw narrows enough.

Removable appliances work only while in the mouth activating their tissues. They should be kept there as much as possible. All day and night is best, even while eating if tolerable. They need regular brief removal for cleaning of themselves and the teeth they're treating. During active treatment, before the patient's parts have reached what is called a balanced position,while the appliance is out of the mouth the tissues tend to relapse, returning to abnormalcy. The more they're used the sooner their purpose is accomplished. They can then be discarded, or saved as a sentimental souvenir.

BITE BALANCE OR EQUILIBRIUM

The orthodontist straightens teeth so the bite is also balanced. Most people's teeth are generally in relative balance. Balance is the normal fitting of pointed cusps of the teeth of one jaw, into the recessed fissures and grooves of teeth of the opposing jaw. It is a mutual relationship between both jaws teeth working together. When the bite is balanced, each time teeth meet in all of life's toothy endeavors, they perform continued miniature personal orthodontia upon themselves, establishing each other and their supporting jaws in place.

Teeth are also stabilized towards proper balance by surrounding muscles of the head. Within their arches the tongue tends to spread them out. Outside, the lip and cheek muscles bring them back. All this biological behavior automatically acts keeping teeth and bite balanced in equilibrium.

Few if any mouths of teeth are all perfectly balanced. They need not be. When orthodontia is complete the tooth arrangement is usually harmonious and healthy, well balanced. There may be minor imperfections, difficult, time consuming, and impractical to perfect orthodontically. They are improved if necessary by spot grinding bite balancing.

SPOT GRINDING BITE BALANCE ∾ The doctor may make models of both jaws and study how their teeth meet together. He has the patient close his teeth into a strip of ink impregnated paper called Articulating Paper. He asks the patient to articulate his teeth, moving through particular mouth excursion positions. Excessively ink marked tooth surfaces may be out of balance. The doctor carefully grinds these spots away, and repeats the paper biting tests, correcting imperfections until the bite is balanced.

KEEPING THINGS STRAIGHT ∾ RETENTION

Nothing in life is ever completely finished or stays permanently perfect that way. After teeth are straightened active treatment is over but not necessarily completed. The orthodontist works to keep them straight. Children's harmful habits like finger sucking, lip pursing, and tongue thrusting, may have lessened during treatment or even been eliminated by training. Sometimes they still exist. While appliances are worn their orthodontic forces are too strong for harmful habits. At the same time projecting irregularities of the apparatus in the mouth make poking performances uncomfortable. So teeth straighten. If the habits return they can cause trouble when appliances and forces are removed. When necessary orthodontists teach patients habit correction exercises.

Devices are made to correct bad habits. There is actually a gadget used in the mouth which electro-shocks the tongue every time it moves to a damaging position. There are several miniature rechargeable batteries within the apparatus, that enervate electrodes placed at locations of orthodontic undesirability. If contacted by the trespassing tongue it is shocked away, learning to break its habit. And it works. I don't know of any apparatus used in the mouth that chops off the tongue like a guillotine. I don't think one is being developed. Some may wish they were. There is surgical procedure however, more popularly practiced in Europe, used for cutting off segments of oversized overactive tongues. And it works.

RETAINERS ∞ Other factors neither doctors or patients are aware of sometimes exist. Muscle systems of swallowing, chewing, and lip movement, may not be completely coordinated to the new tooth positions. Bone surrounding tooth roots may not be totally tightened. These are more significant in mouths of young people whose jaws are still growing subject to change. To insure retention of the improved arrangement orthodontists use Retainers. Retainers are smaller, simpler, more comfortable appliances that keep tissues as they are. They're made on models of the improved jaws. They fit the jaw corrected as is, exert no changing forces, helping the tissues firmly establish their new place. Retainers are usually removable, worn only at night, at first every night. As tissues adapt tightening they are needed with increasing infrequency. Young people usually use them for a year or more. Adults hardly need them at all.

Keeping teeth exactly in place depends upon a complexity of intricately coordinated biological processes. As the body grows maturing, changing with age, factors we are not even aware of can cause some relapse loss of the ideal arrangement reached by treatment. This is never more than a small part of the great improvement accomplished by orthodontia.

SIMPLER ORTHODONTIA

Not all orthodontic problems require prolonged complicated treatment. Some when studied reveal extensive complex procedures needed, to correct even slight defects. Some simple are simply solved, by intelligent application of simple procedure. Simple equipment may be enough. The same orthodontic biological engineering principles always apply. Refer to Plate 13-3, SIMPLE ORTHODONTIA.

PULLING TEETH TOGETHER ∞ Diastema is excess space between teeth. In young children it often corrects itself. It commonly occurs between central incisors where the right and left skull bones unite. See Plate 13-3, Drawing Series A. It's no problem at all if the person isn't concerned. It can seem serious. A small elastic band stretched over such teeth exerts simple tensile forces pulling them together, closing the space. It's not quite that simple. The larger central space divides to separate into

TEETH TEETH TEETH

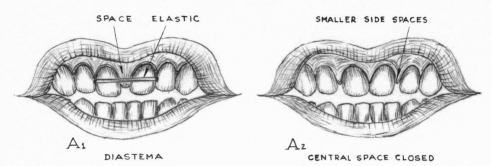

SPACE ELASTIC

SMALLER SIDE SPACES

A_1

DIASTEMA

A_2

CENTRAL SPACE CLOSED

A~ TENSION FORCE ~ PULLING TEETH TOGETHER

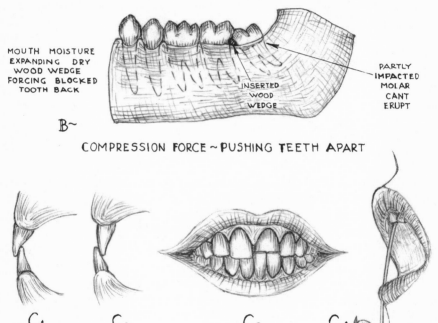

MOUTH MOISTURE
EXPANDING DRY
WOOD WEDGE
FORCING BLOCKED
TOOTH BACK

INSERTED
WOOD
WEDGE

PARTLY
IMPACTED
MOLAR
CANT
ERUPT

$B\sim$

COMPRESSION FORCE ~ PUSHING TEETH APART

C_1

NORMAL
FRONT TEETH
BITE RELATIONS

C_2

CROSSBITE

C_3

CROSSBITE
OF UPPER INCISOR

C_4

SIDE SECTION VIEWS   FRONT VIEW

$C\sim$

LEVER & INCLINED PLANE ACTIVATING A TOOTH

PLATE 13-3

FINGER APPLIED TO WOOD
STRIP MOVES CROSSED IN
UPPER INCISOR OUT~ IF
SPACE CLEARANCE EXISTS

SIMPLE ORTHODONTIA s.G.

TEETH TEETH TEETH

right and left smaller spaces, possibly more acceptable if the teeth would stay that way. If the diastema cause is not eliminated, when the band is removed the larger prominent central space returns. The bite relation may be involved or lip control muscle forces. Professional help is best. Personal treatment also invites dangers. Teeth taper narrowing towards their root tips. Rubber bands placed as described sometimes slip under the gums unnoticed. Neglected such bands have maneuvered deep beneath, causing supporting bone infection and even loss of the teeth.

PUSHING TEETH APART ∾ Compressive forces simply applied may also move teeth orthodontically. Drawing Series B shows an impacted lower third molar. It is blocked from proper eruption by the bulge of the crown ahead under the second molar, and prevented from moving back by the rising jawbone behind. A small soft dry wooden wedge, forced to fit between the molars might help. In position it soon absorbs mouth fluids swelling, forcing the third molar back where it may erupt properly. Several insertions of increasingly bigger wood blocks might be needed.

It doesn't always work that way. The swelling wedge could move down deeper causing serious infection and pain, requiring surgery for removal. If the jawbone behind is especially resistant the wedge expanding forces could work forward, crowding weaker rooted teeth unattractively in front. It's best for dentists to do dentistry.

LEVER-INCLINED PLANE ∾ Simple orthodontic engineering applications of the lever and inclined plane also move teeth. Refer to Plate 13-3, Drawing Series C. Drawing C3 shows crossbite· as seen from the front, of an upper left central incisor going in behind the lower teeth, rather than normally out forward over them. Drawing C1 shows a side sectional view of the crossbite. Drawing C2 shows the correct normal relation from the side.

If adjacent right and left space between the right central incisor and left lateral incisor is wide enough for the left central to pass through the following might work. See Drawing C4. A strip of thin wood like a medical tongue depressor (hard metal could chip the tooth), can be placed inside behind the crossbiting central, and held propped with gentle constant force against the chin. Carefully closing the jaw this way, applies the stick as an inclined plane and lever, tending to move the central incisor forward. Treatment is more involved than apparent. Teeth move slowly. Too high an exerted force could destroy the root attachment causing tooth loss. Each time the mouth is closed without the stick, the lower engaging teeth tend to drive the central back into crossbite. Provision must be made to prevent the teeth closing this way. Dental guidance helps. Once the

TEETH TEETH TEETH

central incisor tip transfers from crossbite, even slightly forward of the lower incisors, normal teeth closing completes the orthodontia.

CONCLUSION

Various orthodontic problems, principles, and types of treatment, have been described. These are only a limited survey of a complex field. Few cases fit any exact category. Each is individual. Some so minor they need no treatment, some of severe disfigurement. The orthodontist plans each case to suit the situation. Patient instructions vary. Periods of adjustment vary. As cases progress the orthodontist sometimes unexpectedly finds need to change treatment techniques. Improved results are worth the efforts.

Orthodontic science engineering is valuable beyond dentistry. Medical orthopedic doctors use similar principles to build Torsion Cable Devices. These removable flexible appliances are worn attached to deformed bodies. They permit use of twisted arms and legs, while constantly applying forces that transform growing those limbs to permanently straightened normal positions.

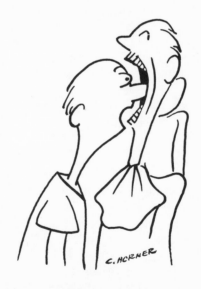

Let me tell you — its Not the Teeth

They're straight — Your Head's Crooked

TEETH TEETH TEETH

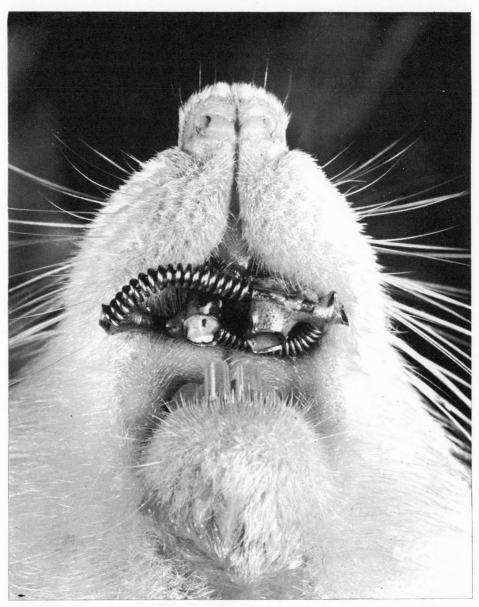

RAT ORTHODONTIC RESEARCH∾At the University of Southern California, researchers Joseph G. Schurter orthodontist, and Lucien A. Bavetta biochemist nutritionist, conducted animal experiments concerning teeth bone movement behavior, related to diet. The one half inch long orthodontic device designed by Dr. Schurter shows it miniature teeth bands attached around the rats upper central incisors spreading them apart. After noting the rats general health they were sacrificed and their tissues examined microscopically.

TEETH TEETH TEETH

APPEARANCE ∞ BEAUTIFUL HANDSOME GOOD-LOOKING TEETH

A-
MOUTHS ALSO APPEAR MORE NATURALLY ATTRACTIVE WITH TEETH OF VARIED FORMS

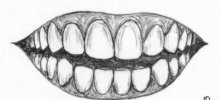

FEMININE TEETH
are often gently rounder

B-
SEX

MASCULINE TEETH
may be blunt-direct

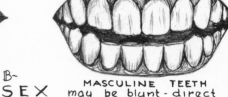
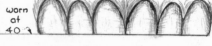

70
60
50
40
30
20

AGE
IN
YEARS

worn
at
40 ?

an extreme though not rare example

LEVELS OF WEAR
THROUGH LIFE

TEETH PLASTIC SCULPTURE REVIVAL AT 40

C-
TEETH WEAR & SCULPTURAL REJUVENATION
Drawn flattened for better presentation

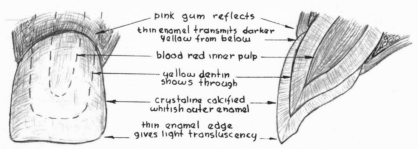

pink gum reflects
thin enamel transmits darker
yellow from below
blood red inner pulp
yellow dentin
shows through
crystaline calcified
whitish outer enamel
thin enamel edge
gives light transluscency

FRONT & INSIDE VIEW

CUT INSIDE SIDE SECTION

D-
COLOR - SHADE BIO-ANATOMICAL ANALYSIS

PLATE 14-1   S.Garfield
SOME TEETH APPEARANCE FACTORS

TEETH TEETH TEETH

14

APPEARANCE ∾ BEAUTIFUL HANDSOME GOOD-LOOKING TEETH

Beautiful is described as that giving a high degree of pleasure to the senses and the mind. Beauty is a quality attributed to forms and proportions, lines colors and textures, the rhythm of motion, tones of sound, expressions of words, and the substance of thoughts. It invokes conception of an ideal. Beautiful is often related to the soft, delicate, graceful, tender, warm, feminine identity. Handsome is a particular realm of beauty more often conceived as masculine. It relates to dignity, impression, virility, eloquence, aggression and strength. Good-looking modifies combining these things.

When objects have such quality, they attract being more desired, wanted by most of us. There are very few who actually prefer being unattractive. When such feelings do unfortunately exist, reasons are usually psychic deeply involved.

Every art object, drawing painting or sculpture, is all its individual components contributing to the total composition. Each part is important, some more than others. Teeth are especially important parts of a person's whole appearance. They adorn the mouth, our primary source of communication. I believe appearance of teeth is often more important than of the eyes.

As people talk more than realized we are all to some extent lip readers, receiving some of our message watching the moving mouth and teeth of the speaker. In a crowded auditorium, few people are content with only hearing the spoken message of the lecturer. Out of our sight we are annoyed, straining beyond interfering heads and posts ahead, to hear and see the talking talking. At home few music lovers are really concerned with watching an orchestra performing on television. The music's sounds are enough. Radio or a record player do as well. Yet when listening to news being little more than recited on T. V. we are not quite content, unless we see the lips and mouth of the speaking commentator. And when we do, we notice the teeth, an important part of the composition of the face, the prime identifying characteristic of the person.

Front Teeth of course are most visible. There are six above, six below, upper teeth more prominently seen lap over in front of the lowers. They've

TEETH TEETH TEETH

been described on frequent appropriate occasion in old Indian, Oriental and Romantic literature as "teeth that looked like pearls". Now that man can culture genuine pearls, more are available and the price of pearls has gone down. Though pearls are still as beautiful such description is used less often.

Many people have the mistaken belief that teeth should be even, of equal length to look best. Just as a flower is more attractive with blending petals of varied size and form, beautiful teeth whether natural grown or dentally made, have individual members of different distinctive sizes and shapes. Colors and shades are added qualities. Refer to Plate 14-1, SOME TEETH APPEARANCE FACTORS, Drawing A.

SEX

There are often differences between teeth of men and women, more distinctive in upper front teeth. Women's teeth generally curve gently. Men's are more angular, blunt, direct. Just as people's personality traits differ in different combinations so do their teeth. See Drawing B.

TOOTH CROWN FORMS AND SIZES

Upper front teeth of both men and women have Central Incisors larger, wider, longer than their adjacent smaller narrower Lateral Incisors. Crowns of Cuspids or canines on each side, sometimes called eye teeth, are sort of oval or egg shaped. They are also wide and pointed longer. The less noticeable lower front teeth are smaller and more regular. Lower central and lateral or side incisors are usually of equal length. Lower laterals may be slightly wider. Lower cuspids are also smaller than their upper mates, longer than other lower front teeth and also pointed at the tip. Teeth usually, both upper and lower, are not positioned directly up and down. Their center line axis tilts attractively from each side, symmetrically right and left slightly toward the center line of the head.

Natural teeth grow in a great variety of forms and sizes and false teeth can be made to match them. Shape variances from gently soft round teeth to squarish blunt, are accompanied by large numbers of intermediate forms. Those provided by dentists, to fill single or few lost teeth spaces between natural teeth, can be made to match their living neighbors. Those used to replace larger areas of missing teeth, can be selected more freely if desired.

TOOTH SIZE ∾ The size of people's teeth are whatever they happen to be. Some would prefer their teeth larger or smaller. Some would like bigger

TEETH TEETH TEETH

eyes, smaller noses and feet. Cosmetic dentistry can sometimes make size appearance improvements in people's teeth, within the range of each person's surrounding anatomical parts. Artificial teeth of removable dentures may permit some size choice. Each person's mouth has a particular proper jaw opening. The dentist cannot use teeth longer or higher than the patient's anatomically determined length, or dentures will not close chewing properly. Chewing teeth width have a less critical maximum dimension. The six front false teeth should fit within the front visible mouth opening. Some latitude exists permitting a range of desired appearances.

Size changes of natural teeth are restricted by added considerations. Jackets which surround entire natural tooth crowns are location controlled by the roots inside that support them. Their width is limited by the boundary of adjacent neighbors. Each jacket can be no wider than between touch contacts with teeth to its right and left. Individual jackets can be made narrower if space is left vacated between, though this is usually less attractive. Bridges of teeth which replace one or more missing teeth, are governed by the same width restrictions between their natural supporting teeth at each end.

Teeth worn short can sometimes be restored in length. This may be more involved than realized. Length of front teeth as they bite are affected by height of back teeth as they close together. Bite relations sometimes demand that teeth in back of the mouth also be increased or lessened in height, to lengthen or shorten those in front. Sometimes either upper or lower front teeth can be lengthened, if their opponents are correspondingly shortened, without changing the height of back teeth.

AGING TEETH

As we age, so do our teeth. They wear away shortening more than most realize. Like cutting edges of knives or soles of shoes, teeth wear at surfaces of use. And just as some people with different walking habits and hardness of shoe leather wear shoes differently, so do people with different tooth qualities and habits of use. Nervous, energetic, determined people wear away teeth quicker. Natural teeth and false too.

Plate 14-1 Drawing C shows upper front teeth at age twenty with their shortening lengths and shapes at successive stages of wear to age seventy. This is a severe yet real case. Such extreme tooth wear is not rare. Looking around at people will find examples of each level shown.

When teeth are normal in form and position, they appear properly good looking to our senses. As they wear with use shortening, teeth look appropriate at each age. As age advances many regret such simultaneous change in their personal appearance. Most prefer youth, it can be prolonged. Each restorative procedure, whether it be medical revitalization of arteriosclerosis or revitalization of teeth, is stimulus towards vitalized life. Art in dentistry can often change appearance of older teeth making them look younger. Just as a sculptor carefully chisels, removing outer portions of a marble block creating his form beneath, the artistic dentist can often sculpture teeth improving them. The same Drawing C shows front teeth worn to age forty, and then sculptured to appear more youthful.

The patient asks, "But doctor doesn't that remove good tooth material." Dr. Art Tisteek, "It does remove material that may be good but is worth it. Good flesh is removed when a nose is remodeled and superfluous tissue as warts. When people's teeth are sculptured to look better it adds feelings of well being. Also as teeth age they become brittle, acquiring fine cracks you can detect by careful study in a mirror. These may chip off especially at corners, sometimes in big pieces causing bigger problems. Artistic blending of these corners deflects forces, lessening accidental fracture."

COLORS AND SHADES

Some people seem to think teeth as white as pearls or even whiter would look best. I don't know how white pearls can be, but absolutely white teeth would look artificially unattractive. Try this. Cut a strip of especially white paper about 1x4 inches. Slip it under the lips in front of around your closed teeth. Before a well lighted mirror spread your lips apart and look. I don't think you'll like it. It could have stage comedy value.

See Plate 14-1 Drawing D explaining teeth color and shade analysis. Young teeth are lighter. They derive whiteness from calcified crystalline enamel surrounding their outer crown. Hard enamel tooth surface when saliva moistened sparkles highlights. Enamel is also transluscent passing light through. Varying enamel thicknesses give shades of gray. At the biting or incisal edge, especially in young teeth where the thin enamel has not yet worn away, a delightful light transparent bluish is created, against the mouth's dark interior background. Dentists call this incisal blue. It can be reproduced in restorative dentistry. Under the transluscent enamel, dentin is light yellow. Showing through slightly it gives yellowish tint to teeth, deepening towards the gums where the enamel thins tapering to an edge. Cuspids or eye teeth are thicker, so that their deeper dentin normally makes cuspids darker yellow.

When selecting shades in dentistry some people recoil at mention of yellow in teeth. This is probably partly due to the excess yellow dirt and tobacco stains collected on neglected teeth. A small amount of properly distributed yellow in teeth adds to natural beauty.

There are also traces of almost undetectable pink, originating internally from red blood of the pulp and outside from gum reflections. A few people have hints of green tints in their teeth, probably from traces of rare minerals. These colors and shades are not obvious, yet all contribute blending to beautify natural and artificial teeth.

Some people's teeth remain light a long time. As most teeth age, in addition to wearing they usually darken. Transluscency lessens, and the incisal blue edge even if not worn, disappears. Dentin darkens, darkening the tooth. Stains from outside also penetrate. They often invade fine brittle fractures as darker vertical lines. Some teeth assume a deep brown. All these teeth appearances can be and are matched by modern dentistry though sometimes perfection is difficult.

Different peoples have different attitudes towards teeth appearance. Primitive tribes ground their teeth to points. Niam-Niam cannibals of South Africa pointed their teeth for use as natural weapons and liked their looks that way. Others preferred teeth that looked like particular animals. Sibnowans of Northern Borneo ground their teeth with quartz to resemble sharks. In Central Africa among Wawira tribes, men pointed their teeth to attract women. In early Japan married women dyed their teeth black to discourage their husband's jealousy of other men. Black teeth became the married woman's status symbol of taboo to others. Until not long ago many black porcelain teeth were made in America for Japanese export use in dentures for married women. Motion pictures still exist showing Japanese women with black teeth.

COSMETIC DENTISTRY

Almost all dentistry affects appearance. Cosmetic dentistry is particularly concerned. Cleaning teeth includes cosmetics. Simple restorative cosmetics, starts with fillings usually in front of the mouth that match natural shades and blend with natural tooth shapes, so they often can't be detected.

Most dental procedures improve teeth appearance. Orthodontic treatment straightens irregular teeth. Jackets protect and improve the outer appearance of natural teeth. Bridges restore ugly spaces of missing teeth. Dentures supply mouthfuls to those without teeth.

For expert professional beauty and teeth opinion, I consulted with Perc Westmore. Mr. Westmore is President of Hollywood Motion Picture and T. V. Make-Up Artists and Hair Stylists. He is a world-wide beauty authority. From the height of motion picture glamour days to present, Perc worked with stars Joan Crawford, Bette Davis, Jane Wyman, Clark Gable,

Susan Clark, Marlon Brando and others, for studios like Warner Bros., Columbia, Universal, A.B.C., N.B.C., C.B.S. Perc is expert at artistically preparing faces for motion picture and television screening in every life emotion, talking, crying, sighing, screaming, laughing, loving, hating. Mr. Westmore said, "The mouth is the most mobile feature of the face. Its moving frame of lips direct attention to their teeth. Beauty demands attractive teeth. When teeth are unattractive, disfigured impression spreads to spoil the person's entire appearance. Criminals and other unsavory characters often are even made up so their teeth look less attractive." Perc added, "Teeth weren't as important in old silent screen days. Today with sound and talking pictures, performers teeth have instant attention. They must look good."

Sometimes with professional performers like actors and any others that care, cosmetic changes are made for the prime purpose of enhancing appearance. More often improvements in appearance are made in mouths suffering severe neglect, needing treatment to save their teeth. At such time, while general dentistry helps dental health, cosmetic dentistry can combine, creating and adding new more attractive small important parts to the face.

The Touch that Adds to Dental Beauty
Converts distress to A Roo Toot Toothy

TEETH TEETH TEETH

15

FIXED PROSTHODONTICS
JACKETS BRIDGES SPLINTS IMPLANTS

Prosthesis are artificial replacements for parts of the body. A mechanical leg replacing one lost, or a glass eye, are both prosthetic appliances. A plastic form added supported externally, replacing a woman's amputated breast, is a removable prosthesis like the leg or eye, and plastic forms inserted internally permanently under flesh, to support remolding existing breasts are fixed prosthesis. Dental prosthesis are artificial replacements of teeth and surrounding tissues. Fixed prosthodontic appliances are dental prosthesis permanently attached to the body. Like plastic inserted to remold breasts they are accepted as an integral part of the person's self not removable. Permanently attached to teeth and jawbone they are one with the skeletal frame. They deliver chewing forces efficiently, like natural teeth, sometimes better, so that patients soon have no consciousness of their existence. Even a simple permanent filling could be considered a fixed prosthetic apparatus and it is, although such minor restorations are not thought of as such. In dentistry fixed prosthesis are more major replacements of the mouth, like jackets which restore entire outer surfaces of teeth, and bridges which supply missing teeth. They are often used combined.

Some dentists who devote their practice to treatment with prosthetic appliances are called Prosthodontists. Prosthetic dentistry is intimately involved with other facets of the profession. Many dentists engaged in other of their profession's important phases also practice prosthetic reconstruction, so that the name prosthodontist is less frequently used as a limiting professional designation.

CROWNS CAPS JACKETS

Dental crowns are replacements for the entire outer surface of the crown of a natural tooth. They are called full coverage restorations by dentists. They provide maximum support and protection to the individual tooth. Early in restorative dentistry crowns were made all of gold and were called "gold crowns" or "crowns," like the outer part of the tooth they covered. They were used back in the mouth and when needed in front of the mouth, sometimes even when not needed. For a time gold visible in the mouth was a status symbol, proudly displayed in broad smiles. For some it still is.

TEETH TEETH TEETH

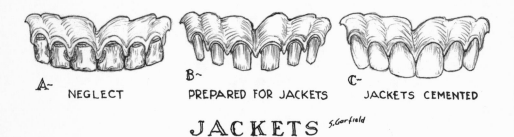

A- NEGLECT   B~ PREPARED FOR JACKETS   C~ JACKETS CEMENTED

JACKETS   *S.Garfield*
PLATE 15-1

FIXED PROSTHODONTICS ∞ JACKETS BRIDGES SPLINTS IMPLANTS

People even had diamonds set in faces of front gold crowns. Other people preferred natural looking teeth, and methods were developed for protecting teeth with gold crowns containing a thin cosmetic layer or veneer, of natural colored material in front to hide the gold. These were called veneered crowns or jackets.

There is no paint of any kind, that can be applied over the face of a tooth or crown which will withstand the abuse of use in the mouth. Techniques for crowning teeth so they are well protected and more natural looking are constantly advancing. Jackets have been made entirely of natural appearing substances like porcelain and plastics. Other names like jacket crowns, caps and jackets arose. They've all grown to mean the same thing, are properly interchangeably used. In some parts of the country the words jackets or caps are used for restorations in front of the mouth, and crowns for those in back. There is increasing tendency with increase of cosmetic dentistry, for the name jacket to be used for front and rear locations.

NEED FOR JACKETS ∞ These replacements of outer tooth surfaces can be made any shape or shades of color within limits. Sometimes with actors and others greatly concerned with their teeth appearance, treatment with jackets is primarily dental plastic surgery for cosmetic improvement.

More usually teeth have suffered severe disease and the dentist said, "Mrs. Jones you've had several fillings over a period of years restoring fronts and sides of these teeth numbers of times. They are decayed again in other places. Some of the fillings though protective are stained and some tooth itself is stained. There is also degeneration adjacent to your gums. There isn't enough healthy tooth structure left to hold new larger fillings together. Even if this could be done and it can't, several such fillings needed in each tooth would be complicated and expensive. Your teeth can only be preserved by jackets which would surround and protect them completely with a material that cannot decay. They would be held together supported from outside like steel rings around a barrel. These jackets would end close to the gum where decay rarely starts, and cover your exposed roots in those areas. While saving your teeth with these jackets there is excellent opportunity to improve beauty as well. We can reshape, recolor and reshade them, to appear attractively youthful. Their new form will also be designed to lessen food entrapment keeping your gums healthier. Perhaps we can even restore some length worn away."

MAKING JACKETS ∞ Jackets can be made for one or any number of teeth. Plate 15-1 JACKETS Drawing A, shows six upper front teeth needing jacket restoration. Not very long ago with old slow tooth cutting equipment jacket preparation was severe experience. Teeth are hard. The continued shock vibrations from rotating edges of relatively soft steel drills was traumatic. Sometimes chisels hit by hammers were used. It was common to take two or three hours and more to properly prepare one tooth. Trauma to even healthy nerve pulps inside was shocking. Many dentists felt it necessary to remove the nerve from any tooth jacketed. Tendencies were far greater to extract such teeth. Jackets can save them.

With ultra speed smooth instrumentation using industrial carbide and diamond cutters, jacket preparation is comfortably far quicker. Far more teeth are preserved. Even today though rarely sometimes unexpectedly, the pulp may later die within a jacketed tooth. If this should occur both tooth and jacket can almost always be saved by endodontic treatment.

JACKET DETAILS ∾ The cutting of teeth is called Tooth Preparation and the remaining cut tooth form is also called the Preparation. To prepare teeth for jackets the doctor examines mouth and X-rays. Anesthesia is used making procedures painless. Dimensions are close and critical. The doctor planning his cuts like a sculptor, removes unattractive excess material from all around outer surfaces, so attractive jackets can be made. Like a dentist he removes decay, leaving a thin protective dentin layer around the live nerve pulp. Like an engineer he cuts, preparing the tooth so that it tapers all around, narrowing towards the tip. The jackets are made in the dental laboratory to have corresponding tapers, so that when cemented on the prepared tooth its margins will fit, sealing the entire tooth border simultaneously. The dentist ends his preparation cuts all around at the gums. This is called the Margin of the preparation.

The doctor has the patient close together, checking to see that enough tooth is removed from the prepared tip, to provide sufficient jacket material between teeth of the opposite jaw. An amount of tooth must be removed from the entire outer crown, so that remaining tooth within and the finished jacket have structural integrity, and sufficient thickness for jacket color shading. Each tooth preparation is individually designed for specific conditions at its site. Like fingerprints no two preparations or jackets in the world are exactly alike. Plate 15-1 Drawing B shows the finished tooth preparation.

IMPRESSIONS AND MODELS ∾ Fine modern jackets require precise techniques, that can be done only in dental laboratories by skilled technicians. To do such work, an exact model of the cut teeth as prepared by the dentist is needed. To make the model, an Impression Tray is selected from a variety of sizes and shapes for upper and lower jaws. The tray is filled with pleasant flavored soft easily flowing Impression Material that looks like dessert pudding. It isn't, though no harm is done if some is swallowed. The dentist places the impression material loaded tray into the mouth, where it intimately fills into every fine detail of the prepared and adjacent teeth. In a short time while the tray is held in place, the impression material sets becoming elastic rubber like.

The tray is removed containing its precise mold of the prepared teeth and jaw. An impression is also taken of the opposite jaw. Models of both jaws are needed, since the jackets made in the laboratory must meet opposing teeth, as they will in the patient's mouth.

BITE RELATION ∾ To assure that upper and lower models are related together in the laboratory as the teeth close together in the mouth, a Bite Registration is needed. The dentist warms softening a small sheet of bite wax, which is placed between the patient's teeth who then bites into the wax, creating a thin wax impression of opposite tooth tips together. In a short time the cooler hardened wax is removed, providing the Wax Bite Registration.

SHADE COLOR SELECTION ∾ Next jacket shades are chosen. Shades for jackets are selected from standardized shade guides, containing many number coded tooth shade specimens, all of which are designed to duplicate natural teeth. Some lighter, whiter, some grayer, darker, some yellower, brighter, some even have stains. Some with more or less translucent tips. The dentist places those considered next to the patient's teeth, who may comment as personal consultant with a mirror. Usually a specimen matches. Sometimes shade selection is difficult. The dentist may make a tooth drawing on his prescription to the laboratory, describing different tooth portions and shades for each. Sometimes shades are so tricky the dental jacket technician is present during selection.

To daylight, candlelight and gaslight, incandescent, fluorescent, and others have been added. Each light has its own qualities. Dentists select shades under lights that satisfy most needs. Only tooth enamel itself will look exactly as it does under every kind of light.

I heard an interesting story, that happened several years ago, of a beautiful girl who had jackets made for her front teeth and she loved them. She was a strip tease performer in a Los Angeles burlesque theater. While enjoying her work, smiling responding to her audience watching, enchanted by rhythmic motions of her attractive facilities, lights in the theater changed, to creat special radioluscent affects upon decorations attached to certain of her developed anatomical parts. These radiated sparkling but her teeth disappeared. They could not be seen. There was a quality in her beautiful jackets making them invisible and her look toothless under such light. Chances are many of the audience never noticed. Since then dental scientists made improvements, so burlesque queens can jacket their teeth in confidence.

TEMPORARY JACKETS ∾ Temporary jackets are placed on the prepared teeth for protection while permanent jackets are being made. They are comfortable and can be quite attractive. Temporary jackets also serve administering dental treatment. They are held in place with temporary cements containing drugs which sedate and medicate the cut tooth.

IN THE LAB ∾ In the dental laboratory, the mouth impression molds are washed of saliva and blood and dried. Model making powder is mixed with water to liquid paste, and carefully poured into the mold to fill every recess. After hardening the mouth models are removed from the impressions, containing every detail of the prepared and other teeth. Using the wax bite registration, upper and lower jaw models are related together as they bite in the patient's head. On these models the technician uses the selected shades to make jackets fitting each of the patient's prepared teeth.

CEMENTING JACKETS ∾ The long awaited last appointment act arrives in life's dental drama of tooth jacketing, when the important, small in size great improvement to the patient, is to be made. Temporary jackets are removed and the area cleaned, so their permanent successors may be tried in place. They are checked for fit and appearance. Anxiously the patient mirror inspects these new tooth parts of themselves, and feels studying their virginal surfaces with lips and probing tongue. Adjustments may be made. They are removed and all is cleaned dry for final cementation. Permanent cement is mixed and applied as the jackets are placed to position, one by one, strongly secured, until in several minutes the cement sets hard. They can be seen in Plate 15-1 Drawing C. Excess is scraped away, some spit out, some unknown will be swallowed. Gums which may have been irritated by less accurate temporary jackets soon heal. If felt, heat and cold sensitivity soon diminishes disappearing. Improved physically mentally and visually, the more attractive patient can smile confidently.

THE IMPOSSIBLE

Years before I dreamed I'd ever become a dentist I was employed as an aircraft designer by Convair, an airplane manufacturer in San Diego, Calif. At the time I was amused impressed, by a sign containing a slogan I felt was an exaggeration, displayed above an entrance to the plant on Pacific

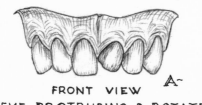

FRONT VIEW A~

SIDE VIEW B~

EXTREME PROTRUDING & ROTATED LATERAL INCISOR

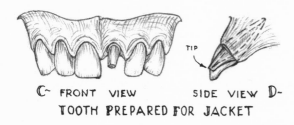

TIP

C~ FRONT VIEW   SIDE VIEW D~

TOOTH PREPARED FOR JACKET

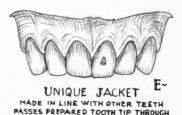

UNIQUE JACKET E~

MADE IN LINE WITH OTHER TEETH
PASSES PREPARED TOOTH TIP THROUGH

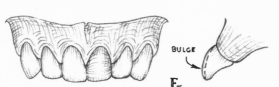

BULGE

F~

COMPROMISE

IMPROOVED OVER ORIGINAL SEEN AT A&B
THOUGH BULGING IN FRONT

PLATE 15-2 A UNIQUE TOOTH JACKET S. GARFIELD

TEETH TEETH TEETH

Coast Highway. It read, "The Difficult We Do Immediately, The Impossible Takes A Little Longer." Since then I've seen the slogan somewhere else, and believe it was only borrowed by Convair. I associate its memory with an interesting story told me by Salvatore Lentini a dental technician in Beverly Hills. The incident happened in New York City where Sal was employed in 1955. Sal was given a set of models and selected shades, for a single porcelain jacket, to be made covering a woman's upper left central incisor tooth. The tooth had been very protrusive, meaning it stuck too far out forward. It was also twisted. This can be seen in Plate 15-2 A UNIQUE TOOTH JACKET, Drawings A & B. Patient and dentist wanted the condition corrected with a jacket, that would bring the tooth attractively normal back in line. The tooth stump tip as prepared by the dentist, and on its identical model, was still too far forward. See Drawings C & D. Sal sculpting his jacket over the model was able to correct the twist. He made the jacket as thin as possible in front, but he had to cover the cut stump, and it was impossible to bring the tooth completely back in line. He did the best he could. The dentist after trial in the patient's mouth complained, and Sal made a new jacket especially thin in front, even sacrificing shading, where the tooth tip stump almost showed through. The jacket still bulged out forward. The patient not understanding demanded better. Sal is dedicated. On his own time, for no compensation, he made what might have been the only tooth jacket of its kind. This newest jacket covered the prepared tooth and was in line with its neighbors. It also had a hole in its face, permitting the out of line tip of the prepared tooth to pass through. Only after this was placed in position could the patient understand. It was impossible to solve the problem perfectly with a simple jacket. The woman selected Sal's first. It did not satisfy completely but did help substantially. See Drawing E. I feel the dentist should have foreseen the complications.

THE DIFFICULT IS POSSIBLE. THE SEEMINGLY IMPOSSIBLE THOROUGHLY STUDIED SOMETIMES REVEALS SEVERAL SOLUTIONS.

This case illustrates an interesting example of dental analysis and planning. The desired more ideal result could have been accomplished in one of the following ways:

1 ∾ Orthodontia might have been used to move the tooth back in line, perhaps even untwist it, so that the original tooth would do and a jacket not be needed. If the final orthodontic position was still imperfect, a jacket would then have more ideally completed the treatment.

2 ∾ The nerve pulp could have been removed from inside the tooth and

its space filled by endodontic dentistry. This would permit more ideal tooth stump preparation whose tip would not stick out. An ideal jacket could then be made.

3 ∾ The protusive tooth could have been extracted and a natural looking attractive bridge replacing it made, permanently attached to adjacent teeth.

Note ∾ All these may have been possible, would probably take more time and be more expensive.

JACKET TYPES

There are different types of jackets. Some better than others. Each has particular values and disadvantages. None are perfect. Neither are any natural body parts. Plate 15-3 TYPES OF JACKETS — CROWNS, illustrates basic principles.

GOLD JACKETS OR CROWNS ∾ About a thousand years before Christ was born Etruscans made primitive tooth crowns. They placed rings of gold around teeth to hold them together, protect and save them. Ever since gold has been used in dentistry. It is inert chemically, keeping itself and surrounding tissues clean. Modern dental gold alloys work well and can be cast precisely. Gold is strong, hard, about the same hardness as teeth, wears well even back in the mouth where chewing force is high.

There is a rather inexpensive type of gold crown restoration called the Shell Crown. See Plate 15-3 Drawing Series E. The gold shell crown has served man many years, saving many of his teeth, although it is not considered a precision crown or the finest. Its use is diminishing. Gold shell crowns are factory made by dental parts manufacturers, from thin sheet gold. They are available in a variety of tooth types and sizes. The dentist selects a shell crown slightly larger than the tooth being repaired, cuts and forms it more closely to size. Over a flame he may add to inside its chewing surface, a low melting point gold solder to thicken the thin shell, so that it will not wear through. He cements the shell crown protectively in place over the tooth. Shell crowns are less expensive, since all the work can be done with the patient in the chair. Little laboratory procedure is necessary. They do not fit exactly as precision crowns and are being replaced by them. They cost less and have preserved many teeth that otherwise would have been lost.

Modern Precision Cast all Gold Crowns are valuable tooth restorations. In the laboratory, on models of the patients cut teeth, they can be more ideally made to fit, sealing the tooth margin against decay, and more ideally shaped to deflect food from trapping between gums. They serve excellently back in the mouth where the large gold mass isn't obvious.

TEETH TEETH TEETH

FIXED PROSTHODONTICS ∾ JACKETS BRIDGES SPLINTS IMPLANTS

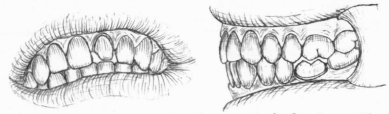

A-
JACKET PREPARATIONS FOR FRONT UPPER INCISOR & REAR LOWER MOLAR

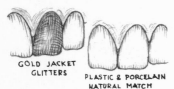

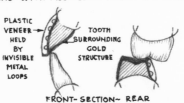

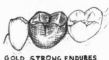

GOLD JACKET
GLITTERS

PLASTIC & PORCELAIN
NATURAL MATCH

JACKET
CEMENT
TOOTH

GOLD STRONG ENDURES
PLASTIC & PORCELAIN MAY FAIL
UNDER HEAVY CHEWING

FRONT TEETH   FRONT-SECTION-REAR   REAR TEETH

B- JACKETS ~ GOLD or PLASTIC or PORCELAIN
EACH FORMED TO BLEND WITH ADJACENT TEETH & PRECISELY FIT ITS INDIVIDUAL TOOTH

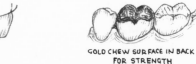

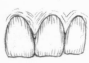

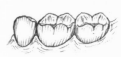

PLASTIC
VENEER →
HELD
BY
INVISIBLE
METAL
LOOPS

TOOTH
SURROUNDING
GOLD
STRUCTURE

THIN PROTECTIVE GOLD
BITE EDGE UNNOTICEABLE~
TOOTH FACE
NATURAL COLOR

GOLD CHEW SURFACE IN BACK
FOR STRENGTH
TOOTH FACE NATURAL COLOR

FRONT-SECTION~ REAR

VENEERED JACKETS -C-
EACH FORMED TO BLEND WITH ADJACENT TEETH & PRECISELY FIT ITS INDIVIDUAL TOOTH

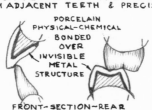

PORCELAIN
PHYSICAL-CHEMICAL
BONDED
OVER
INVISIBLE
METAL
STRUCTURE

ALL VISIBLE SURFACES
NATURAL-DURABLE
PORCELAIN SURROUNDED STRUCTURE

ALL VISIBLE SURFACES
NATURAL- DURABLE
PORCELAIN, SURROUNDED STRUCTURE

FRONT-SECTION-REAR   D-

STRUCTURAL PORCELAIN JACKETS
EACH FORMED TO BLEND WITH ADJACENT TEETH & PRECISELY FIT ITS INDIVIDUAL TOOTH

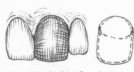

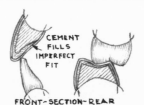

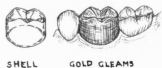

CEMENT
FILLS
IMPERFECT
FIT

GOLD GLEAMS
BULKY

SHELL

SHELL

GOLD GLEAMS
BULKY

E-

FRONT-SECTION-REAR

an old veteran~ THE SHELL CROWN ~ USUALLY MADE OF THIN SHEET GOLD IN STANDARD SIZES
THE SHELL SELECTED FROM A VARIETY IS ADAPTED & CEMENTED

PLATE 15-3 TYPES OF JACKETS ~ CROWNS S.GARFIELD

TEETH TEETH TEETH

Most people object to display of gold jackets in front of the mouth. The all gold precision cast crown is shown at Drawing Series B.

PLASTIC JACKETS ∾ Solid all Plastic Jackets can match natural teeth beautifully. Most are made of methyl methacrylates or acrylics, substances synthesized from petroleum and natural gas. A popular type is called plexiglass. Acrylics are used for windows of high altitude pressurized aircraft. They are strong. Dental acrylics have been improved, yet in most mouths chewing forces towards the back are too high, so solid all plastic jackets there wear through. Acrylics are not as hard as natural teeth, sometimes even wear in time from hard toothbrushing. Acrylics are rather inert but not absolutely so. In some mouths more than others, we don't know why, they may be penetrated slightly by oral fluids, and their original attractive shades may change. They are somewhat elastic, not brittle, rarely break. They do not have high marginal or edge strength, where sometimes slight warpage can occur permitting decay. They've rendered good service to many teeth. All plastic jackets are shown in Plate 15-3 Drawing B.

In the laboratory to make acrylic jackets, the dental technician on models of the patient's prepared teeth carves in wax exact forms of the finished jackets. These individual wax tooth forms are used to make precise molds of the jackets. Using liquids and powders, soft plastics of selected shades are mixed and packed into the mold in blended layers. The mold is closed under pressure, heated and cured until as chemical polymerization occurs the plastic hardens. The mold is opened, the jackets removed, trimmed and polished finished on the tooth model.

Plastic jackets are translucent, permitting some light passage. If the jacket tried in the mouth isn't shaded ideally, colored permanent cements can sometimes be used to improve appearance.

Less precise passably good looking temporary plastic jackets, are sometimes used for the period after tooth cutting while permanent jackets are being made.

Dental scientists are constantly improving acrylics and other plastics in perpetual search for perfection.

PORCELAIN JACKETS ∾ Solid all Porcelain Jackets can match natural teeth beautifully. They are made of glasslike mineral materials, more like natural tooth enamel than any other dental substance known. Their colors obtained by added metallic oxides are extremely stable. Natural adjacent teeth may change darkening in time but porcelain jackets won't. There are pieces of Chinese porcelain art, many centuries and thousands of years old that may have a few tiny cracks in them, but whose colors and finish between cracks are as vitally alive as new.

TEETH TEETH TEETH

Porcelain is especially inert, keeping cleaner than natural tooth itself, providing healthy environment to adjacent soft tissues. Porcelain lined tanks though expensive, are used for that quality in the food processing industry. The Corning Glass Co. once advertising a new porcelain lined coffee brewer, appealed to customers saying "for people who love coffee, for people with coffee in their veins." They explained research had found the porcelains inert surface permitted less adherence of coffee flavor contaminants. Similar finest porcelains obtainable are used in dentistry.

Porcelain jackets do have disadvantages. Like glass they are brittle, can crack. People have been horrified at a bite, to find their porcelain jacket fractured away. People who live in glass houses, with solid all porcelain jackets, shouldn't throw stones, bite steel nails or open bobby pins with their teeth. Solid all porcelain jackets are unsafe for heavy chewing use back in the mouth. Yet millions of people have front porcelain jackets, usually forget it, and they don't break. If they do another can always be made. Porcelain is harder than natural teeth, so when used against them the bite should be adjusted to avoid excessive wear. Great care is needed in tooth preparation for porcelain jackets.

Porcelain jackets are translucent permitting some light passage. If the jacket tried in the mouth isn't shaded ideally, colored permanent cements can sometimes be used to improve appearance.

Working dental porcelains is a special art. Technicians who do such work are called Dental Ceramists. To make a solid porcelain jacket, over the surface of each individual prepared tooth model called the Tooth Die, the ceramist adapts precisely forming a sheet of soft platinum, one thousandth of an inch thick. This die-form-fitting platinum is called the Matrix. Around outside the platinum matrix the ceramist adds porcelain powders of selected shades mixed with pure water in layers. The matrix, platinum melts at 3191°F, supports the porcelain accurately, where placed in a thermostatically controlled furnace the porcelain powders are controlled, to critically melt fusing at 1800° to 2500°F. As porcelain fuses in the furnace it shrinks becoming dense. Vacuum furnaces help increase density. After removal and cooling, additional selected shade layers are added, and blended with additional carefully temperature controlled furnace firings, at diminishing temperature for each layer, so as not to disturb those before them.

Between firings and shade layer additions, the ceramist grinds the jacket as it increases in size shaping it. When the finished product of shape and shade is reached, the sculptured jacket is placed into the furnace for a brief final firing, glazing its outer surface smooth. After checking on the original tooth die, between its adjacent teeth and for bite relation with the opposite

TEETH TEETH TEETH

jaw model, the thin inner platinum sheet is carefully peeled out. The jacket is ready to be cemented in the mouth. The All Porcelain jacket is shown in Plate 15-3 Drawing Series B.

VENEER JACKETS ∾ When a single material cannot satisfy all needs, good engineering combines the better qualities of several substances, to design better products. Gold's strength and hardness is valuable for supporting teeth and chewing, while layers or veneers of softer natural looking plastics can be used over visible areas, where force is low hiding the gold. This is accomplished with the plastic Veneered gold Jacket. Most prominently seen dental parts, are front surfaces of front teeth. When these teeth need the structural support of gold, and it is desired that they look natural, plastic veneered jackets can serve.

Plate 15-3 Drawing Series C, shows a side sectional view through an upper front veneered jacket in the mouth. Gold surrounds completely supporting protecting the prepared tooth. Like many other metals gold has great tensile strength even thin. With teeth closed as at Drawing C, only a small amount of tooth behind needs removal, to clear the lower tooth tip. In front also only a thin gold layer is needed. Over the thin front gold, natural looking plastic covers. Plastics do not bond chemically to gold. They can only be held by retention or holding. The precision casting includes tiny wire loops on its face, and undercut locking ridges along its edges, to hold the plastic securely. Along the incisal or bite edge of front teeth little or no gold need be seen, yet it approaches close behind, supporting the edge like a knife for biting. Precision cast gold also has advantage, fitting the margin close strongly.

Value of natural colored plastics over gold has limits. It is difficult to perfectly mask hiding the gold beneath, so that esthetics may sometimes not be as ideal as with weaker all plastic jackets. Drawing C shows further back in the mouth a lower molar with a plastic veneered jacket. There gold also covers the chewing surface, since molar chewing forces are too high for plastics, which would wear through in most mouths. The molar face if seen during speaking and smiling, is still attractively plastic covered. Its occlusal gold covered surface is visible but not prominent on back teeth. Plastic veneered jackets are popular. They are more expensive than gold or plastics alone. In the laboratory, both gold and plastic separate processing procedures are needed.

THE STRUCTURAL PORCELAIN JACKET ∾ A structure of metal, precisely surrounding protecting the entire prepared tooth crown, whose outer surface is high temperature bonded, firmly securing an attractive covering layer of natural looking porcelain, is a jacket considered by most dentists to be the finest. It is superior for combined beauty strength and hygiene of the mouth. Such jackets are called different names in different places. They're often identified by trade names, given by different manufacturers of precious metal alloys and porcelains used to make them. They've also been called "baked on porcelain jackets." This has some descriptive value, but lacks the dignity deserved by such a fine dental restoration. The name "Structural Porcelain Jacket" is more appropriate.

Any tooth, in any part of the mouth, no matter how unattractive or severely degenerated, if salvagable, can be restored with a structural porcelain jacket so that it will serve its owner well, looking as natural as if it were the original healthy tooth grown in the mouth. The structural porcelain jacket has its entire outer surface of porcelain looking like a natural tooth, chemically bonded to a strong internal structure of precision cast metals alloy. All advantages described under "Porcelain Jackets" are utilized, with almost total elimination of any dangers of porcelain fracture. Strength of the combined parts increase, beyond that of the already strong casting itself. Porcelain lacks tensile strength. When reinforced by bonding beneath to an internal metal structure, its utility increases tremendously, like reinforced concrete with internal steel bands, used for prime structural components of major construction projects. The engineering principles are the same. There's only difference in size. Porcelain is hard, when bonded this way can safely cover any part of a tooth, including chewing surfaces any place in the mouth.

Plate 15-3 Drawing Series D, shows two structural porcelain jacketed teeth, in cross section and as seen visually. One is an upper front incisor tooth. The other is a lower rear molar.

Each prepared tooth is covered with a precision cast metal alloy. For accuracy this must have a melting point higher than porcelain, which later is fused to it. Pure platinum won't do. Its melting point at 3191°F and casting accuracy are satisfactory, but platinum is not strong enough, and porcelain will not bond to it. The metal structure must also expand and contract equally with porcelain, through extremities of mouth and making temperatures, or the porcelain could crack from internal stress. All these complex needs have been met by metallurgists, with what are called Exotic Dental Alloys. Major constituents of most are gold, platinum, palladium, plus smaller amounts of iron, tin, sometimes ruthenium and other rare metals. Each metal, high or low in price, is used only for the particular physical and chemical properties it contributes. These exotic dental alloys are very expensive. In industry, porcelain has been fire bonded to iron-steel alloys for years, to chemical tanks, kitchen pots and pans. Attempts are being made with some success, to develop related dental alloys, using stainless steels chromium and cobalt.

TEETH TEETH TEETH

It isn't known exactly what bonds porcelain intimately strongly to certain metals. The most popular theory is that an interchange and unison takes place between the porcelains and metals oxides.

To mask the metal from showing through, first an opaque porcelain layer is added and fired. With certain delicate shades sometimes desired for the front of the mouth, it is sometimes difficult to mask the metal perfectly. In such cases, if the ultimate in esthetics is demanded, the more fragile all porcelain jacket may be preferred. After the opaque porcelain has cooled, in successive stages, porcelains of different colors and shades are added blended and fired in layers, arranged similarly to layers of dentin and enamel in natural teeth. All of the jacketed tooth is usually covered with porcelain, except for a thin band of metal, thickened for strength, at the inside gum margin invisibly behind the tooth.

The structural porcelain jacket as seen in Drawing Series D is very adaptable. If the bite were very close, porcelain could be omitted from behind the front jacket where unseen, and a thin protective layer of metal would suffice for contacting opposing teeth. If desired for dental design detail technicalities, any part of the jacket can be made with a metal or porcelain surface.

Just like solid all porcelain jackets the surface of structural porcelain is harder than enamel of natural teeth. The bite should be balanced carefully to avoid excessive wear. This extra hardness can be used to great advantage. If structural porcelain jacketed teeth as shown in Drawings D oppose each other above and below on both sides of the mouth, their hardness helps preserve all the teeth. Like bearings applied to heavily loaded parts of a machine, the opposing hard porcelain surfaces act as stops, to minimize wear of other teeth in the mouth.

FIXED BRIDGES

Dental bridges for mouths are designed using the same basic engineering principles as those carrying roads over rivers and canyons. Certain requirements of bridges crossing from one tooth to another, are more critically exacting than of bridges crossing mountains, spanning chasms of space to sides of other peaks. Both must be designed carefully. Each considers factors of supporting structures and loads they carry. All can be made beautiful. Fixed dental bridges supply missing teeth, transferring their chewing forces by structural union to existing teeth, through rooted attachment to bones of the head. They are permanently fixed in place, need not and cannot be removed.

Nature favors dental bridges. Animal and human research experimentation have shown, that when additional bridge span loads are

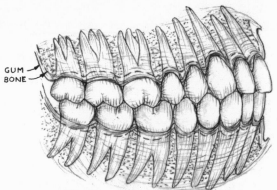

GUM
BONE

A— TOOTH STABILITY MAINTAINED BY ADJACENT SIDE CONTACTS & UPPERS AGAINST LOWERS.

NORMAL TEETH & SUPPORTING STRUCTURES

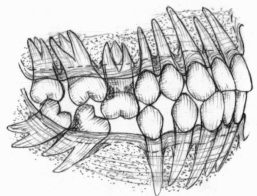

B— NEGLECT TO REPLACE A LOST TOOTH

PROGRESSIVE PERIDONTAL DEGENERATIVE DISEASE

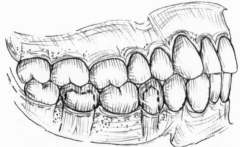

BRIDGES PRESERVE SPACE WITH REPLACED TEETH ATTACHED TO SUPPORTED BY ADJACENT TEETH

C— THE BRIDGE

PLATE 15-4 WHY BUILD DENTAL BRIDGES S.Garfield

a bridge in time may save nine

TEETH TEETH TEETH

delivered to supporting teeth, their rooted bone grows denser stronger. Their chewing muscles also strengthen to meet the new need. The fixed bridge force stimulii are sensed by the nervous system of the skeletal frame as though they were original teeth. Patients have no more awareness of them.

WHY BUILD A DENTAL BRIDGE ∞ The art of training fleas, the only creatures small enough and independently capable is declining, may disappear. No fleas I know of have ever been been taught to walk over dental bridges to get to the other end, and they could easily leap across from one tooth to the other, if that was where they wanted to go. Dental bridges however have great value to people. First is the obvious one of replacing missing teeth. Bridges also prevent more serious dental degeneration, which most people are unaware of, often leading later to loss of additional teeth.

Let's study need of a bridge. Refer to Plate 15-4, WHY BUILD DENTAL BRIDGES. Drawing A shows a full set of normal dentition, rooted in jawbone seen from the right side, teeth closed. Every tooth except the last molars are supported in contact on both sides by adjacent teeth. Chewing surfaces of upper and lower teeth interdigitate. These all help keep the teeth properly positioned. Drawing B shows progressive peridontal degenerative disease, of the teeth and surrounding gums and bone, from prolonged neglect to replace a single missing lower first molar. This could all have been avoided with a bridge.

Failure to replace the tooth resulted as shown in Drawing B. The upper first molar unopposed, moved down into the vacant space. A lower tooth would rise up into space above. As the widest part of the upper molar crown departed from its supporting side contacts with the upper second molar behind and second bicuspid in front, they both tilted unrestrained, towards the narrower exposed softer root of the dropping first molar. Food trapping pockets were created susceptible to decay. Loss of contact caused the drifting bicuspid and molar to create other food traps and decay.

In the lower jaw of Drawing B, the second bicuspid in front and second molar behind also tilted into the vacated space creating traps. Simultaneously these tooth tilts caused other traps at other opened spaces. All these food collecting places are hard to clean, more susceptible to infectious decay of teeth gums and jawbone. The tooth tilts also increase irregularity of the bite relation, so that the teeth are driven over even further by each chew action. The disease progresses as loss of contacts causes teeth loosening.

In the upper jaw, the first molar if unattended, may be the next candidate

TEETH TEETH TEETH

for extraction followed by degenerating additional teeth. This would all be avoided with a fixed bridge as shown at Drawing C. The bridge would attach to the lower second molar and second bicuspid, supporting between them a replaced artificial first molar tooth.

SOME BRIDGE INFORMATION ∾ To build a bridge, the dentist engineer examines the construction site and surrounding areas of his patient's mouth. He uses X-ray survey prints, and if necessary makes mouth survey models for study. Mouths with neglected missing teeth often suffer disease of other teeth, gums, and bone. Existing teeth degenerated beyond saving are removed, also to be replaced by bridge teeth. Diseases of surrounding gum and bone are then treated, so the bridge will be built on firm foundation. It would be foolish to erect a fine house on a swamp.

No two projects are exactly alike. The dentist evaluates every factor. Relationship of the missing teeth region to its opposite jaw. The patient's chewing direction path and length of bridge span needed. The restored chewing surface area, and magnitude of forces upon it. The strength of supporting abutment teeth, their root length engagement in jawbone, and quality of that bone. He designs the bridge. The dentist is especially concerned with crowns of supporting teeth, since some natural tooth structure must be cut away to provide for bridge attachment.

Miss Wanda Know asks, "You mean doctor, some good tooth material must be cut away to make the bridge." Dr. Chief Engineer I. N. Formed answers. "Yes Wanda, you could say so, if necessary, but it is tooth structure well spent. If no bridge is built to replace the missing teeth, your remaining teeth will break down, not immediately but in time. The amount we would cut away now might later decay, even more. The supporting teeth themselves might be lost, making a new needed bridge even bigger. This loss could include your health and looks. If we cut the teeth to support the bridge your mouth and you will be better preserved. I a dentist with my knowledge and experience, would want such a fixed bridge for myself or loved ones if indicated."

"But doctor, I hate having a good tooth cut." Doctor, "Wanda, tooth parts cut away to support a bridge aren't always good. In neglected mouths, abutment or supporting teeth are also often decayed, so that the very part needing removal and repair may be used to attach the bridge. The restoration material is stronger than the natural tooth substance it replaces and it can't decay. It can be shaped more ideally for deflecting food keeping the area cleaner. Its sole weakness is the margin, where it ends cemented and the adjacent natural uncut tooth begins. Here the bridge must

TEETH TEETH TEETH

FIXED PROSTHODONTICS ∾ JACKETS BRIDGES SPLINTS IMPLANTS

be kept especially clean. Regular maintenance prevents problems."

Wanda asks, "Doesn't it harm the tooth, cutting it, removing some." Doctor, "Well you might say Wanda, that the actual cut is a small actual harm. A small temporary one however, whose restoration is usually better than new. The healthy abdominal wall needs to be cut harmed, to enter for major corrective surgery like removing a tumor. When wooden foundation of a house is rotted or termite infested, the carpenter removes all defective lumber plus some additional, which you may say was harming perfect parts for attaching his new repair material to good strong wood." Whether Wanda is delightfully cute or not, the doctor probably won't with a gleam in his eye pinch her cheek as she says, "Yes, I guess you're right." "In rare cases Wanda, under a heavily operated bridge supporting tooth, the pulp or nerve may die. In rare cases this even happens inside teeth without any decay, that have never been cut or otherwise treated. We don't always know why. If such a pulpal nerve should die, both tooth and bridge can usually be saved by modern endodontic pulp therapy."

Wanda Know intelligently asks, "Could a fixed bridge be supported without cutting teeth." Doctor, "Not really. The supporting abutment teeth must be securely gripped. If they were surrounded around outside they would be bulky unattractive. A layer over their chewing surface would prevent proper closure with the opposite jaw, and some of the tooth has to be cut adjacent to the next natural tooth, for surrounding material to pass through."

Wanda Know wants to know. "Is there any way to avoid tooth cutting." Dr. I. N. Formed, "Yes Wanda there is. If natural teeth adjacent to the vacant space are in perfect condition they need no dental cutting to restore them. They can be used to support a bridging dental appliance, but not one permanently fixed in the mouth. A removable bridge can be made. The removable bridge also replaces missing teeth, and is secured by clasping support around the outside of existing natural teeth. These clasps can usually be seen, sometimes very obviously. The denture needs regular daily and even more frequent removal for cleaning. Their chewing sometimes does not feel quite as natural as with fixed bridges. Most dentists consider fixed bridges finest. Some people have mental reservation concerning removal of what seems a small unattached part of their body for cleaning. They feel less than completely whole. The appliance to them is somewhat of a tiny crutch and they feel a bit crippled. It's less romantic. Such feelings vary from person to person. Some love their removable dental apparatus, are hardly aware of their existence in the mouth. Removable appliances are sometimes less expensive, since fewer exacting procedures are needed to make them."

TEETH TEETH TEETH

BRIDGES

Most mouth bridges like those over rivers are supported at each end. Their natural supporting teeth, like bridge foundations at each side of a river, are called Bridge Abutments or Abutments. The actual bridging structure connecting the abutments, delivering the bridge loads to them, is called the Span of the bridge.

Spans of bridges over land and water are rather uniform in section along their length. In large bridges like that over San Francisco Bay, spans contain roadways of steel carried by cables, also conveying electrical and plumbing lines. Such bridges are expensive. They are periodically professionally cleaned and painted to protect them from the weather. Spans of dental bridges are shorter of course, most less than two inches long. They are expensive. They need no painting, but should be periodically professionally cleaned to protect them from the weather.

DENTAL BRIDGE DETAILS ∾ Dental bridges are not uniform in section. They consist of individual connected tooth segments. Though made as one structural piece, each tooth is shaped to look natural separately individual. Those which are artificial teeth replacing missing teeth, are each called Pontics or an older name dummy. Pontis in Latin means bridge. These comprise the Span of the bridge. Those which attach to the natural supporting teeth are each called abutment restorations or Abutments for short. They transfer bridge loads to the abutment teeth, from the span of the bridge. Each individual pontic and abutment restoration is a Unit of Dental Bridgework. A bridge supported at each end by a single abutment tooth, restoring one missing tooth between them, is a three unit bridge. A bridge supported at each end by a single abutment tooth, restoring three teeth between them is a five unit bridge.

BUILDING DENTAL BRIDGES ∾ Building dental bridges requires special skills. The natural teeth cut to support them must be precisely prepared, so that in the dental laboratory on models of these operated teeth, the bridge can be made to fit. Each supporting abutment tooth must be reduced by the dentist so all its cuts taper towards the chewing surface. Each rigid abutment restoration replacing removed parts must fit precisely to place. Requirements are compounded by additional demands. Bridges are of strong structural material, to carry loads of teeth they bridge. All natural tooth supporting abutments at opposite ends of bridge teeth they replace, must also be cut as a unit tapered related parallel to each other, so when the bridge is cemented to place, each tooth support is simultaneously sealed by its attaching restoration. It's not easy. Perfection is difficult in

FIXED PROSTHODONTICS ∽ JACKETS BRIDGES SPLINTS IMPLANTS

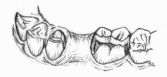

TEETH PREPARED TO SUPPORT BRIDGE

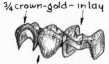

¾ crown~gold~inlay

replaced tooth may be
all gold, partly natural
part gold, or all natural

THE BRIDGE

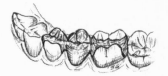

CEMENTED FOR USE

A~ PARTLY EMBRACED SUPPORTS

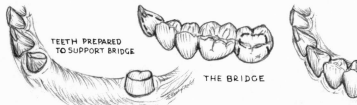

TEETH PREPARED
TO SUPPORT BRIDGE

THE BRIDGE

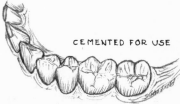

CEMENTED FOR USE

entire bridge~support & replaced teeth may be all gold, or natural looking porcelain or plastic
revealing some gold structure, or all natural looking porcelain with an inner invisible structure

B~ FULLY SURROUNDED, COVERED & PROTECTED SUPPORTS

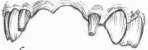

C₁
TEETH PREPARED TO SUPPORT BRIDGE

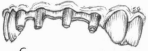

C₂
INNER STRUCTURE CEMENTED

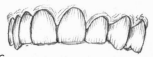

C₃ JACKETS INDIVIDUALLY CEMENTED
natural looking porcelain or plastic

C~ JACKET BRIDGE

Rear view
PIN FACING
porcelain or plastic
with metal pins

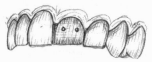

GOLD BACKING STRUCTURE
embracing & cemented
to adjacent teeth

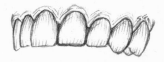

FACING ADAPTED & CEMENTED
natural looking
may reveal protective gold borders

D~

PIN FACING

Rear view
RECESSED SLOT FACING
porcelain or plastic

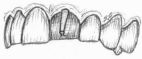

GOLD BACKING STRUCTURE
embracing & cemented
to adjacent teeth

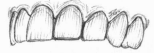

FACING ADAPTED & CEMENTED
natural looking
may reveal protective gold borders

E~

RECESSED SLOT FACING

PLATE 15-5   S. Garfield

DENTAL BRIDGE DESIGN DETAILS

VARIED DETAILS MAY BE COMBINED IN A SINGLE BRIDGE

TEETH TEETH TEETH

any endeavor. Absolute perfection may be impossible. These are exacting demands for the fixed bridge builder dentist. It tries judgment and skill.

Few realize the manual dexterity demanded of dentists doing such work. I have an eminent respected orthopedic surgeon as patient, who watched in a mirror while I prepared several of his teeth, explaining as I worked. He was amazed at considerations and precision required, saying it far exceeded demands of major bone surgery.

There are instruments, available as miniature copy models of industrial precision universal movement milling machines, sometimes used to help. The tiny apparatus is rigidly attached in the patient's mouth, to other teeth not involved with the immediate operating procedure. The dentist places his drill into a receptable, which keeps the revolving cutter centerline parallel, while cutting in any location. Using a tapered drill to cut, he can move from tooth to tooth, removing outer walls or other parts, assured all cuts everywhere have parallel constant tapers. If added bridge foundation grip is needed, the same device may be used to drill tiny parallel holes into supporting teeth, for insertion of miniature metal pins, just as a pile driver drives long structural steel columns into foundations for supporting skyscrapers. These precise little mouth operating dental machines, are made available by our precision machine making industry, so dentists can work as skilled machinists of the mouth. Ours is cooperative society.

COSMETIC AND STRUCTURAL DESIGN CONSIDERATIONS ✖

Appearances of bridges traveled by auto, train and truck are important. Except for engineering designers of such bridges, civic architects, administrators, and a casually interested public, probably more people are personally concerned with appearance of their own dental bridges. The looks of dental bridges are affected by their structural design. Fixed bridges attach to natural supporting abutment teeth, with tooth restorations similar to those used to repair teeth. The larger the loads they carry, the more securely they must grasp their abutments.

Plate 15-5 DENTAL BRIDGE DESIGN DETAILS, illustrates several basic principles. Refer to Drawing Series A. The simplest satisfactory bridge abutment restoration is the gold inlay. While inlays restore inner chewing surfaces of teeth, they can also help attach artificial bridge teeth to them. Gold inlays are excellent restorations of individual teeth, though somewhat limited as bridge supports. When limited to the tooth they lay in restoring, they receive only forces applied to that tooth. When supporting a bridge attached to them, they also take their added loads. Long bridges of artificial teeth, deflect under high load within elastic limits, just like bridges over rivers. Such deflection may loosen inlays. Carefully designed inlays can satisfactorily support small lightly loaded dental bridges.

TEETH TEETH TEETH

FIXED PROSTHODONTICS ∾ JACKETS BRIDGES SPLINTS IMPLANTS

Drawing Series A shows a 3 unit fixed bridge. One unit, is the rooted bridge supporting first bicuspid in front. One unit is the replaced missing second bicuspid. One unit is the rooted first molar in back. All three units of the bridge are a single rigid piece. Cemented in the mouth each tooth appears anatomically separate, naturally individual. The rear bridge supporting unit, attaching to the first molar is a gold inlay. It does not involve the back or face of the tooth, leaving natural tooth seen in front. It embraces the first molar's central chewing surface, passing down gripping the tooth unseen on each side, adjacent to the second molar behind and the artificial second bicuspid or pontic in front. The front bridge supporting unit attaching to the first bicuspid could also be an inlay.

Here the dentist designer desiring greater attachment strength, or because the bicuspid was decayed in back and in need of greater restoration used a 3/4 crown. This 3/4 crown or jacket, surrounds 3/4 of the tooth's four sides, both sides and back. The front tooth face in good condition is left uncut looking natural. Three-quarter crowns are popular bridge abutment restorations. They grip teeth rather securely, and where the tooth front is perfect leave them uncut looking natural, while supporting bridges substantially.

Seen from the front, gold behind the first bicuspid is hardly noticeable. For those especially fussy as the mouth moves talking, the 3/4 crown of the bicuspid and the inlay in the molar may be seen as yellow gold. Their appearance cannot be changed except perhaps to whiter gold.

The size and shape of any supporting metal restoration less than a jacket fully surrounding the tooth, must reveal its metal surface. Such a restoration, is sort of a tiny complicated tooth gripping metal beam, whose every bit is needed for strength. If excessively loaded it could bend, losing its sealing fit. None of its material can be afforded to be spent, by outer replacement with weaker natural colored non-metallic covering substance. There is nothing known, thin strong enough, useable as a paint coating which looks natural and will survive the use of mouth abuse.

In Drawing A the bridge is all gold. The replaced artificial second bicuspid is seen all gold gleaming. Such a tooth is as serviceable as any other, though its bold display is considered unattractive glaring unnatural by many. Some like it.

As bridges lengthen and their forces rise, more substantial bridge attaching tooth restorations are needed to support them. The strongest dental bridge abutment support, is a jacket fully surrounding the entire outside of a tooth. This also gives esthetic advantage, since replacement of a tooth's entire exterior, makes change improvements possible to the outer shape of the tooth. Sometimes jackets are needed to restore badly degenerated invididual teeth. They can also support longest bridge spans.

TEETH TEETH TEETH

Drawing Series B shows a five unit fixed bridge. Jackets surround the prepared cuspid and second molar rooted abutments, supporting three artificial pontics, replacing the missing first and second bicuspids and the first molar. The artificial teeth loads are transferred to the jacketed rooted attachments. This bridge could be all solid gold. Not usually made this way, serviceable, fine if you like it.

The jackets superior engineering value lies in its continuous encircling complete tooth embrace. When metal like a ring, completely surrounds confining the tooth, even a paper thin layer is enough to safely secure highest bridge loads, just as small thin walled steel tanks can hold gas confined under thousands of pounds of pressure. The jacket's inner thin gold layer, leaves remaining thickness available for natural colored tooth covering material.

THE PLASTIC VENEERED GOLD BRIDGE ∾ The plastic veneered gold bridge is similar to the all gold bridge, except that faces of the teeth, like individual plastic veneered jackets, have a covering layer of natural looking plastic hiding the structural gold. The teeth chewing surfaces are also gold. Plastic though able to withstand lighter loads encountered along tooth faces, isn't hard enough to survive the heavy chewing of most mouths. Since front teeth have narrow biting edges they show little gold there, sometimes none is necessary. Over the hard chewing wide surfaces of the back teeth, gold is needed and visible. Jacket supported plastic veneered gold bridges can support long bridge spans. The Plastic Veneered Bridge is within specifications shown in Drawing Series B.

THE STRUCTURAL PORCELAIN BRIDGE ∾ The structural porcelain bridge has an invisible internal structure of metal, encircling each supporting abutment natural tooth at its opposite ends. These are connected to each other, by an invisible internal beam of metal spanning the missing teeth space. Like individual structural porcelain jackets, this internal bridge structure is covered by natural looking inert porcelain, high temperature fused physically and chemically bonded to the metal. This combination of hard porcelain over an inner metal core, strengthens the bridge like reinforced concrete with internal steel bands, as used for prime structural components of major construction projects. The engineering principles are the same. There's only difference in size. Jacket supported structural porcelain bridges can carry long bridge spans.

Porcelain's hardness permits covering all surfaces, so even heavily loaded back teeth may be made to look natural. No metal need be seen. Porcelain's inert quality preserves its natural shades, keeping itself and adjacent tissues hygienically clean, even better than natural tooth surfaces.

TEETH TEETH TEETH

Structural porcelain bridges are considered the finest. All porcelain bridges made in one piece without an inner metal structure wouldn't work. Pure porcelain though satisfactory for individual jackets is too brittle for bridges, would crack. All plastic bridges look good but are too soft for permanent use. They would soon wear through. They are used as experimental and temporary bridges during more extensive treatment. The Structural Porcelain Bridge is within specifications shown in Drawing Series B.

PORCELAIN JACKET BRIDGES ∽ Porcelain jacket bridges replace missing teeth with individual jackets, like those cemented over individual natural rooted teeth. The bridge consists of an unseen internal metal structure, and individual porcelain jackets each fitting cemented over it.

Plate 15-5 Drawing Series C shows a jacket bridge. C1 shows right and left lateral incisor teeth prepared to support a porcelain jacket bridge. Drawing C2 shows the metal structure cemented in the mouth. At both ends it embraces the prepared lateral incisors, surrounding each with a thin precise encircling metal collar. These are connected with a thin structural beam strip, which provides two projecting posts located to secure the central incisor jackets. Drawing C3 shows all four porcelain jackets cemented over their posts in place. When the bridge is completed no metal is visible. The teeth match their natural neighbors.

Porcelain jacket bridges like everything else have advantages and limitations. They require fine fabrication, are expensive. With some natural tooth shades, better results can be achieved with cemented all porcelain jackets, than with porcelains which are fire bonded to their metal structure beneath. They're weaker than structural porcelain bridges, cannot support long spans. They're not safe for chewing back in the mouth. However while their individual cemented jackets might break more easily, in front of the mouth they rarely do, and they're much easier to replace if they should fracture.

Jacket bridges could be made with plastic jackets which couldn't easily fracture. Sometimes they are. Plastic however is softer, might wear at the biting edge and doesn't maintain the perpetual lifelike shade vitality of porcelain.

With increasing perfection of shades of porcelain bonded to metal, porcelain jacket bridges are less popular, being replaced by the structural porcelain bridge.

FACING BRIDGES ∽ Facings are artificial fronts of individual teeth. They're not the entire tooth, only the front facial part of the tooth, like a face mask of a tooth. Some tooth manufacturers specialize in facings. They are made both porcelain and plastic, in a large selection of tooth types, sizes, shapes, and shades. Facing bridges have metal usually gold, as a structural beam behind them over the area of missing teeth, attached at each end to natural rooted supporting teeth. The facings are fastened in front for esthetics. The dentist selects those closest to the patient's needs from an available variety, and may reshape them more ideally.

There are two basic types of facings. Refer to Plate 15-5 Drawing Series D. Pin Facings have two tiny parallel wire pins projecting from their back, which fit into precisely located holes of the bridge structure. Recessed Facings, see Drawing Series E, have recessed slots behind them which fit over, onto precise projections coming out from the bridge structure. When the facings are cemented, held in place by their pins or slots, the bridge is an integral solid unit. Each tooth looks separate and individual. Facing bridges usually reveal gold along their front teeth's biting edges, and sometimes slightly between the teeth towards the gums.

They're usually less expensive than bridges with artificial teeth completely custom made. In front of the mouth esthetics may be less ideal with facings, than with bridges all of whose teeth are individuallly sculptured. Yet many facing bridges are made, rendering attractive functional satisfactory service. Despite lower cost they seem to be diminishing in popularity, probably because of improvements in individually created bridge teeth technology.

COMBINING BRIDGE DESIGN DETAILS

Sometimes varieties of bridge teeth are combined in a single bridge, using each type to best advantage for its particular place in the mouth. In the short bridge shown in Plate 15-5 Drawing Series A, the gold aritficial second bicuspid could be plastic veneered in front, or even have all its surfaces natural, as a structural porcelain pontic or false tooth most ideally matching the supporting teeth on both sides. Sometimes long bridges are made plastic veneered or porcelain covered towards the front, while back areas not prominent are made all gold.

SOCIAL ASPECTS

In the office Willie Know, another patient, overheard the doctor's conversation with Wanda Know. He seemed interested. He was definitely interested in Wanda. Anyone seeing Wanda would know any man would be interested in Wanda Know. They had never seen each other before. They were not related at the time. The same last name was simple coincidence. Here the dental bridge assumed a new role in society, that of Cupid. It brought Willie and Wanda together and now they have a new

TEETH TEETH TEETH

little Know, though Willie never changed Wanda's name. Though often wondering whether Will was really interested in bridges I'll never know.

At the time he asked, "Which do you recommend doctor." I answered, "Well Will, of course price is a factor. The all gold bridge is usually lowest in cost. Functionally it serves as well as any. Most people dislike its glaring gold expanse. The plastic veneered bridge looks natural from the front. As the mouth moves talking, its further back gold is sometimes prominently seen. In some mouths it's hardly noticeable. Plastic veneered bridges are more costly than those all gold. The quantity of precious metal replaced by the plastic is far lower in price than the greater added cost needed to process natural looking plastic over gold. The structural porcelain bridge looks most natural, shows no metal and is best. It's most difficult to make, costing the most. Its especially inert porcelain surface keeps cleanest."

MORE BRIDGE DESIGN FEATURES

The Florida Keys, extending as a long line of little dots of land, curving slightly southward into the waters, turning far to the west to Key West, is a series of thirty nine small islands connected by a continuing number of bridged roadways. The bridging road is not a single long inflexible rigid assembly. That way it would crack. To allow for subterranean shifts of the island abutment supports, and the bridge's yielding under heavy moving traffic loads, and temperature expansion contraction, the bridges are segmented with a scientifically designed collection of flexible joints for absorbing the changes. The dentist engineer when necessary uses similar principles designing bridges for mouths.

Complex major dental projects sometimes have only a few remaining teeth, scattered at random locations around the jaw. This may demand special dental engineering considerations. When forces apply to teeth, they first transfer to a thin cushioning membrane between the tooth root and bone socket. This acts as a shock absorber. Every tooth normally moves a minute amount, within the limits of this cushioning tissue called the peridental membrane. In addition to this the bone also may yield compressing slightly, responding to the exerted force. These are all tiny dimensions, in some mouths almost immeasurable. In some mouths teeth and bone yield significantly.

X-ray and clinical study sometimes leads the dentist to build a bridge all in one piece around the entire jaw. Sometimes biological conditions are such, if a heavy force were exerted on one side, the supporting teeth and bone might yield more than a single piece rigid fixed bridge would, along its length around to the other side. This might pull opposite abutment restorations from their supporting teeth, cracking the cement seal. Dentists sometimes use joints called Stress Breakers, to interlock sections of dental bridgework, so forces applied are transferred in desired directions and yield, relieving other loads.

Sometimes rooted supporting teeth at opposite ends of a missing teeth space are so differently angulated, that a single piece rigid bridge, cannot slip over both simultaneously. The dentist engineer then designs his bridge in two sections. The first cemented to its supporting tooth, contains a female recessed slot parallel to the angle of the opposite supporting tooth. The second bridge section contains a parallel projecting male engagement. Cemented the second section fits its tooth as its projection slips into the slot, interlocking both sections securely.

Dental bridge materials are such that within the range of mouth temperature, expansion and contraction changes are safely within biological limits.

CANTILEVER BRIDGES ∾ Cantilever bridges are supported at one end only. The loads of their projecting span are carried by a single abutment that should be especially strong. They're not made as long as bridges anchored at both ends. In the mouth where fixed bridges are supported by rooted teeth and chewing force is high, cantilever bridge length is especially limited. Sometimes they're used in front of the mouth, where loads are low. The upper lateral incisor is the smallest tooth in the upper jaw, exerting little force. It lies between the central incisor in front, and the cuspid also called canine or eye tooth behind. The upper cuspid usually has the longest root in the head. When the lateral incisor is missing, it can often be replaced with an artificial tooth attached as a cantilever span, to the single strong long rooted cuspid.

Sometimes there are teeth in front of the mouth and a little way back. Yet all teeth behind unfortunately have been lost. A short additional rear span may be enough to help chewing and prevent opposite jaw teeth from drifting. With no rooted tooth available behind the space to support a double ended fixed bridge, it would otherwise be necessary to use a removable dental appliance. For people who resist thought of daily taking out and replacing even a small removable denture, a cantilever bridge may be possible.

If the needed bridge tooth behind were attached as a cantilever span to the single tooth forward, heavier chewing forces towards back of the mouth might loosen the supporting abutment, causing its loss. When possible and necessary, a rear cantilever span of limited length, can be supported by a structure joining or splinting two or more forward teeth together, as a multiple tooth united abutment.

TEETH TEETH TEETH

FIXED PROSTHODONTICS ∾ JACKETS BRIDGES SPLINTS IMPLANTS

SPLINTING

When the single tooth at either or both ends of a long span of missing teeth isn't strong enough to support a bridge attached to it, if available two or more adjacent teeth may be joined or splinted, as a stronger supporting unit. Splints are defined as appliances used to protect, keep in place, or hold parts together. Dental splints join individual teeth as a unit, so all benefit mutually from the strength of each, and all together form a firmer foundation. In union there is strength for states and teeth.

Each tooth splinted to support a bridge, also benefits itself from support of the splint. Splints help all teeth they tie together. When teeth are neglected, disease around gums often causes the bone to shrink away. Just as soil washed from the surface, leaves less supporting engagement holding a pole in the ground, so bone lost around a tooth leads to its loosening. As jaws in action come together, the full force of closure delivers to the first tooth hit. Teeth with less root attachment may become looser than normal, and subject to loss. They can be secured and preserved by splints. Just as an individual fence post in earth has little restraining strength, when two or more are tied together above by cross rails, their resisting rigidity increases tremendously. When teeth are joined above the bone by dental structures called splints, any blow struck is shared as smaller amounts, distributed to each united member.

SPLINT DESIGN DETAILS ∾ Any structure that ties teeth together acts as a splint. The simplest splint is of thin stainless steel wire, twisted tied around each tooth of the arch, holding them together. Thin wire is flexible. Teeth joined with wire can move slightly within it. Wire splints aren't considered permanent. When removed, the teeth almost invariably are tighter than when applied. X-rays show that supporting bone has tightened around them. If causative factors aren't corrected after wire splint removal the teeth loosen again.

Teeth may be splinted by cutting a continuous channel strip along through them, often through areas that are decayed needing removal. This channel can be filled with a continuous strip of plastic tooth matching filling material, reinforced inside with wire. Such a plastic splint is more rigid and permanent than stainless steel wiring alone. Unfortunately there is no plastic filling material of substantial tooth sealing strength. A stronger system of fixed splinting is with continuous gold strip inlays, made all in one piece, cemented as a single rigid unit along the teeth's chewing surface centers.

TEETH TEETH TEETH

Fixed splints have been made, cutting less tooth structure than needed for fillings or inlays. Thin gold castings are made to fit accurately around the inner teeth surfaces towards the tongue. The castings have tiny holes for inserting screws or cemented pins engaging each tooth. While less tooth needs cutting for the screws or pins, tooth enamel is brittle and may fracture failing around the fine attachments. There is also danger of damaging the inner pulp chamber.

Often teeth whose roots have loosened invisibly inside the bone, also suffer disfiguring degenerative decay around their outside. Full tooth covering splinted restorations can correct all these defects. All outer tooth surfaces are removed and restored with full jackets, splinted by small indiscernible connections at all adjacent contacts. The splint though one structural piece, appears as if each tooth were separately individual. The new tooth crowns can be shaped with healthier food deflecting contours. Structural porcelain covered splints can be made looking natural as original teeth, while its inert surface maintains maximum cleanliness.

BRIDGE MAINTENANCE

Fixed bridges and splints need little extra attention. They get professional inspection during regular dental prophylactic appointments. Home toothbrushing is important, though they also deserve special sanitation services. The prime hygienic difference in appliances of teeth joined above the gums, is lack of access between those teeth. This helps keep dirt out, and dirt that does get in harder to get out. The flesh covered missing teeth area spanned by artificial bridged teeth is called the Saddle of the bridge. This can be cleaned by passing dental floss under the span, from one side through to the other. Holding one end in each hand, the floss should be stroked along the saddle, from one bridge end to the other, giving extra attention adjacent to the span side of both natural tooth supports. If getting the floss through is difficult, a short length of soft thin wire can be doubled, using the bent end as the eye of a needle, and the free doubled end to pass the floss between the flesh and bridge. Gum flesh may be stuck at first, but the technique is soon accomplished. Confined areas between adjacent splinted teeth often maintain themselves. If dirt collects try toothpicks. Any gum damage bleeding from cleaning is well worth the trouble, soon heals. Permanent damage from dirt left deep is far more severe.

Power pumping hydraulic tooth cleaning equipment, which forces high pressure jets of liquid cleaning solutions into deep recesses between teeth and gums, is especially helpful.

TEETH TEETH TEETH

REPLANTS TRANSPLANTS IMPLANTS

Replants and transplants are not prosthetic or artificial body part replacements. They involve use of natural tissues.

Replants are separated natural body parts, replaced and reattached at their original site of growth. Teeth replantation also called reimplantation, can be successfully accomplished when the wrong tooth is extracted or a tooth accidentally knocked out. Teeth are rarely though sometimes even intentionally removed for access to complex inner areas, treated outside the mouth, and then reinserted to grow attached replanted.

Transplantation is the transfer of tissue from one body location to another, or to another person's body. Skin removed from an area for grafting, to cover a damaged site is a transplant. Inserting the heart of a deceased person into the body of another is a transplant. Transplantation of mature teeth rarely succeeds. Attempt is made difficult by the unavailability of healthy tooth material, with the almost impossible combination of two teeth ever having the same exact size and form of crown and root. Some success has been accomplished with the transplantation of unerupted teeth in young people. Partly formed third molars developing in less desirable areas, transplanted intact in their dental follicle sac to more valuable regions like the site of an extracted first molar, often re-establish blood circulation and develop to erupt for function.

IMPLANTS

Implants suggest possibility of revolutionary advances in dentistry. In areas where tooth loss leaves jaws toothless, implants supply support through to the bone, for attachment of permanently fixed dental appliances, where otherwise dentures removable daily would be needed. Implants are prosthesis or artificial body parts. Implants of surgical metal alloys holding broken bones together and replacing lost bone, are successfully inserted in orthopedic surgery. Their alloys are especially inert, well tolerated by human tissues. Medical implants have fewer biological demands put upon them. Implanted they are completely confined internally, entirely surrounded by body tissues. Dental teeth support implants are subject to greater trials. They must serve penetrating from inner bone support, through gum flesh to outside. This is not as radical as it seems. Several natural organs serve somewhat similarly. Outer dead skin layers, hair from heads, toe and finger nails, and natural teeth, some parts of which are also normally not alive, extend from inside the body to the outside. For people who've lost too many teeth and recoil at thought of wearing removable dentures, and those whose toothless jawbones shrunk beyond the form

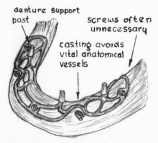

denture support
post
screws often
unnecessary
casting avoids
vital anatomical
vessels

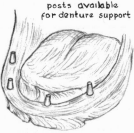

posts available
for denture support

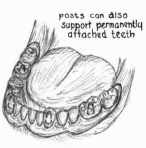

posts can also
support permanently
attached teeth

PRECISION CASTING OVER BARE BONE   GUMS HEALED OVER BONE & CASTING BASE   REMOVABLE DENTURES SHOWN IN USE

PERIOSTEAL-AROUND BONE~RESTING DIRECTLY ON BONE SURFACE~IMPLANT
can also support teeth for upper jaw~ Contributors- Dr I.Lew N.Y.,N.Y., Drs.A.Gershkoff & N.I.Goldberg Prov.R.I.~others

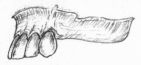

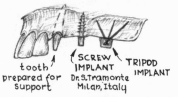

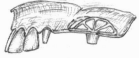

REAR TEETH LOST
no bridge support available

tooth
prepared for
support

SCREW
IMPLANT
Dr.S.Tramonte
Milan,Italy

TRIPOD
IMPLANT

PERIOSTEAL IMPLANT ALTERNATE

INTRAOSSEUS~INSIDE BONE~IMPLANTS
driven or screwed into drilled holes~ can also restore upper & lower entire jaws~contributors around the world
SEVERAL DETAILS OF MANY ARE SHOWN BELOW

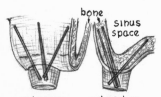

bone
sinus
space

side view   end section
TRIPOD IMPLANT
Dr.J.Scialom ~ Paris, France
Pins inserted individually
avoid sinus spaces.
Joined outside by the post to
form united support.

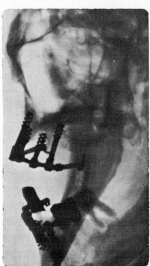

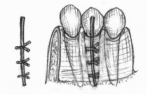

POST   IN USE
CROSSED PIN POST
Dr.T.C.Lee S.F.,Calif.
Placed into extracted tooth root site.
Stabilized until bone grows in
around the post. A tooth jacket
is then permanently cemented.

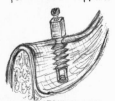

VENT-PLANT
Dr.L.I.Linkow N.Y.,N.Y. Lower vent
opening is for bone filling growth.
Screw shown to secure denture is
optional & also used by other contributors

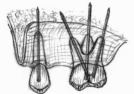

X-RAY~UPPER & LOWER IMPLANTS
Dr.R.Chercheve~Paris,France
Chercheve screws-open threaded
for bone entry regrowth

IMPLANT PINS
several contributors
Driven thru drilled short rooted teeth
to lengthen & strengthen support

PLATE 15-6   S.Garfield

TOOTH SUPPORT IMPLANT DESIGNS & DETAILS
transferring chewing forces of toothless areas through soft gum inside to skeletal bone
VARIED DETAILS MAY BE COMBINED TO SATISFY CONDITIONS OF A SINGLE CASE

TEETH TEETH TEETH

needed to stabilize removable dentures, implants may eventually be the answer.

Dental implants attach to jawbone beneath the flesh, where they have a tooth necklike neck penetrating the gum, providing a structural post, by which natural looking artificial teeth can be supported or even permanently united. Implants transfer chewing forces directly to jawbone just as natural teeth do. People who've lost all their teeth and have dental implants chew as securely as originally.

Implants aren't new. They've been tried by imaginative men since early times. Carved wood and bone pegs have been placed in lost tooth root sockets. Animal teeth, and human teeth sold by self sacrificers, or extracted forcefully from victims, were also inserted in lost tooth sockets, sometimes fitting fairly or put into jaws drilled to fit them. Their life of utility was limited. Recently some reasonable success with surgical metal alloy implants is being realized. In many parts of the world pioneering private practitioners, dental universities, and affiliated hospitals, have conducted animal experimentation and as result of success, human application upon people anxious to try. Many experience excellent satisfaction. Some who couldn't tolerate removable dentures resting on their soft gum tissues, have been using artificial teeth implant supported dental appliances several to even many years, which they say feel like their own grown. They love their implants, though hardly aware of them. X-ray and clinical examination show all tissues in excellent health. Yet cases occasionally fail in varying shorter periods of time. All reasons aren't known.

The prospective implant patient's medical health is carefully evaluated. Mouth tissues are examined, X-rays and mouth models made. Bone needs structural integrity to support attached appliances. If X-ray reveals poor bone quality implants are not indicated.

Refer to Plate 15-6 TOOTH SUPPORT IMPLANT DESIGNS & DETAILS.

PERIOSTEAL IMPLANTS ∾ There are different kinds of implants. Periosteum is a tough fibrous membrane surrounding bone. In the mouth it attaches gum over jawbone. Periosteal implants sometimes called Subperiosteal implants, made of surgical metal alloys lie directly on bone, under the gum and periosteum. They do not enter the bone. They spread over the surface as an open metal network embracing the bone intimately, resting over a large area like snowshoes supporting Eskimos in the Arctic. From central locations of the periosteal implant web or shoe, small round metal implant necks rise, perforating the gum entering the mouth, spreading shaped as structural posts, for denture or bridge support.

TEETH TEETH TEETH

To make a periosteal implant, the surgeon with knife point slices through gum to bone. Each side of the slit he peels the attached gum away, like thick skin from an orange. Familiar with jawbone anatomy, he avoids damaging vital vessels entering and leaving the bone surface. The gum flaps are held apart stitched to adjacent tissues, or retracted by a surgical assistant, exposing the bare jawbone while an accurate impression is taken. Gums replaced, sewed together, the patient leaves with comforting medications prescribed if necessary. In the dental laboratory, on the jawbone models the periosteal metal implant is made. At a later appointment the tissues are reopened and the implant put in position. Periosteal implants usually secure by precise fit alone. Tiny screw holes may be incorporated should the surgeon feel them necessary. The gums are returned together, stitched around the necked perforating post, now available in the mouth for support where teeth were lost. Under the flesh, through the implant web openings, the gums periosteum sutured regrows, reattaching to the bone. Removal of stitches leaves the implant available for normal use.

ENDOSSEOUS IMPLANTS ∾ Refer to plate 15-6. Endosseous also called Intraosseous implants enter inside bone. Endo and intra in Latin means inside, osseous means bone. There are different types of endosseous implants also made of surgical metal alloys. Many are specialized screws. They are inserted by screwing into toothless areas, where dental appliance support is needed. The screw head usually square for turning in with a wrench, is left above the gum for denture support use. Below the square head the implant is necked smaller, round for the region passing through gum. Below the neck inside bone the endosseous implant screw is a screw much like most. Some with thin shafts tapered to a point like wood screws, have thin widespread bone engaging threads. Some with parallel threads like machine screws, may be hollow from their end inside permitting bone to grow entering. Some have holes through their sides for bone to grow through. Studying the patient's X-rays, mouth, and mouth models, the dentist selects the ideal implant for the site, drills an undersized hole into the bone, and with wrench or pliers screws the screw to designed depth.

Tripod implants consist of three long thin round pointed pins, joined above the gum, from where they spread penetrating through, extending into the bone. At the selected toothless site, the dentist first drills through gum, in X-ray determined direction, a short guiding hole through the outer hard bone layer. Using his drilling equipment holding the outer implant pin end, he force twist drives the thin pin into the bone leaving a little extension. At the same site closely, two additional pins are driven, in chosen diverse spreading directions. Above the gums, using soft dental restorative filling type material, the pins are joined together. After hardening, like cutting a natural tooth, the dentist shapes the rigid pin-united unit to a structural post, for supporting the dental chewing appliance.

Different types of implants more ideally meet different bone conditions. Natural existing teeth if present may combine with implants to support dental appliances.

Implants should be kept especially clean around their soft gum tissue perforating metal neck. Failures that have happened usually start at these sites, with irritation and infection spreading inside to loosen bone attachment. Sometimes treatment can correct the defects. In some cases it has been necessary to remove implants. Failure reasons aren't all known. If implants are removed, conventional dentures though less desirable are still available.

Like everything progressive, implants are criticized by some. Such dental criticism serves as valuable conservatism restraining overzealous enthusiasts. Like with all pioneering scientific projects, some failure factors aren't yet understood. Like with new incompletely proven medical remedies, general professional acceptance is properly withheld. Yet despite some failures, slowly increasing numbers of others desperate from frustrated years of uncontrollable removable dentures have been helped. With advancing dental implant technology answers for the faults will be found.

Repair Restoration of our Chew Machine
Keeps All Attractive, Young, Less-Mean

TEETH TEETH TEETH

16

PARTIAL REMOVABLE DENTURES

Some people seem lucky to have everything. Some to have nothing, no things at all. Most have a part, large or small. All desire fulfillment, not necessarily a thing related thing. Some find it, all should try, others sadly prefer to cry. Mental attitude is important. One could say, "Unfortunately when part of the teeth of a jaw are lost, and unfortunately only part of the teeth remain." It's better to feel and to say, "When fortunately teeth are only partly missing and fortunately part remain." It's best to take the better point of view. Facts are whatever they are. Facts plus their worry doubles troubles. Mathematic axiom states, "The total is the sum of all its parts." Dental fact states, "Partial removable dentures replace the part of the teeth of a jaw that are missing and attach supported to the teeth that remain. Together these parts make the mouth whole."

Teeth for removable dental appliances are made of natural looking porcelain or plastic. They are held together by a thin foundation structure, made of plastics or metal or both. They contain Clasps or other attaching devices for grasping, holding on to the natural teeth growing in the jaw. They're also called Partial Plates, Partial Dentures and Partials. Some people call them bridges. In a sense they are since they transfer loads from one part of the mouth to another. As dental bridges they're more properly called removable bridges, like larger portable military bridges that modern armies transport from one river crossing to another. In dentistry the name bridge is more usually applied to fixed bridges, which are permanently attached to natural rooted teeth, and stay permanently fastened in the mouth. Partial removable dentures should be removed from the mouth regularly for cleaning. When in place accompanying their natural teeth, partial dentures combine to restore mouths in appearance and chewing efficiency. They help maintain teeth of the opposite jaw in proper position.

Partial denture chewing forces are transferred to the jaw they occupy, by the teeth that support them and the soft gum covered bone they rest upon. Partials that deliver chewing forces to natural teeth are called Tooth Borne or Tooth Supported. Partials that deliver forces to gum tissue over bone are Tissue Borne or Supported. Most partial removable dentures are both tooth and tissue borne. Partials for the front of the mouth are called Front or Anterior Removable Dentures or Partials. Partials for one side of a jaw are

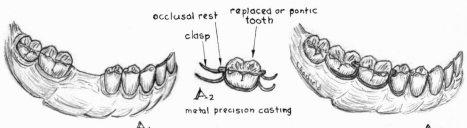

occlusal rest
clasp
replaced or pontic tooth
metal precision casting

A — THE SITE A₁ — THE REMOVABLE BRIDGE — IN USE A₃

UNILATERAL~SINGLE SIDE~REMOVABLE PARTIAL DENTURE~TEETH BORNE OR SUPPORTED

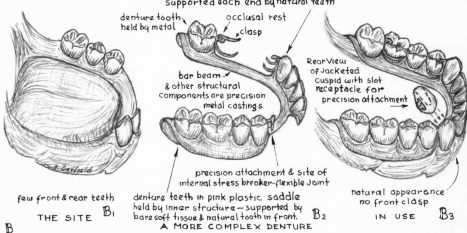

denture teeth in pink plastic saddle
held by metal structure
supported each end by natural teeth

denture tooth held by metal
occlusal rest
clasp

bar beam & other structural components are precision metal castings

RearView of Jacketed cuspid with slot receptacle for precision attachment

precision attachment & site of internal stress breaker~flexible joint

few front & rear teeth
THE SITE B₁

denture teeth in pink plastic saddle held by inner structure ~ supported by bare soft tissue & natural tooth in front. B₂
A MORE COMPLEX DENTURE

natural appearance no front clasp
IN USE B₃

B
BI-LATERAL~BOTH SIDES~REMOVABLE PARTIAL DENTURE~TEETH & SOFT TISSUE SUPPORTED

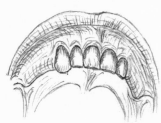

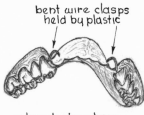

bent wire clasps held by plastic

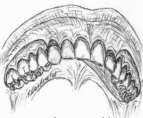

several front teeth
THE SITE C₁

entire denture base of pink plastic structure covering palate & toothless ridges both sides
THE DENTURE C₂

front clasps visible
IN USE C₃

C
A SIMPLER PARTIAL DENTURE ~ENTIRELY SOFT TISSUE SUPPORTED

PLATE 16-1
S. Garfield

REMOVABLE PARTIAL DENTURE DESIGNS & DETAILS
TEETH ARE PARTLY LOST IN INFINITE RANDOM PATTERNS & CAN BE RESTORED MANY WAYS

TEETH TEETH TEETH

called Unilateral dentures. When made to replace missing teeth on both sides of a jaw they are called Bi-lateral.

TOOTH BORNE PARTIALS

Partial removable dentures to be totally tooth borne, must have natural rooted teeth at each end of the space they span or fill. When natural teeth do exist at each end of the missing teeth area, there is often a choice of fixed permanent bridge versus the removable bridge or denture. The fixed bridge is permanently cemented to its adjacent end rooted teeth supports. The removable denture needs frequent regular removal for cleaning. Removable bridges or dentures are usually less expensive. Less dental office and laboratory procedure is needed to make them.

Refer to Plate 16-1, REMOVABLE PARTIAL DENTURE DESIGNS & DETAILS, Drawing Series A. Drawing A1 shows a lower right jaw, missing its first molar. Behind the missing tooth space there is a rooted second molar, serviceable as a supporting or abutment tooth. In front of the space is a rooted second biscuspid abutment. Drawing A2 shows the removable partial denture or bridge. It supplies and supports the false first molar denture tooth. False teeth of dental bridges are called pontics or dummys. Pontic comes from an old Latin word pontis, meaning bridge. This partial has a structural base of metal, which holds the pontic molar and extends to double clasps at each end. The forward double clasp grasps the natural second bicuspid tooth from behind. The rear double clasp grasps the second molar tooth from forward. Each double clasp consists of an outer clasp arm for gripping its grasped tooth along the lip or cheek side, and an inner clasp arm towards the tongue. Each double clasp has above a small strong projecting lug called an Occlusal Rest. The occlusal rest rests over the chewing surface of the clasped supporting abutment tooth. The occlusal rest transfers vertical chewing forces from the bridge span to the natural teeth that bear or support it. The small area of the natural tooth, upon which the occlusal rest rests, and transfers its forces is called the Occlusal Seat. To design a removable bridge the dentist must see that space exists for the occlusal rests, when the jaws are closed together. If no space was available and rests were put over the supporting teeth, upper and lower jaws would prematurely contact there, and could not completely close together.

When such space is not available the dentist cuts a small depression into the supporting tooth creating an occlusal seat. He could also cut away a small part of the opposing tooth of the opposite chewing jaw.

To use the denture the patient relates it to position, pushing the clasps over their abutment teeth until stability is felt, as the occlusal rests are felt

TEETH TEETH TEETH

to stop, seated securely in place. The mouth may be closed gritting for assurance that the denture is ready and available for action. Drawing A3 shows the partial removable tooth borne denture in position for use. Compressive vertical chew forces are transferred to the natural teeth by the occlusal rests. Chewing is not all directly up and down. There are substantial side forces. The grasping clasps in addition to holding the denture, also transfer side forces to the natural teeth. For people disturbed by denture clasps seen around their natural teeth, clasps can be made invisible. Such refined dentures need additional dental office and laboratory procedure making them more expensive.

Tooth borne removable partials can be made to replace many combinations of missing teeth conditions, provided natural teeth are present on both ends of their spanned spaces to support them. Tooth borne removable dentures work best in short spans. If their length is increased to replace many missing teeth, side forces may become so high, their end grasping clasps might be insufficient to resist the side chewing forces. If their length or span is increased to carry larger loads, the engineer dentist may provide a structural extension around to the other side of the mouth, and grasp other natural teeth there for added stability, just as a small pontoon at the end of an outrigger canoe beam stabilizes the principal vessel in rough water.

Life is unpredictable, the far future even more. None know what is to be. It is unlikely, but could happen, that in years ahead when dentistry has surpassed its present status and removable dentures are no longer needed or made, an accidental unusual quirk of social historical cultural interest could arouse collectors, to acquire then rare antique removable partial dentures of the Twentieth Century. They might even be valued far more than diamonds, which are already being made artifically. Outer space inhabitant collectors of the future, should be aware of fake antique partial denture frauds, claimed to have been those of prominent persons, presidents, and other leaders of Earth.

TISSUE BORNE PARTIALS

Sometimes partial removable dentures are designed so that chewing forces are completely tissue borne, or carried by the soft gum tissues over the jaw. This is usually when few teeth or only weak teeth remain in the jaw. The denture relieves these teeth of much of their load, helping preserve them. The denture foundation resting on flesh is called the Base Plate or Saddle. When teeth of such a denture chew, their forces transfer to their foundation saddle, which slightly compresses the soft yielding gum beneath. The gum tissue transfers its load to bone of the jaw. Occlusal

TEETH TEETH TEETH

rests, transferring vertical loads to the few remaining weak teeth, could soon loosen them causing loss. In such cases where it is desired to preserve the teeth for mental gratification and denture stability, their use is limited to help keeping the denture in place. Clasps are designed without rests, so as to exert only minimum loads needed to hold the denture in position. The patient soon, aware or subconsciously, learns to also use cheek lip and tongue muscles as added stabilizing aides. Such dentures should be removed frequently for cleaning, with special attention given to the natural remaining teeth. Plate 16-1 Drawing Series C shows a tissue borne partial denture. This is a simpler partial removable denture. Its pink plastic large base matches the natural gum tissues, and transfers chewing loads to a large part of the upper palate. Its replaced teeth match the natural remaining front teeth. Its supporting clasps are of thin stainless wires, bent to embrace the natural front teeth at each end. They help hold the denture in place and transfer minimum loads to the rooted teeth. Such dentures are quite popular, less expensive and rather satisfactory. Partial dentures are also sometimes made with their plastic base extending as thick gum matching pink plastic clasps, and sometimes without any securing clasps at all.

TEETH AND TISSUE BORNE PARTIALS

Most removable partial dentures transfer their forces to the jaw through teeth they grasp to hold them, and beyond that through soft gum tissue they rest upon to bone beneath. Part of the partial denture is tooth borne, supported by teeth. Beyond the supporting teeth, the denture extends resting on gum covered bone, with no teeth available at the other end for support like a bridge. Such dentures also need regular removal from the mouth for cleaning.

Since back teeth are more heavily loaded, and more trouble to care for, they're usually lost first. Since many people are more concerned with prominently seen front teeth they're generally kept longer. Most partials attach to remaining front teeth and replace missing back teeth. Dentists call them Distal Extension Partials. Distal means remote or back from. Anatomical definition of distal, is away from the place of attachment, or from the center of the body.

Back teeth, bicuspids and molars, are really more valuable biologically than front teeth. They have broader chewing surfaces and are multi-rooted spreading wider in jawbone, to take the heavier chewing loads they're subjected to. They act as stops, determining the vertical height of the face. Closing the jaws attentively demonstrates this. When back teeth are lost and not replaced, chewing muscles soon pull the lower jaw up ahead, squatting face and lips like old Popeye the Sailor man, and many old women that could look younger, and some young teethless women that look flabby face older. The lower front teeth normally overlapped above as they should be, by the single rooted upper front teeth forward of them, frequently drive the uppers even further out front bucked, squatting lips flat even pouting. If front teeth were lost and back remained, their strong roots and crowns could easily support natural looking front dentures, often even permanently attached, for chewing efficiency and facial beauty. If back teeth have been lost, replacement with distal extension partials will help general appearance and health, and preserve the life of remaining front teeth.

AN INTERESTING CASE

Refer to Plate 16-1 Drawing Series B. Drawing B1 shows a lower jaw needing a removable partial denture. This case illustrates several interesting denture design considerations.

There are only five remaining teeth, the right cuspid and lateral incisor, the left first and second bicuspid and first molar. This jaw doesn't look like much. Mark Twain once compared mouths with few remaining teeth to old cemetaries with neglected toppling gravestones. Drawing B2 shows the restoring partial denture. This partial denture has a metal foundation structure, precision cast of dental alloys. This could be yellow or white gold or a whitish metal stainless surgical type steel. Gold is more expensive. Often it doesn't matter which metal is used. Steel is stronger, more brittle, less flexible. Gold is certainly strong enough. It can be cast into finer accurate details, very important for some cases.

Over the jaw ridges where teeth are missing, this metal structure has an inner invisible webbed network to which a pink plastic saddle is cured. This saddle rests over embracing the toothless ridge and supports the false teeth. The pink saddle matches the shrunken gum it replaces. Denture teeth are available in great variety and selected to match their adjacent natural members. On the left side the denture structure extends back or distally behind the first molar, to support and replace the lost second molar. Third molars or wisdom teeth are rarely restored in dentistry unless needed for special considerations.

In the front an attached pink plastic saddle replaces the lost gum, and supports replacing the missing left cuspid, lateral and central incisor, and right central incisor. The long distal extension saddle on the right side behind the right cuspid, supports and replaces both first and second bicuspids and molars, four back teeth. This jaw containing five remaining rooted teeth supports a well designed partial denture containing nine.

TEETH TEETH TEETH

Together they restore the jaw to wholesome function and the patient's pride in personal appearance.

Let's make a detailed analytical study of this denture. On the left it is held securely in place, by embracing clasps on both sides, of the natural first bicuspid towards the front and first molar towards the rear. Vertical chewing forces are transferred to these teeth by occlusal rests. On the right side of the partial, only the cuspid is grasped. Its root is long, strong. Clasps could also be used to attach to the cuspid. It is not shown here that way. Clasping the cuspid would be satisfactory and less costly, but the clasp would be prominent on the cuspid which is a front tooth. Refer to the Rear View of Drawing B3, from inside the mouth looking at the back of the cuspid, as would be shown in an engineering drawing for clarity. Here the rooted cuspid is seen to have been restored with a fixed full surrounding jacket, which incorporates towards the back on the right side a tiny recessed slotted receptable. This female slot precisely mates with a small precise male projecting device on the denture, so that combined male and female parts are called a Precision Attachment.

Well designed dentures and well prepared mouths, like any well matched couple get along well together. The denture is comfortable in the mouth. The female with a poor attachment for her companion prefers being without him. She probably keeps her partial in her purse, or in a drawer at home with her husband. When a partial denture is held with a precision attachment no clasps are seen. Forces, both vertical in chewing and from the sides, are efficiently transferred to supporting abutment teeth. Precision attachments could also be used in one or both places back on the left side. It's less important there since that area is less visible. It would be more expensive.

Now let's consider support of the artificial teeth. Back on the left side, behind the last natural tooth first molar, the short distal extension metal saddle carries a single false second molar. Its loads are uniquely transferred to the jaw. To a small extent they may be carried to the flesh beneath by the saddle. Mostly the second molar acts as a short cantilever bridge supported one end only. Its forces go directly to the first molar through the occlusal rest and clasps, which are also stabilized by the strong metal bar, transferred around to the front of the denture and jaw. This bar runs around inside the jaw, comfortably located under the tongue out of the way, joining the entire denture together.

The four front false teeth are predominantly tooth borne, also supported by the bar, as the main structural beam member, of what amounts to a removable two ended bridge portion of the denture. This four tooth bridge part, transfers its forces to the jaw on the left, by clasps and occlusal rest to

TEETH TEETH TEETH

the natural left first bicuspid. On the right side, the bar beam carries the four teeth loads passing behind the right lateral incisor, and transfers them by means of the precision attachment, to the natural rooted right cuspid.

The right jaw side has the least favorable functional factor, its long distal extension span going back, carrying four chewing denture teeth. This patient unfortunately suffered the neglect of teeth loss, so that no natural tooth is available further behind to support the free end of the saddle. During dining the soft tissues beneath yield depressing. Little can be done about that. This kind of chewing isn't natural, doesn't give quite the same secure control. Yet people enjoy such partials far better than none. Some hardly know they have them. Most chewers favor one side of their mouth and this person would heavy grind on the left. The right saddle helps chew softer stuff, also keeping right upper teeth properly related. The right saddle forces are also carried forward through attachment into the long rooted left cuspid. As the right side chews the saddle depresses, sometimes pumping food particles annoyingly beneath.

Such dentures need frequent cleaning. Like saddles over hard driven horses, denture saddles sometimes make their bone ridges sore. Both horses and jaw ridges need rest. Even properly made denture saddles may sometimes hurt. Modern dental materials keep their size and shape. Natural soft body tissues beneath may change even during a single day. A head cold or other illness, or high liquid intake can cause them to swell. Loss of body water retention could shrink gum tissues, causing a temporary misfit sore abrasion.

As the saddle depresses, its grasping clasp or attachment to the supporting cuspid tends to move, rocking it. Strong rooted support abutments resist. Prolonged neglected disturbances of this kind could loosen, even cause loss of the tooth and use of the denture. Where conditions indicate need there are tiny engineering accessories for such problems. Miniature dental shock absorbers are available, like those helping automobiles over bumps. They're called Stressbreakers. So tiny they're unnoticed in the mouth, they're installed within the denture at the supporting tooth site. Their precision installation adds to the cost. Stressbreakers come in varied designs, some better for certain denture conditions than others. Some are tiny hinges, some compression springs, some wire leaf and torsion springs, some even contain miniature universal ball joints and springs, designed to absorb shocks from different directions of mouth motions. Some shock absorber designs are incorporated within the precision attachments. Some are made for use with clasps. The engineer dentist selects the most appropriate for the site. They're not always indicated, but are valuable when needed, and help preserve supporting abutment teeth.

TEETH TEETH TEETH

OTHER DENTAL POSSIBILITIES ∾The partial dentured mouth can also be helped by improvements to its natural existing parts. If the dentist felt the individual supporting cuspid tooth was too weak for its denture load, he could distribute those forces, connecting the supporting cuspid tooth to its rooted neighbor. If the jacketed right cuspid were splinted, or united as a unit by dental restoration with another full jacket surrounding its adjacent right lateral incisor, the two together would supply far superior structural support. These jackets could also improve the outer appearance of both teeth and help preserve them.. Though joined they would be made to look separately individual. This of course requires added detailed dentistry. Other dental design possibilities exist.

If the remaining natural teeth were weak needing support, or for psychological reasons, all seven teeth within boundary of the right cuspid around in front including to the left first bicuspid, could be made as a natural looking permanently fixed bridge, non-removable. The person would feel and see themselves as more whole and secure, with teeth always permanently there in front. They could more confidently kiss their lover or lovers. The needed partial removable denture would be correspondingly smaller, still making the mouth whole. The jaw's full restoration this way would be more expensive. Usually more complex dental procedure is needed for permanently attached than removable appliances. They usually cost more.

MAINTENANCE

Keeping partial dentures working requires diligent care of their surviving natural teeth. Both are needed to fulfill mouth function. You can't keep one without the other. The denture should daily, and more often, be removed for cleaning and brushing remaining natural teeth. Special attention should be given to the supporting teeth, and especially recesses adjacent to grasped attachments, which are subject to more abuse. They must be kept clean. Special denture cleansers are available, though even mild kitchen cleaning powders used carefully will do. Clasps and other attachments should be scrubbed gently. Accurate fit demands cleanliness. Although strong when positioned in the mouth, denture attachments are delicate and could be bent if carelessly handled. Thorough scrubbing should be over water. Dropping dentures into hard sinks could chip porcelain teeth. Regular dental examination and prophylaxis are needed, to keep the mouth and denture working together and good looking.

Fewer teeth remaining in the mouth, need more care to keep them there. Neglected , they're lost, leaving mouths toothless, bare.

TEETH TEETH TEETH

RELINING PARTIAL DENTURES

Eventually linings of even fine garments wear needing replacement. Partial dentures also need relining though they don't wear away. The lining of a partial denture is the plastic surface saddle, which rests over the soft gum tissue covered jawbone ridge, supporting artificial teeth. It doesn't wear away. The natural tissues beneath shrink away. As chewing forces depress saddles the soft gum tissues yield. There is also a natural jaw bone tissue shrinkage with age. When partials are first used their new actions toughen the gum and bone. The tissues may contract in time with a loss of spacial fit. With such continued shrinkage, chewing deflects the denture saddle so its displaced parts may bruise the soft tissue. Extreme saddle displacement could also loosen the supporting teeth, even causing their loss. Neglect if prolonged might even damage the bite relation, and cause excess wear of the jawbones hinging joint in the head. These defects can be corrected by relining the denture saddle, with an added plastic layer which replaces the lost tissues.

RELINE PREPARATIONS ∾ Saddles should be relined when their supporting tissues are healthy. Irritation from misfit denture saddles bruise swelling their ridges from normal. For recovery the denture should be kept from the mouth for a day or more before, up to the reline appointment, or as directed by the dentist. Head colds can cause mouth tissue swelling, appointments should be postponed until recovered.

MOUTH MOLDED RELINES ∾ To reline a partial denture the mouth must be clean. The ridge to be relined and adjacent parts, may be wiped with a thin protective film of petroleum jelly to prevent smarting. The denture saddle surface is cleaned and an excess of self curing soft plastic mix, added to the reline area. The dentist places the denture in the mouth seeing all clasps, rests and attachments are properly positioned. He may ask the patient to close gently together. The soft plastic intimately fills all spaces between saddle and jaw. Excess squeezes from around the borders. As the patient holds his jaws positioned the shrunken jaw acts as a mold. The plastic curing hard in the mouth may be felt warming. In a few minutes curing is complete. The dentist removes the denture with its relined layer bonded to the denture saddle. While the patient waits, excess plastic is ground away and polished smooth. The relined denture fits for comfortable eating. Minor adjustments may be needed. Mouth mold relines are done in a single appointment. They are satisfactory, though their material isn't as dense inert as plastics processed in the laboratory. They may serve well for years.

TEETH TEETH TEETH

LABORATORY MOLDED RELINES ∞ Reline plastics cured outside the mouth in the laboratory under pressure, are more inert, keep cleaner, last longer. They require two separate dental appointments with laboratory processing between.

At the first appointment the dentist adds a soft impression material to the denture saddle. He places the denture in the mouth seeing that all clasps, rests and attachments are properly positioned. He may ask the patient to close gently together. The impression material fills all shrunken space between the saddle and jaw. When the impression has set hardened the denture is removed. The patient leaves without the denture unless lucky enough to have another. Denture patients have an advantage over those with natural teeth that don't need them. They can depart from their teeth, which can even be damaged severely without them being hurt at all.

In the dental laboratory, a mold is made of the denture with its attached reline impression. The impression material is removed. Soft plastic is packed or injected into the mold, which is closed under pressure and cures hard. After curing is complete the denture is removed and finished polished.

At a second appointment the relined denture is inserted in the patients mouth. Adjustments may be needed. Laboratory processing leaves patients without extra dentures, dentureless while work is done. Close dental office-laboratory coordination, can do relines in a day. The added laboratory procedures add to the cost.

PARTIALS FOR BEAUTY AND PARTIALS FOR BEASTS

COSMETIC VENEER DENTURES ∞ Cosmetic veneers are thin plastic formed tooth shape faces, made to fit over the front of natural teeth, and improve appearance. They're removable. Within the range of their thin thickness, they can change sizes shapes and shades of teeth. They're sort of little teeth masks.

Impressions of the patient's teeth are taken, from which accurate models are made. Over the model of the patient's less attractive teeth, in wax, the dental artist carefully sculptures, usually a one piece thin wax layer, just thick enough to cover the irregularities and supply the new desired tooth forms. This wax model is used to make a mold in which selected shade plastics can be cured hard, making the cosmetic veneers.

Cosmetic veneers can be used in some cases, as a temporary model slipped over a patient's teeth, just to show what new front teeth dental reconstruction can create. They have been used as regular removable dentures. In place they present new attractive teeth. They do protrude out a little, usually unnoticeably, improving appearance. They may be seen thicker at their biting edges, so that wearers consciously avoid such head postures. They usually can't be used to bite with, since they're insecurely held. Sometimes tiny wire holding clasps can be cured in, but veneers are so thin even this could detract from appearance. They're held to place merely by ideal fit and spit. Fine adhesive powders and lip maneuvering stabilization helps. They can't be used for much more than being seen. They may dislodge by biting, drinking, kissing, even careless smoking.

Before modern fixed jacket techniques, during peak of the motion picture industry, they were popular and called Hollywood Veneers. Many motion pictures have been filmed with veneered performers.

VENEERS FOR A BEAUTY ∿ Eleanor Powell, beautiful motion picture star, tap dancer supreme, told me the following story. Eleanor was born and grew maturing properly, except for her irregular upper front teeth. Eleanor's employer Metro-Goldwyn-Mayer Studios wanted her teeth perfected. At the time certain technicalities made full teeth reshaping jackets impractical, and Eleanor was fitted with cosmetic Hollywood veneers. This was before she became my patient and friend. "Syd," she said, "I was known for my beautiful smile and felt uncomfortable about it. My audience saw the veneers."

Eleanor told me, "They drove me crazy. You don't know the special filming considerations involved. I couldn't eat in scenes, was afraid of being kissed or tapping my teeth. Things other people hardly think of. I was even afraid of drinking water, they might float away. I had to carry the darn things in a little box all the time." Mother Powell told me, "Sydney, when she'd leave for location I'd always call, 'Ellie don't forget your veneers'."

Eleanor had especially delicate veneers. They were two separate small upper incisors, providing pretty forms for twisted teeth beneath. "They wouldn't hold," she said. "I always had to push them back with sticky powders." Director, "Cut! Stop shooting camera-man! Miss Powell, Please! Keep your veneers in place." She was always conscious of stabilizing them with her lips. "They felt like a wad of gum. I could smile beautifully sometimes but only a certain way, otherwise I half smirked."

Especially interesting drama occurred when Eleanor was honored by invitation to lunch in Washington, D.C. at the White House by an admirer Franklin D. Roosevelt, President of the United States. "Syd," Ellie said, "I was never so horrified in my life as when those veneers fell off."

Dental technology has made it possible to permanent jacket improve Eleanor's teeth. She smiles proudly, laughs unrestrained and eats with ease. They don't shake off as she dances.

TEETH TEETH TEETH

PARTIALS FOR BEASTS OF THE JUNGLE ∾ Some may consider all animals beasts. I don't think partial removable dentures have ever been made for jackals, giraffes, tigers or kangaroos, but could be if the animals were restrained so the dentist could work. I once made a denture for a parrot named George. George was from South America, a Double Yellowhead Amazon more gentle than most. I never thought of George whose name might have more properly been Georgeane as a beast. The denture wasn't a removable denture but permanently fixed to his skull. Parrots are psittacine birds, members of the Family Psittaciformes, of cockatoos, macaws, parrots, parrakeets and others. One of their distinguishing characteristics is, that different from other birds and animals with only a lower hingeable jaw, both their upper and lower jaws and beaks hinge movably.

Though George loved sardines and ate all kinds of candies, I do not relate its consumption to his dental difficulties. George had lost almost his entire hooked down upper beak, and like some humans some of whom are beasts, suffered physically and mentally. He couldn't eat and lost weight. Using ordinary dental technical methods, and rather unusual professional technique, I made a plastic replica of George's upper beak with little holes around its base. While a surgical assistant held George with heavy toweling, matching holes were made in his small natural skull stump remnant. Care was taken to avoid damaging the brain and other vital parts. With thin orthodontic wire the beak was attached to George. Projections and holes were sealed with dental plastic. Minor adjustments were made. After several quizzical turns side to side, and others in which George looked towards the ceiling, using each eye separately, he stretched both beaks wide three or four times and accepted his denture like real. He didn't seem to mind the imperfect color match. He loved the admiration of visitors and probably appreciated the work though he never paid a fee. The beak served well while being worn and was repointed by me at the tip. Spontaneously, unexpectedly after a while, probably from stimulation use, a new real beak grew back.

PARTIALS FOR BEASTS OF THE SCREEN ∾ Partial dentures supply fiendish fangs for mythical beasts of imaginative horror movies. They're not for chewing ordinary food. They do seem necessary, at periods when the moon is in particular phases, for grasping soft delicate throats of kind hearted tender young beautiful girls, especially those loved by good, devoted, handsome men of honorable intention. Stories with monsters, orgres, demons, werewolves, Frankensteins, King Kongs, and Mr. Hydes of Dr. Jekyl fame, often advantageously use grotesque teeth to shock audiences in recoil at the beast they may fear within themselves. The entertainment industry portrays all this with removable partial dentures.

Some typical tusks may be made directly in the actor's mouth, like other simple dental parts. For finer fiend's fangs, an artist collaborates with the production director, and may sketch on tracing paper over the actor's full faced photos, the new fiend face tooth affect. A dental consultant is called in. Impressions are taken of the beast actor's upper and lower jaws for exact working models. The models are related to hinge open and closed like the actor's mouth. Modeling clay may be added for the lips.

Fangs generally protrude through and beyond lips from the mouth, uppers hook down, lowers thrust up. Longer fangs for proper affect taper broader to the base. Length and angles of thrust are in direct proportion to horror reaction desired. Authentic imaginative frightening pictures feature all these facts to present their fantasy. To get all that fang stuff going in the right direction, the actor's bite and mouth must be opened to clear the lips for fiend fang passage. If uppers and lowers cross outside for added grotesqueness, the bite needs even greater opening. This of course may cause saliva drool, which is usually considered desirable.

When proper jaw model opening is established, the denture is designed and sculpted in wax, over the actor's real teeth models. Wire clasps are incorporated to grip the teeth for acting retention security. Sometimes actual animal fangs if suitable and available are added. Sometimes they're carved of wood. Sometimes dentures are made without wire clasps. Provided with sockets for fitting over the natural teeth holding that way. When the model satisfies the picture director it is processed in the laboratory. They are tried in the actor's mouth and adjusted for fit and bestial fiendification. They need not be removed from the mouth regularly for cleaning.

At the Haunted House in Hollywood, at a meeting of the Count Dracula Society, I met writers and actors of mystery terror and intrigue. During an annual awards' dinner I discussed fang dentures with Lon Chaney. His father Lon Chaney of the silent screen was The Man of a Thousand Faces, The Phantom of the Opera, The Hunchback of Notre Dame. Lon Chaney is a master of extreme emotion. I still sometimes remember his gentle sensitive beautifully awkward portrayal of feeble minded misfit Lenny in "Mice and Men." Mr. Chaney told me of his role as The Wolf Man for Universal Studies, in which on the screen from a human man he transformed, while fangs were seen growing from his lower jaw to a wolf man.

It took twenty two hours of studio filming time, under bright white hot light and six sets of increasing sized fanged dentures, each of which had many pictures taken at changing increasing denture and lip positions for lengthening his tusk lengths, to produce one minute of motion film fang

TEETH TEETH TEETH

growing. Universal felt it worth the cost. Chaney said, "Those fangs fit too darn good. It was hard getting the damn things off for the short relaxation times between all those tiring shots."

Partial Dentures Are Better Than None
The Wholesome Self enjoys more Fun

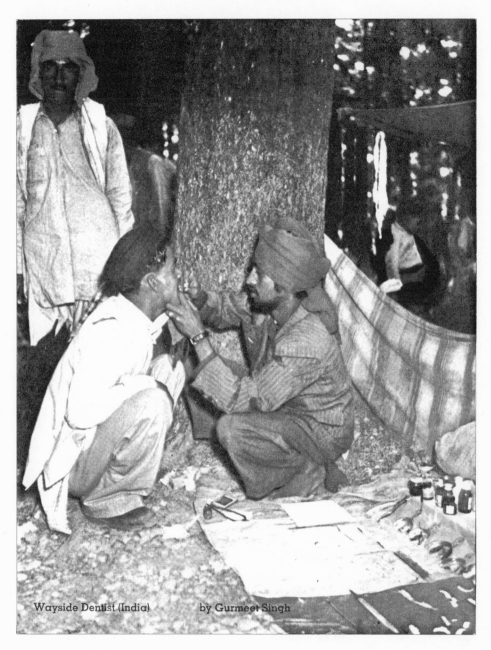

Wayside Dentist (India)   by Gurmeet Singh

Though modern methods reach primitive places refinements are not yet available to all. This outdoor dentists spread contains some medications, forceps for pulling teeth, impression trays for making models of teeth lost jaws, and artificial teeth for dentures to restore them.

TEETH TEETH TEETH

17

FULL REMOVABLE DENTURES

Some things are better bigger. They are certainly more impressive that way. Some people try to get the most of everything they possibly can. Some things are best avoided. The best dental restorations are those so small they are nothing at all. The biggest are full removable dentures. It's best to avoid needing them. When however, all the teeth of a mouth are lost, they are needed and indeed very necessary. Full dentures replace all the teeth of a mouth, and are held together by a structural base, which replaces lost supporting tissues shrunken away. Upper dentures replace teeth and tissues of the upper jaw, lower dentures those of the lower jaw. They are sometimes called dental plates, upper plates and lower plates, also grinders and choppers. Most dentists call them, full removable dentures, full dentures, or dentures. Any dental appliance could be called a denture. A set of full dentures consist, of an upper and lower coupled as a pair. When properly mated they get along well together, in the mouth of their host, who likes what they do there and loves how they do it. They often go to bed together. They may separate briefly at times, but always go back together again. When improperly matched there's lots of trouble for them and the patient.

With teeth gone, bare tender gum covered jaws must close closer for soft food, often the only stuff they can handle. Eating pleasure lessens; digestion, health, emotions suffer. Mouth lips cheek and chin squat flat, jutting up forward, folding to wrinkled creases. Age wizen withered faces around the world are often those of people without teeth. They can all be improved with dentures. Pleasure, health and emotions restore proportionately.

AN ANATOMICAL TRIP

Let's study the mouth. First, the structural bone frame of the mouth used in chewing, the structures supporting teeth which when lost are expected to support dentures. Let's learn a lesson in anatomy. The most available anatomical specimen is our Self. I as your guide will take you on a journey of personal exploration of your parts. We will use our fingers as research investigators and our tongues. It's an exciting educational trip, revealing new unknowns. Voyagers attracted to particular places may linger longer if desired.

TEETH TEETH TEETH

FULL REMOVABLE DENTURES

The upper jaw is scientifically named the Maxilla. It has a horseshoe shaped bone ridge around the front, within the lip beneath the nose, going back right and left inside the cheeks on both sides. This can be felt from outside through the lip and cheek. It is better felt with moving forefinger, around under the lip, back each side to behind the last teeth. The upper ridge is like a down directed retaining wall. It supports upper teeth rooted within growing down out. Feel ridge and teeth between thumb and forefinger moving around and back.

Inside the upper front teeth, just above and behind them, rising along up back towards the roof of the mouth, little hilly flesh corrugations called Rugae can be felt. Few people know they have them. Touching the tongue to rugae and even coming close, gives people an unaware valvelike air passage control, for forming certain speech and singing sounds. They also provide an extra delightful taste touch sensation when certain textured foods are spread between. Within its inside, the upper jaw or maxilla arches curving up as a roofed dome, providing tongue space closed on top by bones of the Palate. This can be felt by fingers and tongue, though on some far back places nerves related to swallowing, may cause tickling. Explore moving around probing, Know thyself. Our cute tongues can do so many wonderful things. God blessed them. The horseshoe shaped upper jaw opening in back, above over the tongue going through, provides passage for food going to the throat.

The lower jawbone or Mandible is the largest strongest individual bone of the skull. It also is horseshoe shaped open in back. It has to be open for the tongue to come up through, forward to its tip, talking and tasting, while its broader muscular base behind is available, for guiding and moving food after being chewed, back down through the throat swallowed. The lower teeth root down in the upward ridge of the lower jaw and grow up to meet chewing surfaces of upper teeth coming down. You can intimately explore all this with fingertips, feeling teeth opening, closing together. Enjoy your personal investigation.

The approximate surface where upper and lower teeth meet is called the Bite Plane. It is not really flat but curves back upwards from the front slightly, as seen from the side. It is in line with the lips slit opening, a convenient arrangement for food entering mouths. This system is responsible for man's creation of slicing machinery, so slivers of ham, cheese and salami, can be conveniently shaped for between bread slice locations, combined to slip into mouths. It is also cause for horizontal attitudes of mustaches.

Opposite teeth closed together contacting act as stops, keeping jaws apart a distance which determines height of the face. The central prominance in front of the lower jaw or mandible is the Chin. Touch it for familiarization

TEETH TEETH TEETH

if you like. The mandible goes around back both sides, where near the right and left middles of the neck, it turns up behind into the head. Feel its borders around each lower edge of the face. The level part of the horseshoe which holds the teeth, is called the Body of the mandible. Back on each side where the body turns up into the skull, is called the Angle of the mandible. Feel your angles on both sides. Each part on the right and left rising from the angle, is called the right and left Ramus of the mandible. Going up each side on top, each ramus bone extension, ends under the flesh in the skull, as a hard bone ball-like knob called the Condyle of the ramus or just condyle. There is a right and left condyle. Through thin flimsy flesh on each side, you can almost feel each condyle inside the head, in front of the ears, while the jaw hingelike opens and closes. Try it. This is an especially explorative searching side trip for each fingertip.

The condyles upper surface on both sides as the jaw drops open, moves turning down forward, in a socket depression of the upper temporal skull bone called the Mandibular Fossa, right and left on each side. Fossa is a medical term meaning depressed cavity. The jaws' right and left condyle bones do not touch the bone walls of the fossa each moves in. They are separated by layers of resilient cartilage, acting as shock absorbers to biting forces. These are all held related together, around their outer anatomical regions, by a strong encircling curtain of flexible ligaments. All these things together involved in jaw hinging connection movements, are called the Temporomandibular Joint. It's quite a joint. It's not easy to get into. To enter the temporomandibular joint you need inside information, and affiliations acquired with long training and experience as surgeon of the head.

Right and left temporomandibular joints connect by the lower jaw as a unit, moving hinged within them. The joints permit more than doorlike direct angular opening and closing. Encircling elastic flexible ligaments around each joint condyle keep it there, at the same time permitting within limits, an extended range of many motions, coordinated right and left for side excursions. Try that swinging your jaw side to side, rhythmically with music if you like. Within these ranges of jaw motion limits, open, side, close, lie all actions of chewing, talking and other mouth movements. It's quite complicated, more sensitively controlled than any joint of any machine made by man. Sometimes it dislocates as the condyle slips forward out of the mandibular fossa, and the horrified patient cannot close his mouth. As muscles relax it may slip back in, or need controlled guidance down to be forced back up by a dentist. At worst the joint fusing together fails in arthritis, so the lower jaw becomes rigid, unopenable, unclosable, needing surgical correction.

TEETH TEETH TEETH

FULL REMOVABLE DENTURES

MUSCLES AND MOVEMENTS

We will study jaw movement. The lower jaw bone or mandible has a series of muscles attached to its surface, from back near the angle where the ramus rises, and along the ramus near the condyle of the hinging joint, which make the jaw move. They are called Muscles of Mastication. Masticate in Latin means chew. These muscles from the mandible radiate many directions, attaching their other ends at particular places along surrounding skull structures, and through inner regions of the neck and throat. They accomplish their movements by contractions only or shortening, when they receive signals from the nervous system. These signals cause man's muscles to contract, just as frog muscles shorten when stimulated by electric currents in biology laboratories. The muscles are balanced in opposing pairs, so that when muscles receive opening signals to shorten pulling the jaw down, their opponents simultaneously are signaled to let go, relaxing yielding to stretch.

No muscles have any pushing power. Opening muscles actually pull the jaw down and also pull their opposing relaxing muscles apart. Closing muscles shorten to pull the jaws up, and also stretch lengthening their relaxing opponents. It's quite a complex system, working somewhat like strings activated by a puppeteer manipulating marionettes, only many millions of times more involved.

Mouth opening muscles are far inside, rather difficult to demonstrate by finger feeling. One, the External Pterygoid can be felt tightening by the tip of the forefinger, placed far back on either inside of the throat, past the last molar tooth. You can feel it tighten as the jaw stretches widening apart. In some mouths this is near a group of nerves that activate automatic swallowing. When touched, by the finger instead of food, this probing may induce tickle, or with very sensitive people a tendency to gag.

Muscles of closing for chewing, are necessarily more powerful. They have to crush food, sometimes very hard. With natural rooted teeth up to 100 or even 200 pounds and more can be exerted. There is a broad muscle band, attached to the forward upper border of the rising ramus of the mandible, spread wide along each side attaching above to the skull towards the temples, called the Temporalis muscle. If the palms are placed forward of the ears, over their area of action they can be felt, relaxing as the jaw opens and tightens with closing. Pressing teeth harder tightens them more. These and other muscles pull moving jaws to all positions, open, closed, right, left, forward, back, and combinations of all those directions.

TEETH TEETH TEETH

JAW RELATIONS AND BITE BALANCE

When jaws normally close together with opposite teeth touching, they are in what is called Centric Position or relationship. In most of life's living, upper and lower teeth are not touching. Teeth touch with conscious effort as in chewing, and may also occur at times of tension. Usually jaws are relaxed with their teeth a short distance apart, at what is called the Rest Position. Relax, try this, fingers aren't needed. Talking teeth leave and return to rest position, normally never touching.

Certain muscles can pull the lower jaw back a bit from centric position, to what is called Retruded Position. You can detect this slight movement, holding a fingertip against closed front upper and lower teeth. Try it. In retruded position cartilage lining the rear of the jaw hinging joint is slightly compressed. It's easier using other muscles to pull the jaw jutting forward into what is called Protruded Position. The lower jaw can swing right and left, into what are called the Right Lateral or Side Position and the Left Lateral Position. As a jaw swings right, its condyle in the skull on that side goes slightly back, while the left condyle moves forward. When swung to the left lateral position, the reverse occurs. You can feel these hinge movements with fingers, touching the temporal joints on each side.

When teeth are in centric, both sides closed contacting, they are also said to be in Centric Balance. All muscles of mastication are balanced, as opposing teeth tips fit into each other. When jaws touching move side to side, as tooth tips of each jaw mutually slide along in recesses of teeth of the opposite jaw, this coordinated with the muscles moving is called the Balanced Bite. When bites are balanced jaw forces distribute among many teeth, rather than being concentrated on one or few. These balanced positions and jaw working combinations, are used by jaws doing jaw jobs, and when these jobs are done muscles and jaws relax apart, returned to their Rest Position.

MOUTH LINING TISSUES

When a mouth ordinarily opens most obviously seen are teeth. When teeth are lost, their root vacated space heals, fortunately filling from the tip up with growing bone. The local jawbone level shrinks a little towards the bone fill, leaving the healed ridge unfortunately a little lower. Surrounding gum grows closing together, covering the voids where the teeth before loss came through. What was once tooth territory is now all bone, covered with a blanket of bare soft gum. The thin gum cover assumes a new role as a bearing or supporting surface, for enduring chewing forces delivered by covering dentures. Gums toughen to the need as they adapt transferring

TEETH TEETH TEETH

force to their jawbone beneath. These endurable forces are far lower than can be exerted by natural teeth. Rooted teeth can apply forces of one hundred pounds and much more, removable dentures hardly over twenty.

Let's study the soft tissues around the inside of the mouth, the only tissues available for supporting and controlling dentures. The vestibule to a building is its entrance passageway. If the upper or lower lip is pulled forward, what is called the upper or lower Vestibule of the mouth is seen spread open, between inside the lip and the front gum of its jaw. You can see this in a mirror. The vestibule continues around back on each side, between the gum covered jaw and cheek. Usually the vestibule of the mouth is closed contact surface, with tissues of lips cheeks and gums touching. The vestibule opens in front to some extent while speaking, more in pouting, and even more all around if the lips are held tight together, and the cheeks blown up like for filling a balloon. If a finger pointed up is run along the upper vestibule, it must stop on top by what is called the Muco-buccal fold. This is the place inside the mouth around the outer jaw surface, where the gums reflect turning back, becoming lining of cheeks and lips. The same can be felt by a finger directed downward in the mouth, around the lower outer jaw. This flesh fold is where cheek and lip support and controlling muscles, attach to bones of the jaws.

The muco-buccal fold is of little significance to people with their own teeth. Sometimes it traps food, cleanable if within the range of long snaky tongue tips, others use a finger. For people without teeth the muco-buccal fold location is more significant. It also sometimes traps food. More important than that, it limits the depth of extension of the outer or vestibular jaw embracing border of the removable dental appliance. It limits outer ventures of removable dentures. When jaw ridges are high, like a high dam holds more water, the deeper larger outer denture border more securely grips the jaw, for stabilization against side chewing denture dislodging forces. It also provides more frictional surface against slipping from place.

From the muco-buccal fold borders of the mouth vestibule, the rear inner wall of the vestibule rises all around the jaw, as the front gum covered bone Ridge or wall of the jaw. Passing from the front jaw wall, we come to the rounded toothless top edge of the jaw, called the Crest of the Jaw Ridge. With the toothless mouth closed, upper and lower gum covered ridges both face each other around the jaw arch, like the chewing surfaces of their teeth did before they were lost. From the crest or edge of the jaw ridges, we pass into the mouth cavity, over to the inner gum covered jaw walls.

It is these projecting jaw ridge walls with their jaw crest or edge that lost their teeth, which must internally support and stabilize the removable dentures, which replace those teeth around them.

TEETH TEETH TEETH

Inside the upper jaw the rising hard palate domed bone roof also covers with gum. Behind the hard palate, extending, the soft palate continues as a movable flap of flesh. It acts as a flapper valve during swallowing, sealing inner nasal air passages from food. This area has nerves which when touched by food moving back, starts automatic swallowing reflexes. In sensitive people's mouths, when impressions are taken for dentures the nerves sometimes cause gagging.

Within the lower jaw the most prominent part is the Tongue. It is an important organ of speech, supplies sensations of taste, though taste buds also exist other places in the mouth, and for those who so desire tongues can be cleverly used in specialized kissing techniques, even with removable dentures. If a finger is run down along inside behind the lower jaw ridge, towards the base or root of the tongue, while the tongue moves stretching, its attached muscles can be felt tightening. These tongue attachments limit extension ventures of the inner borders of lower removable dentures.

Under the tongue at the center of the mouth, there is a thin ligamentous band, tying the tongue bottom to the floor of the mouth, called the Tongue Frenum. This frenum restricts extension of tongue tips to some people's regret. It can easily be finger felt. When especially short it may limit tongue action causing a speech impairment called Tongue-Tie. This can be corrected by surgery. The frenum also affects the design of lower dentures whose borders must clear its anatomical movements. In the front center of the mouth of both lower and upper jaws, there are smaller frenum bands attaching the jaw to inside the lips. These are all considered by the dentist anatomist designing and building removable dentures.

MAKING FULL DENTURES

Let's follow construction of a set of dentures considering function and appearance. The information concerning both upper and lower appliances as a pair, applies similarly to either an upper or lower denture made individually, if that alone were needed. Refer to Plate 17-1, DENTURE-SKULL-RELATIONS. Since dentures are activated by their jawbone structures, the drawings are shown of bare skull bone with flesh removed for clarity. Drawing A is a side view of normal jaws containing natural teeth, closed together with the bite normally related. Drawing B shows the jaws with their teeth lost, held kept positioned similarly related. They are separated now by space needing full removable dentures.

To make dentures, the dentist needs models of the patient's upper and lower jaws. To relate those mouth models to each other, measurements are needed of the jaw's relations to each other, and of both related as a unit to their jaw hinging joint in the head. These measured recordings are used to

TEETH TEETH TEETH

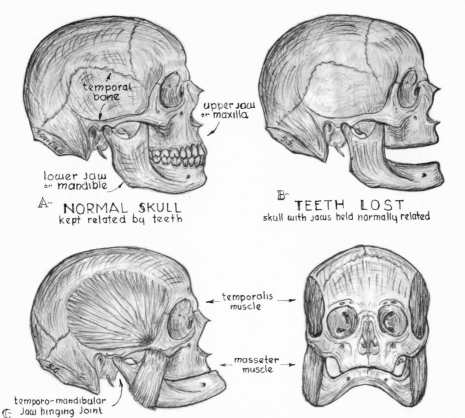

A~ **NORMAL SKULL**
kept related by teeth

temporal bone

upper jaw or maxilla

lower jaw or mandible

B~ **TEETH LOST**
skull with jaws held normally related

temporalis muscle

masseter muscle

temporo-mandibular jaw hinging joint

C~ TOOTHLESS SKULL SHOWN WITH MAJOR CHEWING MUSCLES PULLING THE JAW UP FORWARD

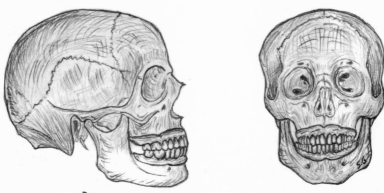

D~ DENTURE RESTORATION

PLATE 17-1 **DENTURE~SKULL~RELATIONS** S. Garfield

TEETH TEETH TEETH

FULL REMOVABLE DENTURES

mount the models in an adjustable insturment called the Dental Articulator, which reproduces patients chewing actions as they occur in heads. In the laboratory on these articulated models the dentures are made.

THE DENTAL ARTICULATOR

Let's study the dental articulator. Articulators are much like industrial assembly jigs and fixtures, used to manufacture complicated machines like automobiles, whose moving working parts require precise relations. Articulators are used in all phases of restorative dentistry. They are described here for convenience. There are many types of articulators. Some as simple as an ordinary hinge, satisfy simple dental problems. There are articulators costing thousands of dollars, containing many precise adjustment features, for reproduction of the complex combination of patient's jaw skull related movements. We will examine an instrument satisfactory for many dental services.

Plate 17-2 THE DENTAL ARTICULATOR is a pictorial view of such an articulator seen looking down from the front and side. The instrument consists of two hinged portions, upper and lower, for holding models of the respective jaws. They are connected at right and left by a movable mechanical joint, which acts much like human's right and left temporomandibular jaw hinging joints. Upper and lower jaw models may be mounted on the articulator, within a large range of positions occupied in human heads, related to each other as they are to human head chewing joints. The instrument can easily be opened and closed as the mouth does. A patient seeing one said, "Dr. Garfield it's an imitation jaw!" It is an imitation jaw. An imitation that can be adjusted as a dental tool to work like real jaws.

The articulator shown provides for side jaw movements similar to those performed by people. It has adjustment for controlling bite opening distance. In life a person's lower jaw with head erect as usual, opens down. As dental articulators rest on laboratory benches, their upper jaws are swung up instead. The difference doesn't matter since the instrument is designed so its jaw movements have the same related geometric path. Dental technicians often hold articulators in their hands, moving its jaws different directions for study. Upper and lower articulator parts may be easily separated, for working access inside either denture. They readily snap back when desired to the patient's adjusted relationship, for that phase of work, so the finished denture product will properly function in the living mouth. Dentistry would be easier and cheaper, if dentists could do this directly with their living patients heads.

TEETH TEETH TEETH

FULL REMOVABLE DENTURES

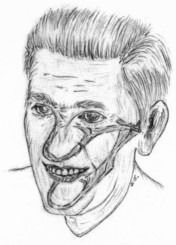

ARTICULATOR PORTRAYED IN THE HEAD
IN THE JAW RELATED POSITION

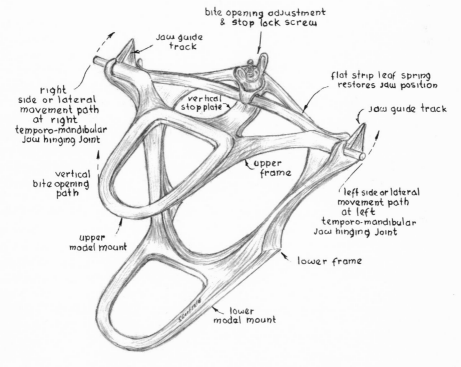

bite opening adjustment
& stop lock screw

Jaw guide
track

right
side or lateral
movement path
at right
temporo-mandibular
Jaw hinging Joint

vertical
stop plate

flat strip leaf spring
restores Jaw position

Jaw guide track

vertical
bite opening
path

upper
frame

left side or lateral
movement path
at left
temporo-mandibular
Jaw hinging Joint

upper
model mount

lower frame

lower
model mount

PLATE 17-2 THE DENTAL ARTICULATOR S. Garfield
A DENTAL ASSEMBLY-JIG-FIXTURE INSTRUMENT
FOR BITING MOVEMENT RELATIONS OF JAW MODELS

TEETH TEETH TEETH

DENTURES ALONG THE WAY

There are many ways of making dentures. The simplest sometimes satisfies and even more. Just as a simple camera with few or no adjustments, may take a prize winning photo of an average subject, if the light is right about average, and the subject an average distance away, holding still. To take even a reasonably good picture, of horses galloping around a mudded track curve, through slashing rain, perhaps even including lightning flash, requires fine photographic equipment, special knowledge, experience, and skill. If patients have well formed substantial toothless jaw ridges, are tolerant, and not too demanding, simply made dentures may seem ideal. Difficult denture cases demand finer advanced techniques. Here some popular procedures which demonstrate important principles are explained.

IMPRESSIONS ∾ After examination and discussion of patient needs, the dentist takes impressions of upper and lower jaws, for making mouth models. When ill fitting dentures are worn they irritate bruising tissues. Dentures made on models of such jaws wouldn't fit. Patients are asked to leave old dentures out for a tissue recovery period. Mouths heal quickly. Often being left without dentures through the previous night and daytime until the impression appointment will do. Impressions shouldn't be made while suffering severe head colds, or other disorders which also distort mouth tissues. Impressions of jaws are taken with individual impression trays, upper and lower, formed to fit around jaws. They have a handle for placement into the mouth. Lower trays open horseshoe-shaped in back, to clear the tongue. From a standard variety, trays slightly larger closest to the patient's jaw size are selected, and may be more ideally adapted. Impressions of both jaws are taken, one at a time. After seeing the mouth is clean, the tray is filled with soft pleasantly flavored impression material, and carefully located to place. Excess squeezes out around the jaw borders. Bulk back towards the throat if disturbing is instantly scooped away. The material soon sets, gelling around its jaw, and is removed from the mouth as a reverse mold. In the laboratory dental plaster powder is mixed with water, and poured filling into every detail. Within an hour it sets hard. The hard models are removed and trimmed as duplicates of upper and lower jaws. Patient's name and impression dates are recorded on each.

Studying these models the dentist may consider them adequate. Sometimes he feels finer detailed models are needed for denture construction. If so, the preliminary or study models are used to make individual custom made impression trays, more ideally suited to take impressions of toothless patient's jaws.

TEETH TEETH TEETH

MUSCLE TRIMMING IMPRESSIONS ∾ Impressions are desired of the largest muscle free jaw area possible. Within this region, the gum covered bone foundation has no disturbing moving muscle action. The region ends around each jaw close up to its borders, uninvaded by normal or stretching movements of attached lip, cheek, tongue muscles, doing any of the things they ever do; talking, yawning, sneezing, wrinkling, curling, snarling, laughing, swallowing, puffing, anything. Dentists taking such impressions use detailed knowledge of the intimate behavior of the mouth's anatomical parts. While the impression tray with still soft impression material is in the mouth, as impressions are being taken, patients may be asked to move their lip, cheek, and tongue parts different directions, deflecting their muscles, forming confines of the impressions borders as it hardens. This is called Muscle Trimming.

If the denture ends within its own borders, as close to those boundaries as possible, it will cover the largest territory available without special patient consciousness. Dentures with larger bearing surface areas, can carry more chewing load and deliver more force. Also, since removable dentures are not attached to mouth tissues, only resting accurately upon them, getting some suction and frictional help, the bigger the denture base the greater its stability, if it avoids trespassing on muscle territory. Dentures and muscles are like neighboring nations, they get along better when one does not intrude upon the other. If a denture border extends into, interfering with a muscle attachment, it is resented. It irritates the attachment, annoying the muscle, which in its actions moves, to resist dislodging the denture as a foreigner. When they respect each other's borders, they can help each other, to the mutual benefit of both. The closer denture bases get to their neighboring muscles without disturbing them, the more they can cooperate as patients learn, adapting to their dentures, automatically using lip, cheek, tongue muscles, to grip and control them. It's a close tricky relationship. Dentists taking impressions must act like careful diplomats and ambassadors. Perhaps we need more dentists in our nation's foreign services. Perhaps diplomatic training should include dental impression taking.

FIT ∾ When impressions are first taken they sometimes fit so intimately, removal from the mouth is difficult even with powerful pulling. Replaced only moments later the fit is good but not as ideal. The impression hasn't changed. The mouth has, during the tiny time taken putting the appliance back. As accurate impressions are replaced, their soft lining gum supporting tissues are displaced, yielding to frictional resistance forced from place. Also gum covered jaws often have fine deep wrinkles in them like their hosts faces, even more. Accurate impressions reproduce the

TEETH TEETH TEETH

wrinkles. Unfortunately it is impossible to replace well fitting dentures with such wrinkles, each into its own recess. The denture wrinkle projections themselves push the adjacent soft gum away, causing their own misfit, irritating the soft tissue which like rubber may push the denture away. The doctor using skilled judgement decides which projections to remove for the finest final fit.

DENTURE MAKING CONSIDERATIONS ∽ So that dentures coordinate biting and chewing together, after accurate models are made the dentist must determine the patient's jaw relations as they meet, upper and lower jaws working together.

Teeth rooted jaws are kept properly related rather securely. The jaw hinging joint confined behind in the skull, stops the lower jaw from moving back. Upper front teeth lapping over lowers, and other opposite interlocking tooth surfaces, also keep lower jaws from moving back or frontward. With neglected tooth loss, formerly teeth occupied barren jaws having little left to stop them swing up forward. In fact bare jaw hinge path movements are such, that toothless people can only bite and chew the little they can, with only their front toothless ridge areas. In many teethless mouths the back won't even meet. People with little else to grub food, force their lower jaws even further forward. Such unfortunates and negligents must munch, gumming gums, maneuvering lips, ruminating like rabbits. Their chewing muscles distort adapting to meet the need. Dental objectives are to restore normal balanced biting postures, which more efficiently operate dentures.

BITE RELATIONS & DENTURE DESIGN

Making dentures for difficult cases is sometimes very involved. Understanding the steps that follow may take careful concentration.

ONE OF SEVERAL METHODS ∽ To transfer bite relation measurements from the toothless mouth to jaw models, dental tooling devices called Bite Bases are used. Bite bases are thin sheets of rigid material, sometimes a hard wax, often plastic, formed to fit the jaw models, upper and lower, as they will fit their patient's toothless jaws. To take bite relation measurements of how teeth bite and chew, wax blocks are attached to the bite bases along their jaw ridge areas, occupying the space held by teeth, somewhat taller than the denture teeth are expected to be. Bite bases with wax occupied tooth positions are called Bite Blocks. They're sort of experimental removable dentures with wax instead of teeth. These bite blocks fitting toothless jaws, may be used by dentists to

TEETH TEETH TEETH

determine the shape of outer borders of dentures, the location and length of denture teeth, the gum surface form around the teeth, and the toothless mouth's proper vertical opening. Sometimes patient's biting chewing movements dictate the location and length of their denture teeth. They can't be anywhere else to work well. Sometimes the upper bite block may be used within limits, to determine the most attractive tooth positions and amount of teeth showing beyond the lips.

When older dentures aren't available as guides, one method starts inserting the upper bite block on its jaw. The doctor and patient studying upper lip positions, at rest, talking, laughing, can form the wax, to decide how much upper tooth surface would be most attractively seen. Marking that length as the upper teeth's bottom edge line, the bite block is removed and the dentist carves excess wax off to that line. He may trim the wax continuing back on each side, establishing the Bite Plane or chewing surface location, of the upper dentures back teeth.

The upper bite block with its established occlusal or chewing surface plane, is inserted in the mouth. Then the lower bite block wax along its upper surface is heated, softened, and also inserted. The patient is engaged in active conversation. Magazines may be given for reading aloud. Special oral exercises may be recited. Patients left alone sometimes feel silly sort of talking aloud to themselves. While their mouth moves articulating varied sounds, the hard upper bite wax drives its soft lower opponent flattened, to meet the bite plane surface. The dentist removes the soon hard lower bite block, trims off the flatted excesses while preserving its talking determined plane level.

During normal speaking people's teeth do not quite touch, they come close, but slightly short of meeting. To establish the lower teeth height as they will be in the denture, having observed the patient's mouth movements, the dentist shaves a thin wax layer from the talking leveled lower plane At this lowered level, slightly past the opposite teeth talking approach, the denture teeth will meet chewing. These denture heights, the upper dentures down to its bite plane, plus the lower dentures from the bite plane down, total the mouth's measured proper Vertical Bite, or closed together height.

When old dentures are available, though outworn in chewing efficiency, they're often valuable aides as dental tools, to help establish the vertical bite opening. Their existing teeth are a basis for considering changes in the new denture teeth. All these procedures which may or may not seem simple explained, sometimes involve unexpected complexities, which can only be appreciated experienced by the dentist and patient.

TEETH TEETH TEETH

FULL REMOVABLE DENTURES

LIP CHEEK FACE FORMS ∾ The same bite blocks may also be used to create within limits, attractive living forms of adjacent outer lips and cheeks. Around the wax blocks outer surfaces, additional wax may be added and removed shaping, trying inside the mouth for the faces outer appearance, filling tissues here, removing wrinkles there, while the dentist sculptor of life forms the wax, until the result desired if possible is achieved. This wax bulk if patient tolerable, can be reproduced in the finished denture for the same affect.

Bite blocks like full dentures they're used to make, are of such size, though both fit the mouth in use together, only one can be inserted or removed at a time. The jaw related bite blocks, must be made to interlock each other in the mouth, so that after removal both will meet in the same exact related position. The dentist removes the upper bite block. With a pointed knife, centered along the wide wax chewing surface for the back teeth, he cuts on each side right and left, a sharp shallow V-shaped groove. Then in the wax chewing surface, at a couple of places on each side, he cuts short crossing grooves. Both sides bite surfaces with their crossing V-grooves are lubricated with a thin grease film, and the upper bite block is reinserted in the mouth.

To the lower bite block on both sides flat surfaces for the back teeth, in the area opposing the upper V-grooves of each side, with a hot instrument the dentist adds small amounts of molten wax. As it starts to cool slowly hardening, he inserts the lower bite block to place, and asks the patient to close. If concerned that the lower jaw from neglect may have habitually wandered too far forward, with thumb and forefinger the dentist helps guide the jaw back, as the patient closes. The lower soft wax fills into the upper grooves, as the patient closes, stopped at the proper height bite related position, and holds closed. The wax soon hardens. The doctor asks patient to open and close, checking to see that the jaws relate so the lower projecting wax V's fit into their upper grooves. Before removing the bite blocks, the dentist may mark in front a center line below the nose, and the right and left lip opening extremities, as a later guide for teeth arrangement. Out of the mouth, upper and lower bite blocks can now be readily related, in their proper bite position.

JAW RELATION MEASUREMENT VARIATIONS ∾ The described technique for relating toothless jaws satisfies many cases. Sometimes simpler ways work. Sometimes the doctor feels other precise methods are needed. The Arch Tracing may be used. In this method one bite base has attached a small dry inked plate. The opposite base holds a pointed pin centered over the plate. The patient swings the lower jaw to all positions

TEETH TEETH TEETH

possible, holding the jaws closed while the pin rides over the plate. The pin traces a path through the ink which helps describe the jaws related movements, and mount the bite bases related together. There are methods for establishing bite relationship using a tiny squat balloon between upper and lower bases, into which air or liquid plaster is forced expanding against the bases, to help certain phases of getting accurate bite relations.

Sometimes case complexities require instruments to precisely measure the jaws distance from their head hinging joint. Each technique is designed to help different difficulties. Denture construction is sometimes very involved.

MORE ARTICULATION INFORMATION ∽ In the laboratory, the upper and lower bite blocks are attached related together, with their respective jaw models inserted. The assembled unit is mounted in the articulator as in the mouth, lower jaw model at the articulator's lower jaw mount, upper model at the upper mount. The related bite blocks are separated, each removed from its mounted model. Both jaw models are now apart a toothless space, mounted in the articulator at the bite position opening, as established for their patient's head. Dentures made filling that space will fill and fit the patient's mouth. Refer to Plate 17-3 ARTICULATED DENTURE CONSTRUCTION. The individual bite blocks used to help design the dentures, may each be replaced on its articulated jaw as tools to make the dentures.

TEETH HEIGHT OR LENGTH ∽ A method was described which determined the length of upper teeth or the height of the upper denture. From the upper teeth's chewing surface down, the space beneath is occupied by the lower teeth and its denture. The chewing plane surface, between upper and lower dentures, approximates the mouth's lip opening. This total measured articulated distance must be maintained for dentures to work. If upper teeth are made shorter, the lowers must be equally lengthened longer. Sometimes the bite plane division, distributing upper and lower teeth lengths, can be some extent be determined by the desired appearance of the teeth. Often patient's natural chewing actions are such, that for dentures to work best, some appearance sacrifices must be made for function efficiency.

With jaw models mounted in the articulator, holding bite blocks determining the teeth's lengths and their surrounding gum forms, the basic tooling for denture making is set up, and construction almost ready to go ahead. Before completion however certain critical supplies must be secured, the Teeth.

TEETH TEETH TEETH

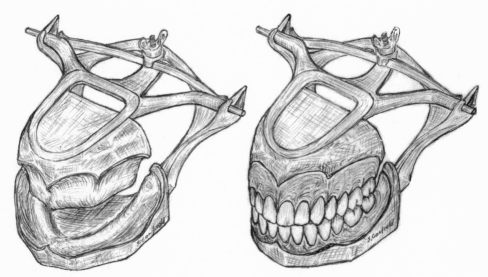

UPPER & LOWER JAW MODELS
MOUNTED ON ARTICULATOR
AS RELATED IN THE HEAD

DENTURES COMPLETED
FUNCTION AT
PATIENTS HEAD-JAW RELATIONS

PLATE 17-3 ARTICULATED DENTURE CONSTRUCTION S.Garfield

TEETH TEETH TEETH

FULL REMOVABLE DENTURES

SELECTING DENTURE TEETH ∾ Removable dentures provide owners with advantage unavailable to natural toothed people, the ability to choose their own teeth. Denture teeth are available in natural tooth matching shades, from lightest lightness to aging stained darker tints. Like natural teeth they contain colors, not obviously apparent, yellows, green, pink, others, which many think unattractive, but are necessary tiny constituents of tooth falsies, if they are to look real.

Some people wanting youth restored, have misguided preference for the lightest teeth possible. They're often more mature people with teeth lost in more neglected years. Teeth should be selected lighter, within a reasonable range of youthful possibility if youth is desired, but shades beyond usually look artificial. Some people prefer that denture teeth match their originals. If photos or other information is available that can be done. It's usually best to select teeth most attractive for the person as they are. They may look better than original.

In many sizes teeth are available in different shapes, to create varied personality impressions, from soft gentleness to massive strength. Dentists have samples to help selection. Denture teeth are made in matched sets, combining qualities of shade size and form. Each is shaped anatomically like the natural tooth it replaces. No two teeth in a denture, as no two teeth in a toothed mouth, are exactly alike. Teeth of identical twins, sometimes are almost identical. Front upper sets contain right and left central incisors, lateral incisors and cuspids. Their lower front teeth have the same named matching to meet them. Back chewing teeth upper and lower, in sets matched to meet, contain right and left first and second bicuspids, first and second molars. Dentures do not use third molar wisdom teeth.

Denture teeth are made of porcelain and plastic. Porcelain are more inert, keeping a cleaner life like sparkle. They're harder, wear better, are more likely to chip if dropped. Plastic teeth are softer, may wear away sooner, though modern plastics are tough, lasting a long time. Their slight yielding resiliency can be helpful to patients with tender gums. They act as shock absorbers, softening chewing forces like rubber heels more comfortable to walk on. The doctor can chose best.

DENTURE TEETH CHEWING SURFACE DESIGNS ∾ Dentists spend little time discussing the choice of back denture teeth. They spend more time than patients realize selecting them. Back teeth are made for denture chewing in a variety of dentally engineered chewing surface shapes. Most look more or less alike. There are small important differences. Natural rooted teeth are equipped to resist most any force they encounter. Dentures merely resting on gum surfaces are more limited. Irregularity in their chewing motion paths could easily dislodge their

TEETH TEETH TEETH

dentures. The dental profession has developed a variety of scientific chewing surface shapes each suited to patients particular needs.

TEETH ARRANGEMENT ∞ In the dental laboratory teeth are arranged in dentures as they are in mouths with added denture considerations. Arranging teeth in dentures is also called Setting Up teeth. To arrange or set up denture teeth, the dental technician has the patient's upper and lower jaw models mounted in the articulator as in the head. Upper and lower bite blocks, each shaped for its denture as dentist determined in the mouth, are on their models. The technician also has the selected teeth and the dentist's prescribed set up instructions.

Starting with the upper wax bite block from the front centered mark, to right and left, tooth sized wax scoops are removed, and beginning with the central incisors, false tooth by tooth each is stuck, placed in adjacent wax that holds it. Each tooth face is positioned at the front wax bite block face, as was determined in the mouth, as each tooth's bite edge is brought to the dentures biting edge, as was also earlier established in the mouth. After all six upper front teeth are arranged, the lowers are set up, located on their bite block to meet them.

After the front teeth are arranged, continuing towards the back, within the boundaries of wax over the jaw ridges where the natural teeth originally were, the dentures chewing teeth are placed. Right and left each side, in anatomical sequence, first the bicuspids then molars are located held in wax. Each tooth's chew surface meets the dentures established plane. Lower teeth are located to meet their uppers. The articulator like a jaw is opened, to work inside around each tooth. It opens and closes, in the determined adjusted for patient's head related position.

Setting up teeth is an art its own. The technician familiar with living mouth movements, uses a flame heated instrument to soften the wax around individual teeth, moving each to more natural appearing better biting places. Particular characteristics asked for can often be created in the teeth held by wax. Since dentures only rest on soft flesh this isn't always easy to accomplish. Sometimes placing denture teeth most attractively for seeing, locates them unfavorably in the mouth for eating. Compromises may have to be made.

After upper and lower teeth are arranged for articulated opening and closing, the technician swings their articulated jaws through side motions, like the living mouth will move. Sometimes the denture teeth need grinding away to clear side movement interferences, just as natural teeth wear away.

TEETH TEETH TEETH

SURROUNDING GUM TISSUE ∾ After the teeth are arranged, the technicians' attention turns to surrounding tissues which can also be made to look natural. Shaping the teeth surrounding wax, while providing the mouth determined lip supporting gum form, is called Waxing Up dentures. Miniature lifelike sculpturing, around each individual tooth and beyond, so the gum looks as if the tooth were growing through, is an added art called Characterization of dentures. Inside the upper denture behind the front teeth, on the forward palatal roof surface, tiny irregular ridges called rugae can be carved, unseen from outside, touchable to the tongue, like those naturally in the mouth to help speech control. The denture models looking rather real, with their real denture teeth supported in tissue pink wax, is ready for trial in the patient's mouth. Plate 17-3 shows the trial dentures completed on the articulator.

THE TRY-IN ∾ Dentures like other technical products are often tested first. The models are tried in the mouth. Faults found can be corrected, desired modifications made, before finishing for the long expected intimate relationship. Doctor cautions patient to close carefully since the teeth are held only in wax. Adjustments may be made.

FINAL LABORATORY PROCESSING ∾ In the dental laboratory molds are made around the denture models. The molds are opened, and except for the denture teeth held precisely in place, all wax and everything else is removed. Their voided space is filled with strong resistant permanent plastic denture base material, colored to match the natural gums as prescribed by the dentist. The finished denture base structural foundation fits the mouth and holds the teeth, exactly as the tested model did.

DENTURE BASE COLORS ∾ Gum tissue color inside mouths is related to the color of people's outer skins. Skin color is controlled by three factors. Skin itself is basically biologically sort of light yellow. Blood beneath imparts a reddish hue. There are cells within skin called melanoblasts, that manufacture a dark coloring pigment called melanin, which masks the natural color of living tissues. Distribution of melanoblasts and their pigments in skin varies among races of man.

Caucasians or fair skinned people, have little color pigmentation in their outer skin, and very little in their gums. Pink in the gums is created by blood in the capillaries showing through flesh tissue cells. An average tissue tone pink denture base matches the gums of most fair skinned people. Lighter and darker pinks are available. Denture bases can be given even more lifelike quality. Fine red plastic threads, usually nylon,

TEETH TEETH TEETH

incorporated in the pink plastic, like capillaries, impart a vital reality.

Black or darker skinned people like Negroes, often have pink close around the tooth necks, with heavily melanin pigmented varied browns further away, sometimes in blotchy patches. This can be duplicated in the denture mold, using pure pink around the teeth, and added browns with slight mixed blues and purples at other areas. For Oriental or yellow skinned races denture bases are sometimes made pink, into which small amounts of lighter purples, browns, and blues, are more thoroughly mixed.

DENTURE ADVENTURE

Wearing full removable dentures the first time, is a personal drama sometimes distressing, though usually only briefly in the life of patients. They are new parts added to the body. Like artificial legs, dentures are prosthesis or missing organ replacements, custom made for cutting and grinding food. No two dentures in the world are exactly alike. Each needs individual care to control. Denture wearers become machine operators of small specialized equipment, their own dentures. Instruction helps, but only patients personal practice results in efficient performance. The infant growing to child takes years of instinctive, gradually needed learning, to use natural teeth. Adults without teeth must and can adapt to dentures. They are often unaware of the technical problems involved, and in these days of quick changing progress, impatiently frustrated at less than immediate complete control. Dentures are far smaller than any person who wears them, but those who fight their dentures can only win limited victory. A dental assistant told me of working in an office where she heard a frustrated man say, "I got so damn mad Doc, I smashed the damn thing with my heel." I wonder if anyone quick on the draw ever shot their denture.

LIMITATIONS ∾ Modern removable dentures help, but can't be expected to equal natural teeth. If patients are reasonably patient they learn to use them successfully. Even the best dentures depend on conditions of their natural supporting structures, mental attitude, and diligently applied dexterity.

EARLY TRIALS ∾ When first worn they may be removed occasionally for rest. Border areas sometimes bruise until the tissues and denture settle. Adjustments by the dentist eliminate interferences. Cheeks and tongue previously filling the missing spaces may be bitten by their new neighboring companion teeth. They learn to adapt staying out of the way. Where mouth corners crease and lips draw thin from long neglected

TEETH TEETH TEETH

toothless years, restoration to the new inner support may take a little longer.

Sometimes the new denture bulk acts as an irritant, or like food bulk stimulates the glands to drool extra saliva. Swallowing will solve the temporary problem. Some patients sense voice changes which sound exaggerated to them. Sounds are affected by size and shape of chambers they come from. The mouth cavity is most of the voice chamber. When teeth have been missing a long time dentures change that chamber closer to normal, sometimes with slight voice changes, which may seem strange at first, and soon improve. Reading aloud helps, and talking at a mirror. Adjustments may improve particular tones.

Eating for the first time with full removable dentures can be trying ordeal. Young and adaptable people may learn in a week or less, some take months and more. Start with small bite sizes of soft balanced diet food, crackers, vegetables, fish, ground beef, vitamins, avoiding sticky stuff. It's best beginning alone at home, and until mouthing maneuvers are mastered avoid busy dinner tables and restaurants. Early awkward lack of chewing control can be discouraging, frustrating, embarassing. Practice with personal determination yields continuous improvement. Family and friends should sympathetically understand, avoiding jokes. Denture eating beginnings are times of trial, especially for those in less than good health.

NATURAL TEETH EATING MECHANICS

To study eating with removable dentures, we will first examine the mechanics of instinctive eating with natural teeth, information hardly needed of things done daily by those who have such teeth. Eating activities may be divided into biting, chewing and drinking. Let's analyse each.

BITING ∽ There are varied bitings, like those which shouldn't be of hands that feed us, and the times some bite the dust. Our biting discourse concerns delivery of a small piece, also called a Bolus of food, passed through into the mouth. A bite can be taken of proper size whole, delivered by fork or spoon. Orientals use chopsticks. Probably most bites are from food held in a hand, separated for the mouth by the front sharp single edged teeth, coming together through, while they often also slice slightly sideways. Sometimes the hand helps tearing, while the head pulls the bitten piece away. Sometimes both join, reversing twists. Less often lower jaws without thinking, jiggle their teeth closely, severing tough things like celery strings. Natural rooted toothers with teeth firmly jaw fixed, hardly think of these things they do.

TEETH TEETH TEETH

As mouths almost thoughtlessly open for biting, their lips lift parting to welcome the food. While the jaws are closing they return, holding as a soft sealing gasket from which almost lost particles may be tongue swept, inside if treasured delicious, fluffed if worth less away.

CHEWING ∾ The bitten bite or bolus is smelled, felt, and tasted, giving those pleasure sensations and tongue manipulatéd rearward, to the right or left back teeth, for single sided sideways chomping like cows chew cud. Most people chew on one side. The crushed stuff squashed squeezing out between, is returned to the teeth by cheek and tongue for fuller pulverization. When synchronized reflexes think particles are small enough for efficient digestion, though these reflexes are often prematurely subdued by desire for another bite, the tongue back wriggling and cheek pulsing, move the fine food finally throatward to swallow.

DRINKING ∾ Liquid consuming by drinking uses gravitational forces, and man made air pressure differences. As the hand delivers the cup tilting to the mouth, the lips outside purse moving to meet wich a smaller opening. Inside the clever tongue sends its tip curving close for better control. When the proper sub-consciously calculated cup content level is reached, the lungs deep inside expand, lowering inner air pressures which transfer to the mouth, where outer barometric conditions cause a tiny soft severe typhoon that sucks such foods in tasty little tidal waves.

DENTURE MECHANICS

SOME PHILOSOPHICAL ASPECTS ∾ Eating with dentures needs learning new unnatural skills. Muscles of lips, cheeks, and tongue, in addition to their ordinary actions, can and must adapt to do things they're not originally designed for. They must hold and control dentures in place while talking, open and close biting and chewing, and moving food back to swallow. At first it's not easy. Patients who wisely determined accept the challenge can learn to use dentures with pleasure.

Learning to operate an automobile the driver bewilders at the need for giving each mechanical control device; foot pedal for speed; hands wheel for steering; hand and foot brakes; transmission shift; a maze of gauges; individual and coordinated attention, while simultaneous alert observations of outer surrounding road conditions are demanded. He is frightened insecure, unsure of himself. With practice, one by one, almost subsconsciously, increased automatic sequence responses are acquired. Reflexes adapt to the close mechanical controls, leaving more relaxed attention available for the unexpected dramas of surrounding people and other vehicles. Confidence grows. Strains lessen, while driving sometimes

FULL REMOVABLE DENTURES

becomes a welcome challenge as a game of skill and personal pleasure. Eating with dentures can also be fun, enjoyed by people as another life trial controlled. And just as nervous impatient automobile drivers harass frustrating themselves to disaster, so can denture drivers.

DENTURE ACTION ANALYSIS

Dentures can deliver actions of biting, chewing and drinking. Let's analyse each. Full removable dentures are limited by lack of any attachment to the inner skeletal frame that activates them. They only rest in place on the soft tissues that support them. They may have some vacuum like adherence, from accurate moist sealing contact with their soft inner tissues.

DENTURE BITING ∾ Biting with full removable upper and lower dentures requires education and experience. A course follows here. Some learn faster than others. Corn can be bitten from cobs and apple through skin and pulp from fruit. Let's see how. As biters close front teeth together, dentures tend to rotate, about the forward jaw ridges like a lever, so that lower dentures in back may flip up out, and upper dentures down. Denturers without special skills should never pull food forward holding, tearing off from the bitten piece. This could jerk the apparatus from its jaws. Biting into apples or other such, is best accomplished by pushing the food with the holding hand, somewhat back into the front teeth, coordinated with the dentures closing. Both actions combine, creating resultant forces tending to seat each denture firmly. The lower as though grasped between fingers and forced down back, the uppers as if held and pushed backwards up.

Some find biting simpler, inserting their food a little to the side. Any who try may like twisting their eaten things off. At the same time, in a short time, or a longer time, teeth apparatus operators also should learn to tighten their tongues, rigidly placed directed forcefully at inner denture locations felt loosening, supplying invisible needed stabilization at that spot. As these techniques are mastered, simultaneously lip and cheek muscles around the dentures, should learn to do their bits, exerting opposing coordinated controls from outside. Adroit denturers are skilled lip cheek maneuvering tongueteers. It can all be done by those who really try, though some take longer than others. The human mind learning, can coordinate all these mouthing muscles to control removable dentures, like autogyros designed by human minds give signals, releasing forces to balancing control surfaces, for stability of ships crossing stormy seas and aircraft scanning skys.

TEETH TEETH TEETH

Some denturers do all their biting outside their mouths, using knives with firming forks against tabled food plates, satisfied with slicing proper sized pieces for simpler service to their dental apparatus. All these ways get food inside for chewing.

DENTURE CHEWING ∾ Now chewing. Another word for chew is masticate. Though meaning the same it sounds strange saying, "masticating the rag" or "masticate tobacco." Here we're concerned with the grinding pulverization of food as done by back teeth, so smaller particles can be tasted better, and more thoroughly penetrated by digestive juices for better nutritive absorption.

While chewing with natural rooted teeth is usually single sided, with removable dentures it often doesn't work that way. When a denturer chews on one side that side's soft tissues beneath yield depressing, deflecting the rigid denture from its jaw position of the other side. Patients sense such loss of control with fearful feelings of insecurity. If the tongue is thrust to stabilize the loosening side, food squeezed from between the teeth is lost from handling control. If the tongue returns for food control denture control is dangered. No tonguers can wag fast enough from right to left, side to side. A few expert manipulators manage with control, combinations of their own, though most denture users shouldn't expect to chew as before. Many learn to use both right and left sides at the same time. The lower jaw is raised rather parallel to the upper, so both sides back teeth meet together while the jaw swings sideways if desired. For some it's easier more directly up and down. At the same time the tongue learns to flatten thin spreading wider, distributing the chewed ground food to both sides inside, while beyond the teeth outside both cheeks cooperate. When the food is finally finely ground, all join moving it back to the throat for swallow.

DENTURE DRINKING ∾ Some denturers sometimes have drinking difficulties completely unrelated to alchoholism. Their lips learn to help hold their dentures by inward exertion, which is rather practical for most of denturers functional duties. When those same lips purse out to sip liquids, leaving their dentures less of that acquired feature of control, some people get awkwardly involved. There are lip, teeth, tongue training practices, that can solve the problem.

Though their lips come closer to purse towards water tea coffee or other liquids, most people sip with their teeth apart. It's natural tendency to separate them opening, for sucking in air to sip with. They're never far apart since their surrounding lips must meet. The denture drinking difficulty answer, is to start with teeth kept closed together. Sipping

TEETH TEETH TEETH

through closed teeth is easy, and the teeth aren't far from where they ordinarily would be. This soon becomes so satisfactory, the tongue with its owner unaware often learns to hold dentures for drinking while their teeth even open a little. It really does'nt matter, either way will do.

All these eat action things seemingly awkwardly difficult at first, with practice can be done indiscernibly.

DENTURE DIFFICULTIES

With teeth naturally rooted inside jawbone ridges, longer broader roots are best, though even the smallest root to bone attachments comfortably carry their chewing loads. When only gum covered jaws remain to support and stabilize unattached removable dentures, it is their size, shape, and surface conditions that count. Biting chewing forces contain components, vertically up and down and horizontally side to side. Denture ridges shaped best to resist such forces, support stabilizing dentures best.

The horseshoe shaped jaw arch form itself, tends to satisfy stability. If jaws also closed across in the back, completely encircling like a ring with an added rear ridge of teeth, such dentures would be easier to control if people weren't afraid of biting their tongues off. Our teeth arches open in back being simpler to insert, more easily slip forward out.

Like the wide top of the Great Wall of China men could march on, broader jaw ridges have wider areas to withstand vertical chew loads. Sharp narrow ridges concentrate forces, and are more easily hurt. Taller ridges like high walls, supply larger side denture flanges to grip them better, resisting side dislodging chewing movements like seated riders gripping horses backs between their legs. Some people are lucky, like heirs of millionaires. Some patients luckily inherit, or for other reasons have ideal denture foundations, so their dentures are easier to operate. Others through fates misfortunes or dental neglect have poor denture ridges. They may be flat with little or no wall to grip. They may have flabbly gums over their bones, so biting squishes their dentures away. Operating dentures over degenerated jaws is difficult.

Lower dentures suffer added disadvantage. Their total supporting area is smaller, an amount occupied by the tongue. And that tongue closely passing through their middle actively moves, postage stamp licking, lip moistening, wagging, laughing, talking, swallowing. And people sometimes have difficulty within their small confined mouths, learning to use the tongue to stabilize a denture one place, while avoiding dislodging interferences at others. I don't think tongues cleverly operative as they are, realizing their special importance will ever organize, unite and strike, against the very dentures that feed them.

TEETH TEETH TEETH

Sometimes dentures loosen temporarily though their size doesn't change. Mouth flesh expands and contracts even within a single day. Head colds sometimes swell. Heat, dry thirsty weather, and water elimination drugs used in weight reduction therapy, can cause shrinkage. Certain kidney and heart ailments more common in older people retains urine, expanding the bodies tissues also in the mouth.

Even properly made dentures which shouldn't, may sometimes clack during talking and at other odd times. Patient with denture manipulation difficulties, without realizing discover a way to stabilize each, upper up, lower down, by bringing their jaws together. After a while it's hard to resist, and teeth closing together become a subconscious denture realignment technique. Some obviously purse lips and cheeks for similar control, while observers outside are unaware of their inside coordinating maneuvering tongues.

DENTURE ACCESSORIES

Many things have been tried. Dentures have been made using compression springs between them, to help keep uppers up. Powerful miniature magnets have been tried, with opposing poles in each side of each denture, for similar purpose. Powerful miniature magnets located for pole attraction have been surgically inserted inside jawbones, beneath flesh opened and healed, for attracting other magnets in dentures to hold them in place. Some have been helped by dentures that have tiny surgical metal alloy buttons, projecting from the dentures tissue side, that snap into small holes surgically sliced in their gums. The holes heal around holding the appliances painlessly in place. They need regular removal for cleaning and snapping back for use. Small suction cups have been used. In infrequent cases people are allergic to particular denture materials. Sometimes nothings seems to help people with removable denture problems. Dentists using all methods available are still sometimes limited by inadequate mouth anatomy foundations. Sometimes patients involve in psychological factors, subconsciously fighting their dentures as some parents unfortunately reject an unwanted child. Some cases seem impossible to satisfy.

AN INTERESTING CASE

Gypsy Rose Lee, famous burlesque stripper queen with other talents, in her autobiographical memoir "Gypsy," Harper Bros. & Dell Pub. Co. N.Y. NY, writes interesting reading. Several relate to dentistry. Gypsy tells of being admired by gangster racketeer Maxey Gordon who generously had her front teeth jacketed. Many have more than one sided personalities.

Maxey was also sort of a modern Robin Hood. He put a poor boy through dental school on to becoming Maxey Gordon's own dentist. Gypsy also tells of friendship and performing with celebrity comedienne Fanny Brice. Fanny had a toothless mouth problem. Though frugal she had three sets of full removable dentures. One was for performance in the theatre which Fanny called her funny face teeth. One was for eating, she called them her choppers. Her favorite set, she called gentile teeth for their dentist maker who was Irish. Fanny said, "I can't eat with the funny face job, I can't make faces with the choppers and all I can do with the Gentile set is look pretty."

DENTURE MAKING TEETHLESS TIME

Most full dentures made are a new set, replacing an old set, outworn being discarded or sentimentally set aside, often with older denture relations, in a drawer for retirement. Many full dentures made as the patients first are fit to the jaws after a long period without teeth, or a minimum of a month or so allowed for healing after the last remaining teeth are removed. During this time the patient is toothless, often in hiding, until the dentist feels healing progressed to such extent the jaws are ready for dentures.

OUT WITH THE OLD   IN WITH THE NEW
IMMEDIATE DENTURES

Immediate dentures are inserted immediately after the teeth they replace are removed. There's no time without teeth. During a single visit, under painless anesthesia, diseased ugly teeth are removed and dentures with attractive new teeth replacing those and others already missing are put in the mouth. It's almost as though the dentist were a sleight of hand artist holding new dentures in his left hand hidden, while his right extracts the teeth, then PRESTO the hand is quicker than the eye, and SWITCH dentures immediately appear in the mouth. Here's how it's done. It isn't magic, nothing really is, it only seems that way. It's accomplished by modern dentistry coordinated in the office and laboratory.

The dentist evaluates his patients dental and physical condition. Mouth models are made. In some cases more teeth need removal than the patient should endure at one time. If so, back teeth are extracted first. Front teeth are left for the denture insertion appointment, so patients can face themselves and others, during the time the dentures are being made.

The dentist studying X-rays and models, can predict rather accurately the tissue response to extraction surgery, and the jaw shape after healing. He

17

plans the final extraction surgery. In the dental laboratory, the surgery planned for the patient is preceded by similar surgery on the plaster models of his jaws. First the plaster teeth are cut off as they later will be extracted. Then model material around the teeth is trimmed, as felt needed to shape the patient's tissues for proper jaw denture form. The dentures are made to fit these laboratory operated models. They will fit the jaws later surgically prepared like the models. A thin transparent plastic template may also be made to fit the model if needed, as a guide for later teeth extraction surgery.

If desired the jaw models are duplicated, and using one with its remaining teeth as a guide, the dentures are made matching the teeth as they were before extraction.

THE MAGIC APPOINTMENT ∾ At the final teeth extraction appointment, the operated mouth model and transparent template are available for surgical reference, with the completed denture ready for insertion. Painlessly the diseased teeth are removed. If in doubt the surgeon checks using the template until the jaw is properly formed. Tissues are sutured and medicated and the new dentures inserted immediately. The patient who fearfully arrived with ugly diseased teeth, though perhaps a bit bewildered, smiles seeing their new teethed self and leaves proud.

AFTERCARE ∾ Surgical aftercare instructions and medication are given. Immediate dentures should not be removed for at least the first full day or as advised by the dentist. As with any surgery the tissues may swell, and patients find dentures first taken out at home, painful to replace. If necessary they're removed and inserted by the doctor during post operative examination treatments. With healing the sutures are removed.

Art Belzer whose father was a Connecticut dentist, is a dedicated dental technician with special interest in full dentures. Art told me of a Bridgeport farmer who had an upper immediate denture inserted, and disregarding instructions failed to return until a year later. He had never removed his denture. His mouth smelled, his face swelled, and he hurt. He said he'd had no trouble at all, didn't think he need bother removing the denture since it hadn't bothered him until recently. Now he wanted to but couldn't get it out. The denture seemed grown adhered to its infected jaw beneath. Under anesthetics, cut into small sections, each piece was pried, torn peeled from the tissues. After healing another was made.

Since jaw regions where teeth have recently been removed shrink radically at first, immediate dentures usually need refitting sooner than dentures made over long teethless time healed-gum-covered jaws.

TEETH TEETH TEETH

ADHERENT POWDERS & PASTES

Dentures properly made from perfect impressions fit their jaws. With passing time the snug fit may become less satisfactory. It's rarely caused by the denture. Modern denture materials change little. Some don't change at all. Their jaws within slowly shrink from original form. As denture control skills increase, early misfit is seldom discernible. With continued shrinkage the dentures eventually loosen. Some denture wearers like filling the voids with Adhering Powders or Pastes. They're different forms of similar substances. Some prefer one over the other. Some dislike the feel of any. Most denture adherents are made of natural colloidal gum exudates like acacia, karaya, and tragacanth, of plants from India and adjacent areas. Colors and flavors are added. The same substances are used as pharmaceutical pill binders.

Each should be applied according to its instructions. In place they swell with mouth moisture, forming a mucilaginous gel, filling small spaces helping dentures stick to jaws. Some people acquire sensitivity to·their continued use, needing dental attention. Adherents may help but won't substitute for a proper fit. Eventually the jaws may shrink to such extent powders and pastes are inadequate, and the denture needs refitting or replacement.

DAILY DENTURE CARES

Dentures may be removed for rest as need is felt. People who feel more comfortable with their dentures constant presence, probably experience better tissue tolerance and need removing them less. General professional attitude is that all should have some edentulous, or toothless periods without dentures, to provide periodic unrestrained blood circulation. Sleeping without dentures is an ideal way, though some feel more secure with them, horrified at the thought of awakening toothless with Prince or Princess Charming.

Physical gymnastics strengthens jaws like lifting weights builds muscles. With teeth lost for toothbrushing, for those with weak toothless gums, finger gum massage is good. Stimulation of gums with as stiff a brush as won't bruise toughens and cleans. Bare jaw chewing gum chewing, hard bread and other foods, help more tastefully. Some dentists recommend regular home gum exercises with dental chewing bags designed for the purpose.

Don't borrow your dog's rubber bone, If you like it get one of your own. Embarrassment shouldn't bother you, Pets have chewed owners dentures too, An Australian's might've been by kangaroo, Yours perhaps in a zoo.

TEETH TEETH TEETH

Adenturers advantage unavailable to rooted toothers, is the ability to brush their teeth while whistling. Dentures should be cleaned as often as needed to keep them clean, inside and out. Brushing with soap or detergents will do. Denture cleansers used as instructed, are usually more ideally compounded for the job. Debris consists of food, tobacco stains, and salivary deposits, thickening if neglected. Accumulations inside affect the fit, creating a soreness irritation causing jaw tissue shrinkage. Scraping with hard instruments could damage the denture. Dentures should be scrubbed over water where if dropped they won't break. When not worn some should be stored in water. Most modern denture materials are extremely inert, so outside the mouth it doesn't matter whether they're wet or dry. The dentist can tell. For ideal care, troubled or not, dentures and jaws should be examined yearly or at advised periods.

DENTURE VARIATIONS

ROOFLESS UPPER DENTURES ∾ Lower removable dentures are horseshoe shaped, fitting over their lower jaw, curved in front, open in back, extending around each side of the tongue. Upper dentures have a similarly shaped supporting ridge. They're usually not open, but closed on top by a domelike roof covering the upper palate. They're not always made that way. Sometimes upper dentures can be made leaving the palate uncovered, open towards the back like lowers. These are called Roofless or horseshoe uppers. Some people get more of a kick wearing them. They provide more tongue space, taste, direct food feelings and temperatures through the exposed upper palate, increasing eating pleasure.

Unfortunately roofless upper dentures can't be controlled by some, since they embrace less jaw. They're more easily dislodged while riding galloping horses. They can only be made when the upper jaw is favorably formed for substantial denture support foundation. Experienced denturers capable of using both and have tried, prefer their upper dentures open.

METAL BASE DENTURES ∾ Almost all upper and lower removable dentures contain teeth in a base of natural looking pink plastic, and serve well that way. They weren't always made that way. Denture bases used to be made of hard dark red rubber. Before plastics and rubber were invented, for the few people that could afford them, denture bases were sometimes made of solid gold which fit the jaws and held the teeth. Gold dentures had a stylish gleam at the time. Like all metals they had advantage of temperature conductivity, so hot and cold foods could be better enjoyed. Gold, an especially heavy metal, has distinct disadvantage as bases for upper dentures. The force of gravity pulls them down. Denture wearers shouldn't blame Sir Isaac Newton, he only discovered the laws of gravity. Of course gravity will help gold upper dentures stay in place for acrobats hanging by their feet. It is of no significance to astronauts in weightless space. Metal in dentures may be slightly helpful gravitationally, holding lowers down.

Modern full removable denture bases are rarely made entirely of metal, especially for the large areas of upper jaws. They are sometimes made combining natural looking plastic where appearance is important, and metal in invisible places, where its characteristics of strength and heat transfer help. Most frequently, a lightweight inexpensive stainless chrome steel surgical alloy is used. It is lighter than gold, far less expensive and heavier than plastic. Dentures with metal structures are less likely to break. As time passes and jaws shrink, it may be more difficult and costly to refit the metal surfaces of denture bases.

Some people with allergic sensitivity to plastics find metal bases more satisfactory. Dental research may be able to adapt industrial technique, for applying micro thin metal, electro-plated coatings to plastics for use in dentures.

REFITTING, RELINING FULL REMOVABLE DENTURES

Bone used less will normally atrophy, experiencing a loss of substance, shrinking in size. Older less active people for that reason and others shorten in height. Jaws without teeth heal shrinking while filling their vacant root sockets, and continue shrinking. Dentures made that fit at first with continued use loosen. The significant change isn't the dentures. Modern denture materials hardly change at all. Loosening of dentures is caused by shrinking jaws inside them. Refitting removable dentures consists of relining, or adding an inner lining layer of denture material, refilling the tissue shrunken vacant spaces.

To reline a denture properly, it must be located in the exact mouth position where it chewed before its supporting tissues shrunk. In this place the shrunken space is properly located for filling, to fit the new jaw surface. While relining toothless areas of partial dentures, the dentists can position the denture accurately by clasping its metal clasps as usually used, to the natural remaining teeth that support it. Refitting full removable dentures to shrunken jaws is more complex, since full dentures have no precise hard locating devices relating them to their jaws.

RELINE CAUTIONS ∞ For best results dentures should be relined when their supporting tissues are healthy. For abused tissues to recover

FULL REMOVABLE DENTURES

from misfit denture damage, they should be kept from the mouth a day or more before the reline appointment or as instructed by the dentist, and brought pocketed or pursed. Head colds can cause mouth tissues to swell, so appointments should be postponed until recovery.

TWO RELINE METHODS ∾ Two most popular reline methods are described.

The Mouth Mold Method relines dentures in a single seated appointment. The shrunken jaw itself is used for molding the reline. The dentures inner surface is immaculately cleaned. A plastic mix is made from fine pink powder called polymer and clear liquid monomer. Mouth mold plastics harden within room and mouth temperatures and pressures. On contact powder and liquid start chemically combining, experiencing a process called polymerization, during which molecules of each integrate hardening in a short time. As the mix thickens the dentist distributes an excess inside the denture. The patients mouth may be coated with a thin film of protective grease, against possibility of slight temporary smarting, while the plastic cures.

The doctor places the loaded denture into the mouth. With knowledge of static and dynamic head-jaw anatomy, he guides the denture to its jaw as excess plastic squeezes from around edges. The dentist studies the patients open-closing mouth movements. He controls the jaw towards closure, directing its relative position to the opposite jaw. When satisfied with the jaws proper denture relation, the patient is asked to keep closed. The reline plastic filling the shrunken void may be felt warming as it cures hard, bonded to the denture, fitting the jaw. The denture is removed.

Excess plastic is ground off, rough surfaces polished, and the denture inserted for comfortable eating action. Mouth mold relines serve well, though their materials are not quite as densely inert as plastics pressure molded in the laboratory.

The Laboratory Mold Method provides more substantial relines. Two separate dental appointments are needed between which the denture is laboratory processed. At the first appointment an impression material is mixed, placed into the denture which is then located in the mouth. As the jaws are guided to position the impression material fills shrunken voids soon hardening. The denture with attached impression is removed and the patient leaves for home, teethless, or if lucky to have one wearing another denture.

In the laboratory a two part mold is made of the denture with its impression. The mold is opened and the impression material is carefully

FULL REMOVABLE DENTURES

removed. A plastic mix is placed inside the denture in the mold. The mold is closed under high pressure. The reline plastic accurately fills the void bonded to the denture. Sometimes plastic is pressure injected into the mold. After an appropriate curing period the mold is opened, the denture removed, irregularities trimmed and polished. At the next appointment the denture is inserted.

Laboratory processing leaves patients without extra dentures dentureless, while the work is done. Close dental office-laboratory coordination, can sometimes do relines in a day. The added laboratory procedures add to the cost.

For those who can afford them an extra set of dentures will insure against the toothless time, or accidental inconvenience of loss or damage.

A single denture sometimes serves many. Tahitians limited to poi, native taro root starchy diet, have terrible teeth. Many lose all at early ages. A patient told me of having his date with a girl in Tahiti rescheduled, while she awaited her turn of the shared use of the family single denture set, made to approximately fit every one of its wearers.

TIME FOR A CHANGE

Refitting relining renews dentures, for fast shrinking jaws this sometimes lasts less than a year. In most mouths relines last years, sometimes as much as many more. In time more refit relines may be needed. In time the aging jaws shrinking surface is accompanied by changes in their moving muscles, and other bone changes at the skulls jaw-head hinging joint. These may be so substantial, original denture fitting relations cannot be restored within denture relining limits. Proper chewing can only be accomplished with a new set of dentures.

DO IT YOURSELF RELINES

There are varieties of home kits and materials, advertised in newspapers and magazines, available on store shelves for denture relining by patients at home, for low cost. It may be practical for some expert at fixing their own leaky plumbing, but I advise against home do-it-yourself relining. I will describe two types. One consists of thin pink sheets shaped to fit either upper or lower dentures. The material is wax impregnated loosely woven gauze sheet. The sheet is adapted in the denture, then inserted into the mouth. Warm tissues soften the wax, and as the fibers slip yielding, the sheet conforms to the jaw, helping fill the shrunken voids. The wax flows to some extent into spaces where needed, and may give the patient a feeling of security. In some cases the material may have some limited value. It could cause serious trouble. Continued prolonged wax contact, under pressure of use may sensitize some peoples delicate tissues. The wax is not firmly fixed to the denture base, though it adheres somewhat by friction. In use in time it may slowly drag flow, changing the bite relation. At the same time the gauze fibers sometimes gather into concentrated masses that may ulcerate soft tissues, causing premature bone loss.

Another type consists of a kit containing powder and liquid similar to that used by dentists for mouth molded relines. Brief instructions and a small piece of sandpaper for adjustments are included. Relining dentures is sometimes complicated. Professional courses are studied by dentists on the subject. The kit material is good. Its application is critical. I myself a dentist luckily have my own good teeth and don't wear dentures. I have taken advanced denture training and successfully made dentures and relines for many. Based on all my experience, if I were to reline dentures I wore, I feel I could do it successfully, but would need use of all my knowledge and acquired skill. It is unlikely that most patients could reline their own dentures properly. They can easily mix the material as told and put it in. After hardening in the mouth the fit itself will be tighter with a sense of immediate security. It is rather unlikely that the patient would properly relate the bite, while hardening took place. An improper bite relation can cause serious damage. Once improperly relined, correction can be extremely difficult even by a dentist.

Some reline kit manufacturers promise to refund patients money if dissatisfied. They cannot restore the natural tissue damage and loss.

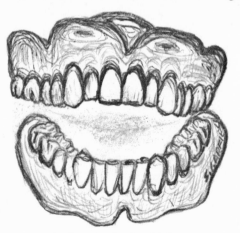

*Im in search of a doctor
to make a less-misfit person
for ME*

TEETH TEETH TEETH

322

18

NUTRITION

Man today both gathers and produces food. Most animals through search or seizure, find collect and gather food in the range they roam. Probably the only other living creatures that produce foods are certain tiny insects. An ant, Atta, and a termite, Nasa Termites, grow fungi in underground narrow canal gardens they fertilize with organic debris. Pastoral ants capture and enslave aphids grazed like cows, on plant leaves and stems, from whose bodies they milk a honeydew for food. Bees collect nectar which they process to honey and store for food.

Early man only gathered or collected food. He ate when hungry and could get it, berries, fruits, roots, insects, worms, eggs, turtles. Learning to use clubs he captured rats and lizards eating them raw. Sometimes alive. Man is the only animal that cooks food. Many other animals prefer cooked food when they can get it.

Probably through lightning or other accidental fire, burnt animals were found by men who tasted and liked them. Charles Lambs' "Dissertation Upon Roast Pig" gives his delightful explanation. In ancient, ancient China, Ho-Ti left his son Bo-Ho watching their home while he went searching for food. Bo-Ho playing with fire, accidentally burnt their house including several young pig pets. In anguish he touched his personal favorite burning his fingers. Bringing them to his lips, Bo-Ho became the first person to taste the delicacies of roast pork. There was a spreading epidemic of fires burning down houses with pigs. Chopsticks and soy sauce came later.

At first finding food was a factor of fortune. Agricultural methods, preservatives, and storage, were unknown. In good weather, plants animals and man flourished and multiplied. Severe winters and drought caused starvation and famines. Sometimes extreme changes of temperature, wind, and moisture, brought insects and vermin beyond control with pestilence and scourges of disease and plague. Travel and transport had not been developed. Some people enjoyed overabundance and waste, unavailable to other hungry starving on opposite sides of seas and mountains.

INSECT EATING ∾ Early man with little choice, took foods available to him. Because their size, shape, color, and noticed actions of motion, caught his attention like lures do fish, insects were common diet and quite

TEETH TEETH TEETH

I	II
Boiled Cod with Snail Sauce	Snail Soup
Wasp Grubs fried in the comb	Fried Sole with Woodlouse Sauce
Moth sautés in Butter	Curried Cockchafers
Braised Beef with Caterpillars	Chicken Fricassée with Chrysalids
Carrots with Wireworm Sauce	Boiled Mutton with Wirworm Sauce
Gooseberry Cream with Sawflies	Ducklings with Green Peas
Deviled Chafer Grubs	Cauliflower garnished with Caterpillars
Stag Beetle Larvae on Toast	Moths on Toast

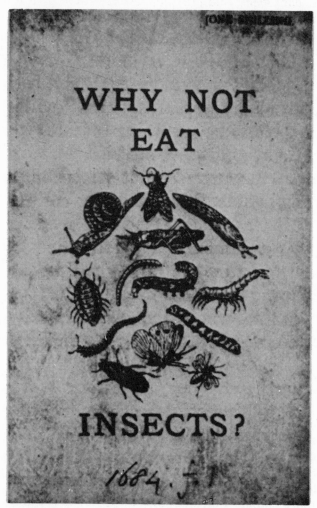

Cover and two insect menus from a serious 99 page booklet by V.M. Holt published in London, England 1885. Holt's motto was "The insects eat up every blessed thing that do grow and us farmers starve. Well, eat them and grow fat." His book cover includes drawings of a snail and slug which may also be repugnant to some but are molluscs not insects.

from "INSECTS AS HUMAN FOOD" a scientific text by F.S. Bodenheimer of Hebrew University, Jerusalem: 1951, W. Junk Publishers, The Hague, Netherlands

TEETH TEETH TEETH

acceptable. In the Bible in addition to Matt, 6:11 "Give us this day our daily bread," we find in the Old Testament, Leviticus, XL:22 "And the Lord spoke--saying unto them--even of these of them ye may eat; the locust after his kind,--and the beetle after his kind, and the grasshopper after his kind." In parts of the highly civilized world today, canned chocolate covered ants, baby bees, and grasshoppers are eaten by a few curious. In parts of Africa today, insects are a prominent part of native diet. In Oaxaca Mexico, I saw large heaping trays of caterpillars, larvae and grubs, alive raw and roasted, for sale in open public markets. They tasted good to me. On the street I was offered what looked like earthworms for sale by a native Indian. In South America forest tribes eat ants, using knowledge of the little things ignorant instincts. They insert one end of a stick into an ant hill hole and the other in their mouth. Disturbed ants leave their nest, walking up the stick into the mouth of the human ant eater. For those repulsed at thought of eating insects, I call attention to the many among them that enjoy eating honey. Every particle of honey ever eaten, has been manufactured in the tiny stomachs of honeybee insects, regurgitated in the nest, and manipulated being worked over by the miniature mouth parts of young worker house bees.

Scientific analysis has found insects high in food value, containing fats, proteins, vitamins and minerals. Some insect eater natives have excellent teeth, the teeth of some are poor. For natives with inadequate other foods insect bodies though offensive to some of us, like eating whole sardines does supply variety of dietary needs, and is valuable to general and dental health. The military forces of modern nations teach their militia to eat insects in emergency if available.

CANNIBALISM ∾ Insect eating is called Entomophagy. Cannibalism is Anthropophagy. Among the few cannibals that exist today the practice is a sacred rite, believing the eater acquires the soul or powers of his victim. People eating people was once ordinary. Stone Age Man caves have been found containing broken and cut human bones, indicating they ate each other for food. Homer the Greek in his Iliad and Odyssey of the period 800 years before Christ, describes human flesh among other food varieties like beef and fowl and fish. Like other young animals, children were considered more choice. For thousands of years humans found each other tasty. It was not until about 800 years after Christ that Charlemagne, first Emperor of the Holy Roman Empire, found cannibalism so widespread through Europe he passed a law against it. This helped only to limited extent. During the 11th to 13th century, Christian Military Crusades for recapturing the Holy Lands from Moslems, prisoners were roasted and

TEETH TEETH TEETH

eaten. Marco Polo the Venetian explorer told of people eating others in Asia and China. Among Fiji Islanders cannibalism of relatives was common. I don't know about mothers-in-law. Twentieth Century war prison camp stories even tell of cannibalism among our civilized selves. Human flesh probably has value approximating beef.

MODERN DIET

In today's world of wealth for more than a few, and much for many, quite a bit is spent for swift flight to other sides of the earth, where unfortunates live that hardly have pennies for food. Their inadequate diet yields poor general and dental health. The same rapid transport delivers edibles of all kinds from everywhere. Part of my research for this chapter led me to several large food shops with a pad and pen for notes. From my eye sides I could see several uneasy employees, concerned with who I might be. Modern markets make varieties available with little concern for seasons. Time was when fruits and fish were identified with weather, and people waited for watermelon. In modern society today almost anything can be had anytime. King crab legs flown from Alaska. Papayas and mangoes from tropics. Oriental food if desired. Beef, pork, lamb, seafoods and fowl. Vegetables, fruits, berries and nuts, in and out of the local season. Exotic cheeses, candies, drinks and delicatessens from over the world. Vitamins for those who aren't sure. With all this, people that get these things and their teeth, are healthier than people used to be, but far from perfect.

DIET SCIENCE ∾ The science of diet is new. Only as recently as 1930 had sufficient knowledge accumulated, for standards of nutritional needs to be established for the first time, by the U.S. Dept. of Agriculture and the League of Nations. Dietary research and knowledge progresses constantly. The balanced diet of proteins, fats, carbohydrates, calcium, phosphorus, other minerals and vitamins, as suggested by the medical dental professions, though they may include and omit yet unknown excesses and inadequacies is best. Specific diets prescribed for specific diseases of the body or teeth should be followed.

TOOTH DECAY AND DIET ∾ The exact cause of caries or tooth decay, is not known yet. Researchers have many theories. Among any given group of people there are differences between individuals in their natural resistance to decay. The reasons are difficult to determine. The exact constituents of the same food substances, vary with areas and times. It is difficult to subject humans to studies requiring carefully controlled food consumption and mouth hygiene. Even investigations among isolated primitive groups in different parts of the world have not established definite conclusions.

Studies of certain areas, where for limited periods in addition to malnutrition a scarcity of sugar existed, has shown a lower incidence of caries than in the United States. During World War II several involved nations, England, Norway, Sweden and Germany, suffered an almost complete loss of refined sugars and starches. Comparisons of the caries incidence, during the prior, war, and post war periods, have been made. Dental research revealed that children of the period without sugar, though they also suffered other dietary disadvantages, had less decay than those of the more sweet satisfying earlier and later times.

Dental experimentation has been done with hamsters, rats, dogs, monkeys and other apes. In several projects, two same animal groups were fed identical well balanced diets plus excessive sugar, in two different ways. One group was permitted to feed themselves as usual with their mouth. The other group was hand fed the same food, through an inserted tube avoiding teeth touch, delivering its contents for digestion directly into the animals stomachs. After the experimental period both groups experienced similar general health. The teeth of the tube fed showed little decay. The self mouth fed animals teeth suffered severely.

Among other microscopic parasites that live in the human mouth, there is a germ called Lactobacillus acidophilus (lac means milk, bacillus germ, acic acid, philus loving). Lactobacilus is frequently found in the normal vagina, intestines, and the vicinity of teeth. Lactobacilli (baccilli is plural for bacillus or germ), in the intestine are harmless, and increase tremendously when milk or its products are eaten. They may even help digestion. Certain strains of lactobacilli are important in the dairy industry, where they help convert milk to other related foods. Lactobacilli multiply rapidly in an environment of refined sugars and starches, which they ferment to lactic acid and in which they reproduce even more rapidly. In the mouth lactobacilli are especially numerous in areas of decay, and unclean tooth crevices, and in the plaque layers of debris which adheres to teeth. There is evidence that the acid produced by lactobacilli and other organisms break down calcium, which is the basic inorganic structural component of teeth. Electron microscopy has shown, that acid decalcified areas of teeth expose certain organic binding substances of teeth to further destruction or decay by germs. The intimate nature of these mouth, teeth, food, bacterial, biological chemistries, are not all known. Theories concerning them differ. Some peoples teeth suffer little damage despite excess sugars and minimum care, they seem to resist decay.

TEETH TEETH TEETH

FLUORINE

Fluorine is a chemical element related to chlorine and iodine. It is extremely active, combining with other elements. Never found pure in nature, fluorine is always found combined or compounded with other elements. The fluorine itself of any compound is always identical, the same in whatever compound it may exist. There is only one kind of fluorine. Combinations of fluorine with other substances are called fluorides. In high concentrations fluorine compounds are poisonous, used to kill rats. In minute trace amounts fluorine is valuable and may be necessary to life. It is found in all plants and animals, and in small quantities is always a constituent of human bones and teeth. It is found in all foods. Most vegetables, meats, cereals and fruits contain .2 to .3 of one part per million (p.p.m.) of fluoride. This means two to three tenths of one single part fluoride, in a full million parts of the food. Seafoods contain 5 to 15 p.p.m. and tea leaves as much as 75 to 100 parts per million.

FLUORINE IN WATER ∾ As early as 1874 Erhardt suggested fluorine was important to teeth. In those days fluorine or fluoride in water wasn't thought of. Whole grain cereals like wheat have substantial fluorine in their outer hulls. This is lost when the grain is refined to white flour. In 1892 Chrichton Brown recommended bread be made of whole wheat and other whole grains rather than new refined flours being introduced. He too felt fluorine was valuable to teeth. There was little interest at the time. In 1914 Cook associated differences in drinking water with differences in the rate of tooth decay, though he was unaware of fluorides in water as a factor. In 1916 mottled enamel patches were described as occurring in teeth of particular geographic regions. An unknown agent seemed to be in the water supply. In 1928 Bunting reported children born and raised in Minonk, Illinois, had fewer cavities than children who came to Minonk after their teeth had developed. He didn't know why. It was later found Minonk water contained 2.5 p.p.m. of fluoride. In 1930 it was realized mottled enamel teeth resulted from an excess of fluoride, and that while such teeth were less attractive, they were far more resistant to caries or tooth decay.

Research established a minimum of 1 part per million fluoride in water as satisfactory. At 2.5 p.p.m. mottled enamel may start to appear in some mouths though such teeth are stronger. At levels of 8 and more p.p.m. a high percentage of people growing in such areas have mottled teeth. Such teeth though less attractive are especially stronger.

Findings that teeth from drinking water areas with 1 and more p.p.m. fluoride have far less decay has been confirmed by investigators in the U.S., Argentina, Canada, England, South Africa, Italy, Greece, Hungary and Soviet Ukraine. The U. S. Public Health Service coordinated with various low fluoride communities to add fluoride, bringing the concentration up to 1 p.p.m. or more. Within reasonable time the caries frequency dropped fifty per cent, compared with the prefluoridated period and nearby communities still using low fluoride water.

FLUORIDATION ∾ For fluoridation, fluorine is added to water in the form of sodium fluoride which is extremely soluble. In nature, fluorine finds its way into waters by the dissolving of calcium fluoride, a prime ingredient of the mineral fluoriite, over large areas of which natural waters flow to fill reservoirs. The fluorine in calcium fluoride or fluorite or sodium fluoride or any fluorine compound is identical. Calcium fluoride is extremely insoluble, that is why through the ages of man it is still around, slowly dissolving supplying fluorine to natural water. If calcium fluoride were used as a preferred natural water additive, tons would be constantly needed by truckload, and its bulk would block the waters. Sodium fluoride because of its ready solubility, is easily controlled in small amounts and cheap. The traces of sodium or calcium in the water with the fluorides are rather unimportant. They are both available in sufficient quantities in other foods.

FLUORINE CONCERN ∾ There was concern whether high fluoride diet that helped teeth might harm other parts of the body. In 1943 two similar small communities, Bartlett and Cameron Texas, 30 miles apart were selected for a survey. Bartlett water had 8 p.p.m. fluoride, Cameron's practically none. Studies were made of 237 typical residents, each had lived in either town at least fifteen previous years. They were 15 to 68 years of age. Bartlett supplied 116 of whom 57.8 per cent were over 55 years old. Cameron 121, with 47.2 per cent over 55. All were throughly examined by physicians. It is difficult to get cooperative human subjects for prolonged testing. Ten years later, 1953, all available were examined again. There was no significant difference in general systemic health between Bartlett and Cameron residents. Many younger from Bartlett had mottled healthier teeth. Among Cameron's people there was a slightly higher incidence of cardiovascular disease. This may have resulted from other factors unrelated to lower flouride water.

MEDICAL EVIDENCE ∾ Dental initiated interest stimulated medical research. Extensive medical investigation in this country and England indicates fluoride may be valuable to skeletal bone and helpful to the remedy of bone diseases. Detailed man and lower animal, microscopic tissue growth and clinical studies, seem to give substantial proof that even doses far higher than used in water fluoridation cause no affects on the soft organs of the body, and strengthen the crystalline bone structure.

It seems every scientific advance is resisted by certain people who unfailingly appear opposing progress. They ridiculed and criticized Christopher Columbus. Some find fault with fluoridation.

PROGRESSION VERSUS RETROGRESSION ∾ After Edward Jenner in 1796 had discovered and demonstrated, that vaccine from a diseased cow could induce a mild reaction which immunized and prevented smallpox disfiguring scars, blindness, and death, to thousands in virulent epidemics around the world, many of his own medical colleagues and the public ridiculed and attacked him.

In 1847, and several following years not much over a hundred years ago, Ignaz Semmelweis a Hungarian physician in Vienna was discharged from hospitals where he protested what was the usual often high as 30% death rate, for women during childbirth. He rebelled against doctors coming directly from dissection and surgery of dead and diseased bodies, satisfied merely wiping pus putrefaction from their hands, then entering the delicate birth canal to deliver children from pregnant women. Germs weren't thought of much yet, infection an unknown word. Despite Semmelweis' own demonstrated far higher proportion of mother child survival, they laughed using explanations of their own, mocking his demands that doctors throughly wash their own hands.

Typhoid fever is an acute infectious communicable disease. Before antiseptics and antibiotics typhoid fever wiped out entire families, often spreading death through cities, hospitals, and armies. Its path was fled with fear. Typhoid invasion caused greater destruction than attack by powerful enemies. Typhoid is a problem in even modern military expedition where it can be controlled with care. In 1856 Budd suggested typhoid was transmitted through sewage contaminated waters.

Addition of up to a maximum of one part excess chlorine to one million parts of water, has practically eliminated typhoid in regions of such supply. Excess chlorine is a small amount left free as insurance, and unfortunately tasted slightly in the water, after whatever quantity testing found was needed as an antiseptic to kill the infective germs. Chlorination of water was first introduced to the United States in early 1900's. City by city as chlorination was proposed, similar local objections were raised, to that of today's fluoridation. Rare cases of typhoid fever that do occur today, are invariably traced to infected food and water of non-chlorinated private sources or non-chlorinated small communities.

TEETH TEETH TEETH

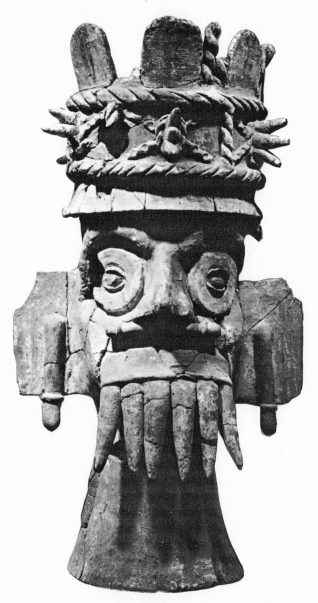

RAIN GOD   **PRECOLUMBIAN**   **MEXICO**
This 49 inch tall terra cotta Mixtec figure found near Vera Cruz symbolized a mythical idol. Teeth from its crown reach to the clouds. Its mouth's up to 7 inch long teeth direct down, to deliver rains of water fertilizing Earth. Harry A. Franklin Gallery, Beverly Hills.

TEETH TEETH TEETH

NATURAL FOODS

From time to time sickness is blamed on modern food. Sickness is imperfection. This fault finding may be an idealistic attitude of people seeking perfection within themselves, relating their disease to outside sources of food provided by others. In the few remaining isolated primitive societies whose only diet is the natural things around them, sickness is common and probably related to demons. Perhaps some sick aboriginals who've heard rumors of far civilations feel sickness is due to the lack of modern foods. Theirs could be. Man's earliest thousands of years old writings, before food processing was even thought of, describe severe and less serious diseases of the body and teeth. Wild animals of primitive jungle and forest are found with teeth decay.

Towards the ending of the 19th century Mummery an Englishman traveled the world for years, studying primitive areas of varied climates and diets, to find why some peoples teeth are better than others. He found caries abundant in most races. Colyer and Sprawson in 1931 London, interpreted Mummery's extensive investigation to indicate diet of primarily animal and fish flesh leaves people freer of decay, than others feeding entirely or largely on vegetable food. During part of the 20th century Price of the U.S. also explored primitive and isolated places, for the affect of nutrition on dental health. His travel included sections of Switzerland, Ireland, far northern Eskimo land, South Sea Islands, Africa, Peru, other places. From all these regions he describes and shows photographs of excellent teeth, which he attributes to natural foods. Often in the same photographed group or family he shows others with very poor teeth, which Price asserts was caused by available refined or unnatural foods eaten by those, but avoided by the others. His stops in each area were limited. Critical analysis might indicate a tendency to favor a preconceived idea. Price visited Lotschenthal, a small confined valley in the Bernese Oberland of Switzerland, where two thousand people at the time lived on diet limited to local products. They were in good health and most had excellent teeth which he related to natural food. Recent investigation in Switzerland disclosed soil and water of Lotschenthal Valley was high in fluorine, while its food was also rich in other demonstrated valuable minerals and vitamins.

Some people have an excessively romantic notion of the values of nature. At one time many sought sunlight as a cure all and God given elixir to health, treasuring its rays, exposing themselves at every chance. It has since been found excess sunlight causes cancers of the skin.

Natural food consists entirely of natural elements. Any food or any other thing made by modern man, except for certain products of recent atomic manipulations, is composed entirely of basic elements originating from nature. No other source of material is available. Food of certain local areas, due to the chance condition of local terrain, may be naturally deficient in substances needed for adequate diet. People whose intake is limited to such sources suffer defects of such inadequacy. Foods of other areas that may naturally happen to be composed of an ideal combination, whatever that may be needed for better health, would contribute to such health of those people who eat them. Medical, dental, and dietary search and science, are finding the food factors needed for health, for use as a guide in selecting and arranging better diets. Sometimes food purveyors in an effort to improve taste sacrifice value. Certain food values are sometimes lost in modern food refinement and processing procedures. Some processing procedures add important needed nutritive values to food. It is claimed some substances added in small amounts to foods as preservatives, may cause some harm to those that eat them. Such additions make food more available to many, and have prevented serious internal infection sicknesses from eating foods that did not have them.

All these defects of modern foods of whatever magnitude they may exist, large or small, are only a small part of the total value man's modern food industry provides. The total value of modern food far surpasses that of the varieties naturally available in any local limited area. This is readily demonstrated by the superior health of modern man, over that of the few primitive groups that still do exist, wherever they may be. Some nutrition factors are still unknown. The problem is complex and occasional errors are made, just as many missiles ours and Russian, failed to reach their targets. Nevertheless all findings combined result in a constant progress, producing tastier better healthier food for man.

Proper Food helps all to Healthy
Body discomfort makes Poor of wealthy

TEETH TEETH TEETH

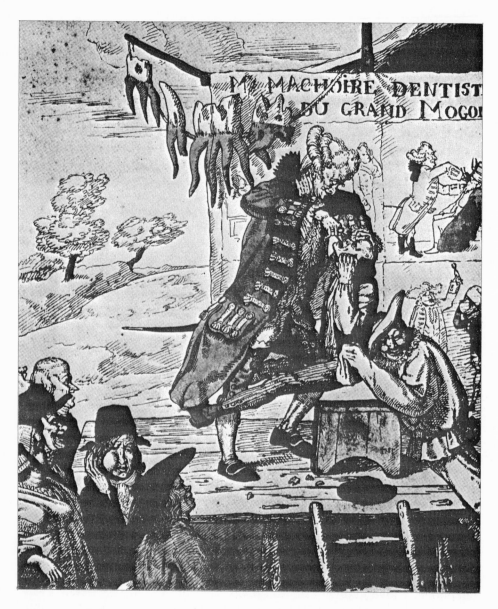

EARLY DENTAL SHOWMAN WITH WAITING PATIENT AUDIENCE

TEETH TEETH TEETH

19

ATWIDOIAS

All The World Including Dental Offices Is A Stage

A play from life in a small representative what could be an unlimited number of acts.

PLACE ∾ Beverly Hills, California, United States of America
SCENE ∾ Mostly Dr. Sydney Garfield's office. An office whose
    prime purpose is the treatment of dental disease.
TIME ∾ Daytime, 9 to 5, Mondays through Fridays, rarely on
    Saturday or Sunday.
CAST ∾ Dentist, Assistants, Patients, Friends.

Many live life dramas as romantically exciting as that of any fiction. Many play such parts unaware of their own starring roles.

This play presents several interesting incidents in the lives of dental patients. Not information concerning their dental treatment. That is thoroughly discussed in other parts of the book. These feature other phenomena of the lives of people dentistry was done in.

All similarity between situations as they happened and are described is real and intentional. Some names have been changed to protect the guilty.

ACT I

I started dental practice with few patients, lots of spare time, delighted to answer a rare telephone ring "Dr. Garfield speaking," and worry about the rent. As my practice increased I learned to take advantage on several occasions of free help offered by a school which trained medical and dental assistants. The girls' education after a lengthy period of class instruction included one month of internship in a dental office for which they were not paid.

It was nice having another person around. I felt more professionally important and relieved not to be interrupted while working to answer the telephone. I love dentistry and its people but detest red tape detail. I hate opening office mail and can't decide what to throw away. I hate keeping records, making appointments, and sending bills, though I do like being paid for my work. As soon as practical I employed the first intern dental assistant I could afford to keep.

TEETH TEETH TEETH

Arlene Torrance was nineteen years old, blond, beautiful, curvaceous, warm and cheerful. Though small and cute she had a clever mature air about her. She was full of charms of male enchantment. She may have enchanted me. Our patients all seemed to like her, I know the men did without exception. Arlene increasingly came in late and sleepy eyed. When I inquired she assured me she was getting proper rest. My practice increased slowly though we had a great increase in phone calls. It was soon apparent as I recognized voices of young and older men, that Arlene's enchantment spread beyond our office and was reaching back inside to disturb its functions. We had a conference. I don't like to interfere with others private lives but demanded that Arlene stop dating patients and suggested that she restrict her courtship associations to younger men. Arlene agreed to stop dating patients but said, "But Doctor Garfield, I prefer older men."

One Sunday at home, I got a call from my office exchange saying a patient Ted Cornette wanted to talk to me. Ted is a forty eight year old actor. "Dr. Garfield," he said, "I hate to disturb you, I may be silly, but I'm worried. I had a date with your girl Arlene for today and she's three hours late. I'm worried about her. Do you have any idea where she may be or how I can reach her. I hope she hasn't been hurt."

I cautioned Arlene strongly the following morning. She assured me it would not happen again. She said the date had been arranged a long time before and she now realized I was right, Ted Cornette was too old for her.

Not long after, a fifty four year old friend and patient George Loftus a builder, called me at home during the evening. George is short, chubby and bald. "Syd," George said, "I don't know how to tell you. I know it sounds funny. I don't know why, I'm over twice Arlene's age but I made a date with her. Don't tell me I'm crazy I shouldn't have, I know that myself. She disappointed me for the second time and I'm ashamed to come to your office. Yet don't want to go to any other dentist. I don't know what to do."

Immediately the following morning I met with Arlene who somehow still captivated me into believing she was a valuable employee. I said, "Arlene - This can never happen again if you want to continue working here. You must under no circumstances ever date any patient - But - If you do make a date," I said, "Darn It, Keep It."

ACT II of ARLENE AND THE DENTIST

TIME • Not long after Act I.

Patient in dental chair - "Dr. Garfield, I believe you are a very good dentist and suggested that my daughter and her husband come to you as patients. He called for an appointment and your girl said there was no time

TEETH TEETH TEETH

available for over two months. I just can't believe that. You're not that busy."

Not long after - Mounting suspicion had been increasing. Investigation led to Arlene's dismissal.

Shortly after that - Opening my own mail, I found a letter from the California Board of Dental Examiners in Sacramento which read, "Dr. Sydney Garfield, since you have failed to respond to our third request for payment of your regular license fee to practice dentistry in California, this informs you that your license to practice dentistry will be revoked." I was terrified. I had never seen or heard anything of even the first or second request and would hate to take the long examination for admission to practice all over again. I called the Dental Examiner's office in Sacramento by telephone and explained my position. I had found Arlene would not make appointments, probably so that she would have less work to do, and apparently sometimes threw mail away unopened for the same reason. Or perhaps after opening some mail would throw it away, to cover up the fact that she had failed to take care of previous related letters. The dental examiner assured me he understood, that my license was still effective, to continue treating my patients. That such things had happened before, but that I would have to pay an added penalty fee for late payment. I did. I've never practiced without a license.

One year later - I received a letter from a dentist in Seattle Washington, asking for information concerning Arlene Torrance. She had given my name as reference. He was considering employing her. I answered telling him of my experience.

Another year later - Office Assistant,"Dr. Garfield, a girl named Arlene Torrance is on the telephone and wants to talk with you. She says it's personal."

Arlene Torrance by telephone - "Hello Dr. Garfield. It's so nice to hear your voice again. I'm back in Los Angeles from Seattle. How are you? I'd like to see you very much. I've always liked you and thought that since we do not work together any longer perhaps now we could go out together. Have a drink and dinner or something." Arlene and I never met again. I wonder whether she would have kept the date. I never found out. She's not quite my type but Arlene was pretty and full of charms of male enchantment.

ANOTHER ACT

Here we see Dr. Garfield's waiting room. There is an abundance of art objects, ancient, traditional, modern, bright, subdued, colorful. Paintings and drawings are everywhere. One large framed oil covers almost an entire wall. Dr. Garfield is an artist himself. The waiting room contains several

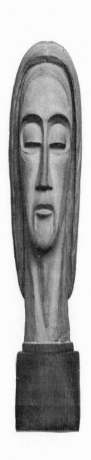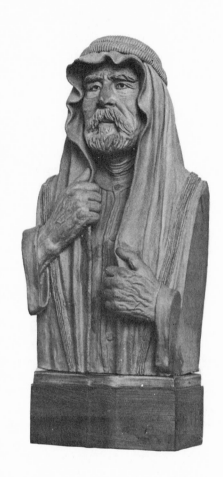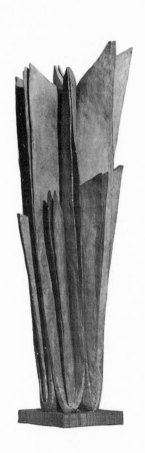

SCULPTURE BY DR. GARFIELD

of his own sculptures. The strongest is classic, an old Sheikh, the wise leader of his Arab tribe, almost lifesize to the waist. Another a modern piece, is the elongated graceful head of a delicate sensitive girl, eyes downcast. In one corner on a shelf we see an abstract sculptural design reaching towards the sky. A fourth is the nude voluptuous body of a woman, lusciously formed in choice natural desirable places.

CAST - Sandra Winters - an especially beautifully faced and figured light olive skinned, long dark haired, young married woman. Sandra has been my patient for several years.

Fred - Sandra's husband.

One day Sandra had an appointment. She arrived at the office alone and asked, "Dr. Garfield could I see you in your private office." As I entered behind her she said, "Will you please close the door." As I did Sandra released her blouse to drop, exposing herself completely nude above the waist, breasts protruding and pointed. Bewildered, though I'd known and respected Sandra and Fred for years, for a moment I felt the closeness of being victimized in some sort of a racket. I demanded, "What is this." Sandra said, "My breasts, Dr. Garfield." I asked, "What about your breasts," starting to relax, relieved. Sandra, "Well, Dr. Garfield, you know I'm beautiful, but I don't think my breasts are perfect and went to see several plastic surgeons about them. I want them operated on and improved, but Dr. Garfield, you're such a great artist and sculptor I wanted your opinion. Can my breasts be more beautiful."

Dr. Garfield - "Sandra I'll answer you. Though first I'd like to say something you didn't ask for. Then I'll answer your question. I myself am a surgeon, familiar with the behavior of human tissues as they are cut during surgical operations and how they heal. I've done delicate surgery of a plastic nature in the mouth. As a surgeon and as an artist I'm now telling you something you did not ask for. I feel you shouldn't have that surgery done. Your breasts are beautiful. Fred is lucky to have you with them as they are. They're not perfect but they're beautiful. To make them more so would require an especially skilled artistic surgeon, and though I have no experience with breast surgery I believe even if the result you desired were obtained, in time the tissues would change again, and your breasts might again lose their perfection. These things are hard to predict. The breast surgeon would be a better judge of that. Now I'll answer your question. Sandra, Yes, your breasts could be more beautiful."

We then discussed details of Sandra's breast design. I suggested sketches could be made of them as they were, with proposed improvements. I told Sandra even if ideal drawings were done, that breasts consisted of muscles, glands and ligamentous tissues, whose finished response was not as predictable as sculptors clay.

TEETH TEETH TEETH

Later that evening at home I received a phone call from Fred Winters.

Fred - "Dr. Garfield, excuse my disturbing you, Sandra told me of asking your opinion concerning her breasts. I hope you understand, it's so important to her, it's all right with me if she wants the operation. I love her any way. We were discussing your ideas Dr. Garfield, would you discuss them with her breast surgeon." Sandra then got on the phone. I told them I'd be glad to but that they should discuss it with him first. That he might resent my intrusion. I would help any way I could.

About a week later Sandra called from a hospital saying the surgery had been completed.

Some time after that Sandra visited our office again. We entered my private room and I closed the door behind me. She dropped her blouse again. Sandra is beautiful and her breasts looked gorgeous. She said, "Touch them Dr. Garfield, they don't have any feeling." I felt I could now touch them professionally. Since a professional evaluation should contain all factors, I include my reactions as a human male. They were hard, cold and impersonally unyielding. As a man I would say they were more beautiful, but less desirable to cuddle and coo. I never saw Sandra's breasts again.

ACT ANOTHER

Much restorative dentistry replaces defective mouth parts. Certain of these dental things are tiny, finely made in the laboratory and sometimes quite expensive. They are finally cemented into the patient's mouth. They're sometimes so small it is difficult for the dentist to hold them in his fingers, or even with special instruments, and deliver them through the mouth for cementing in proper position. As he tries them for fit prior to cementing, the dentist may caution his patient against swallowing the porcelain jacket or inlay if it should slip and fall.

Donald Voyne is a fine dentist and friend of mine. He told me the following story which happened while Don was a dental student. Such stories are not rare. A dental student needs to complete a number of restorative procedures of wide variety to graduate and obtain license to practice. For credit towards graduation an examining dentist checks the fit and quality of each completed part. It is common for dental students to treat courageous members of their own family in the school clinic. One fellow Frank in Don's class, had made a tiny complicated gold inlay of especially precise complex detail for his fiance Eleanor. He'd spent a lot of time making it in the lab, and it fit the mouth models ideally. As he tried it in Eleanor's mouth it slipped, and responding with automatic human reflexes Eleanor swallowed. Usually fine small dental parts can only be

TEETH TEETH TEETH

made once on the model, which deteriorates slightly in the making. If the restoration is lost a lot of procedure needs repeating, which would have burdened, and perhaps endangered Frank's school workload.

Eleanor went to the Student Health Center for full X-rays where the inlay was located in her stomach. Doctors there recommended that she consume smooth bulky food to help the little piece of gold on its organic voyage along the long curving passage, amid flowing digestive juices through her alimentary canal. After close consultation with Eleanor's time schedule they predicted the arrival date for the end of its journey. Frank got Eleanor a pair of surgical gloves and a fine sieve. At the expected time she was ready to meet and retrieve the inlay, upon arrival at her personal port of departure. She was her own customs inspector, happy to catch it crossing her border. The well traveled gold inlay is serving cemented in Mrs. Eleanor Frank's mouth. He graduated.

A LITTLE ACT

This short act involves a child star. It did not occur in Dr. Garfield's office but was told to him by a dentist who prefers not being named.

CAST - Dr. Jones a Pedodontist (child's dentist), the name is assumed.
      Johnny - a five year old boy.

Johnny was seated in a small dental chair being treated, when Dr. Jones detected a straining change on Johnny's face, and recognized an unpleasant odor from the region of Johnny's trousers.

Dr. Jones - "Johnny what are you doing! - don't you think you should go to the bathroom."

Johnny - "I will Dr. Jones, as soon as I'm finished."

ACT STILL ANOTHER

CAST - Mrs. Selle Fishe and Dr. Garfield the dentist. (Mrs. Selle Fishe's name before marriage was Miss Incarne Sciderate.)

After other work, the dentistry needed to complete Mrs. Fishe's treatment was a removable appliance, replacing several missing teeth of her lower jaw. Its basic structure was to be a metal casting which clasped holding on to existing teeth, and showed a small amount of visible metal. Sometimes dental technical detail determines that metal is best as either a yellow gold alloy or a white metal. Sometimes it makes no difference and certain white chrome steels are less costly. They serve as well, in some cases even better. In Mrs. Fishe's mouth it made no difference, and I asked which she preferred showing her examples of each, yellow and silvery white. Specimens of each colored metal were placed in her mouth for personal inspection with a mirror. She chose the whitish as least noticeable. When the denture was completed she liked it. Two or three days later Mrs. Fishe came in saying the whitish color didn't suit her and that she wanted it made over in gold at no extra cost. I pointed out that I'd shown her both examples prior to finishing her case. She insisted she disliked the whitish color, little of which showed.

About a week after that Mrs. Fishe phoned, saying she had accidentally dropped her denture into her kitchen sink disposal grinder, and that it went through, lost. I sympathized saying that now in her new one she could select yellow gold if she preferred. She said she preferred yellow and asked about the fee. I replied this denture would be less expensive since the work of planning and design was already done in making the first. Mrs. Selle Fishe said, "But Dr. Garfield, I didn't get any use from it at all, it's less than two weeks since I got it, such a denture should last for years and I feel you should make me one with no cost to me at all." I could hardly believe my ears. I explained that it was she, not me, that dropped it in the grinder, but Mrs. Fishe kept insisting that she had gotten no use from her denture and should get a new one for free.

ACT OTHERS

A collection of short acts concerning dental appointments, making them and keeping them.

Cathy Crowfoot, a beautiful clever young American Indian girl, talented dancer and actress, has on several occasions driven to our office in a Jaguar automobile, accompanied by her pet African Lion named Tiger. Leaving her Jaguar at the curb, Cathy graceful as a gazelle, walked Tiger the lion, along the street into the building, to enter our office where both waited for Cathy's appointment. I once parted Tiger's lips to examine the lion's teeth. Twice the cat pee'd on our coach and rug. The fun of telling it is worth its trouble.

Mrs. Drippe took her own human cub along on her appointments. Many mothers do and we like them to. Mrs. Drippe was distinctive. On her first appointment the child wet our couch and Mrs. Drippe made a very feeble apology. And then it happened again and again. Mrs. Drippe may have been efficient, she stopped repeating the apologies. We sort of got to expect it all. It was probably an expression of Mrs. Drippe's feelings towards us. It created our impression of her, poor soul.

TEETH TEETH TEETH

ATWIDOIAS

ACT ACT

CAST - Dental Receptionist and Patient, Mrs. Mooney

Telephone rings - Receptionist, "Dr. Sydney Garfield's office."
Mrs. Mooney - "This is Mrs. Mooney. I have excruciating pain in that lower tooth Dr. Garfield warned me about three months ago. I can't stand it. It's driving me out of my mind. I'm in the neighborhood and want to come in to have it fixed right away. Please."
Receptionist, "Of course Mrs. Mooney, I'm so sorry for you, come right over. Dr. Garfield is very busy, but will quickly relieve your pain with medicated temporary treatment, and then we will make another longer appointment since I see from your record Mrs. Mooney, that the tooth is seriously involved and a full hour is needed to complete the restoration."
Mrs. Mooney - "Can't the whole thing be finished right now."
Receptionist, "No Mrs. Mooney, I'm sorry, Dr. Garfield has several patients waiting, and one other is also in pain, but he will stop your suffering."
Mrs. Mooney, "Well then, I'd prefer an appointment for a week after Thursday."

ACT ACT ACT

Dr. Garfield again - Partly on Sunday.
John Lindsay is an architect. I could possibly say we were friends. We had mutual interests. Being both single we went out together several times. Perhaps it was through an exchange of technical ideas that John developed confidence towards me, resulting in his mentioning now and then, over a period of several months, that he'd like me to make a new set of dentures for his mother. She had lost her teeth and never been satisfied with her old pair. She couldn't eat with them and they were increasingly more painful. I was flattered and suggested an appointment, but despite John's repeated references none was made for a long time.
One day John was definite, and asked if his mother could be treated during the evening. She worked during the day. I told John I did not work evenings, only Monday through Friday five daytimes a week. I will come in anytime for an emergency, even Saturday or Sunday or the middle of the night, but am so constituted that I feel capable of performing dentistry efficiently, only during my normal day hours. John asked that I make an exception for his mother which I couldn't do. I've tried making exceptions a few times and became regretfully involved. He offered to pay above my normal fee but I repeated that I wouldn't work nights.

TEETH TEETH TEETH

One Sunday while relaxing at home during the late afternoon, John phoned again saying his mother's mouth was especially painful. Though I made no reference he again volunteered, saying he'd be glad to pay extra for my weekend services. He sounded worried and asked if I could possibly see her. I met them at my office in half an hour where both repeated the desire that I make Mrs. Lindsay a new set of dentures, upper and lower. When I examined her mouth I was alarmed. The upper denture severely misfit, had cut a long bruised opening inside the entire right cheek. It was seriously infected. I was amazed she could wear it that way. I cleansed the area and applied medications. Gently I tried the denture in and out of her mouth and then carefully removed a large misformed part of a flange, which I felt caused the cut and a biting misalignment. Mrs. Lindsay said the denture never felt as good since she got it. I prescribed home care and asked that she come in the next day for observation. She didn't keep her appointment. The following morning we called Mrs. Lindsay at work. She said she felt fine and enjoyed eating with her dentures for the first time. At the end of the month we sent John Lindsay a bill for twenty five dollars. He didn't pay that month, nor the next, nor the next. I phoned him and was told he thought twenty five dollars was quite a high fee for one appointment. Eventually he did pay.

That was several years ago. His mother may still be using those dentures. John himself has never been my patient, though he calls at odd times asking the fee to have his teeth cleaned and examined. He never makes an appointment.

PLAYWRITERS NOTE ∾ The previous acts describing unusual situations present a small interesting part of life. Larger numbers of happenings every day are rather normal, usually involving patients as people that live and meet their obligations in the ordinary way. They would make less spectacular reading, but do deserve this token of recognition.

A SHORT STORY

The following story is a documentary of an exceptional dentist, and tells of a most extraordinary man among his many unusual patients. Dr. E. Ray Brownson is the exceptional dentist. While in high school he made a small steam engine. At twenty three in 1914 after three years of the time's typical dental education, he graduated from the University of Southern California's Dental School. Schooling included tempering and forging steel and making his own instruments. He wound electric coils helping to build the first X-ray machine in Southern California. In a darkroom he cut his own film and wrapped it light tight in small packets, for early use in patients' mouths. He extracted one of his own wisdom teeth. He made major early contributions to full mouth dental reconstruction. He's one of a dentist family. His son Hugh is a dentist. His brother Earl M. Brownson taught the profession for years at U.S.C. Dr. Earl's son Lou Brownson was one of my favorite classmate friends when we studied together at U.S.C. I feel privileged to have formed Dr. E. Ray Brownson's friendship.

His patients included many most famous motion picture people at the height of that industry's peak. Among them were producers Louis B. Mayer and Darryl Zanuck. Stars, Greer Garson, Elizabeth Taylor, Joan Crawford, Spencer Tracy, Margaret O'Brien, Norma Shearer, Hedy LaMar, Lionel Barrymore, Marion Davies, others. One of his patients was the Maharajah of India.

Dr. Brownson's most extraordinary patient was the world prominent publisher William Randolph Hearst. One evening while I was dining with Dr. E. Ray he referred to Mr. Hearst as W.R., the way close friends addressed him. After establishing confidence in Dr. E. Ray's skills, Mr. Hearst asked him to design and supervise the installation of a personal dental office and laboratory at his San Simeon Ranch Castle home. Dr. E. Ray may have been the first flying dentist. He told me of being flown, many times in early 1920's, from Los Angeles in an aircraft owned by Hearst's Los Angeles Examiner. It was a small, First World War, French, single engined, two-seater open cockpit biplane. With his instrument case between his legs, E. Ray told me of cold flying, through heavy winds over the ocean, for few hour flights to San Simeon. At the castle he treated Mr. Hearst with thorough prophylactic scalings, endodontic or root canal therapy, and fine gold inlays. Dr. E. Ray said, "W. R. was very much aware of the importance of teeth, good dental care, and interested in its details." Dr. Brownson occasionally treated castle guests some of whom have been named. His visits were sometimes also spent as a guest during which he would stay several days and usually returned by rail.

APPLAUD SHOUT! HIP HURRAH HOORAY!
Clap Hands to Dentistrys Story Play

TEETH TEETH TEETH

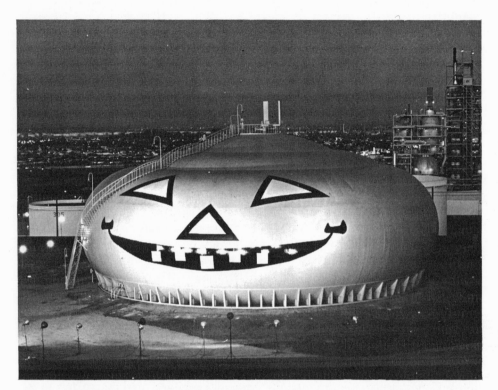

BIGGEST SHOW TEETH IN THE WORLD

This two-faced pumpkin grins through four by four feet square teeth, in both of its seventy-three feet long mouths. One faces the Harbor Freeway to Los Angeles, the other toward Palos Verdes Peninsula into the Pacific.

Presented each year by the Union Oil Co. at its Wilmington California refinery. The pumpkin repainted annually for Halloween, masks a Horton-Sphere shaped steel 80,000 barrel tank containing 3,360,000 gallons of pressure liquefied butane. Quite a mouthful. Though serviced regularly yearly, it's teeth are not restored by a dentist.

TEETH TEETH TEETH

20

DENTISTRY IN SPORTS

Athletes leading otherwise ordinary lives are subject to the usual variety of dental disorders. These if undetected often affect their body efficiency. Sportsmen of highest skill, at times for no apparent reason, have fallen from superiority and routine medical examination could find no cause. Searching dental studies on occasion, revealed diseases of the mouth, which when corrected restored original prowess. Athletic activity of course helps general health. Active participants however, in what are called contact sports, are exposed to accidents to all of their body and sometimes severe damage to teeth. Dentistry repairs such damages and helps prevent them.

Contact sports are competitive athletic activities, whose participants use body contact actions against each other in effort to attain victory, individually and in teams. Wrestling, boxing, football and ice hockey are contact sports. Games like basketball and baseball do not provide for intentional contact between opponents, but in the intensity of play, situations sometimes arise that make personal encounter unavoidable. At times contest reaches spirited peaks, during which while striving to surpass extreme exertions are necessary. In effort to conquer and win, local forces may become especially high, at moments uncontrollable, so that accidents can happen, sometimes serious even on to death.

When such accident does occur some start crusades to stop those games, or invoke rules limiting their behavior. This seems idealistic and may be helpful, but accomplishments of satisfaction always require effort and chance, which unfortunately is accompanied by danger. It isn't much fun gambling for wooden nickles or even real ones. It's more of a thrill when high stakes are risked on the horse that comes in, and even a thrill though disappointed when he doesn't come in.

Accidents can sometimes be lessened, but accidents by definition are accidental and cannot always be avoided. Driving on most perfectly designed freeway, fallen debris from another vehicle could cause skidding, and a small dented fender or major disaster. Babies placed in cribs by careful loving mothers, somehow sometimes crawl over the rail to fall, suprisingly unhurt or seriously injured. Soldiers fighting aggressive invaders are mistakenly bombed by their own militia. Thats how things are. Anything can happen.

TEETH TEETH TEETH

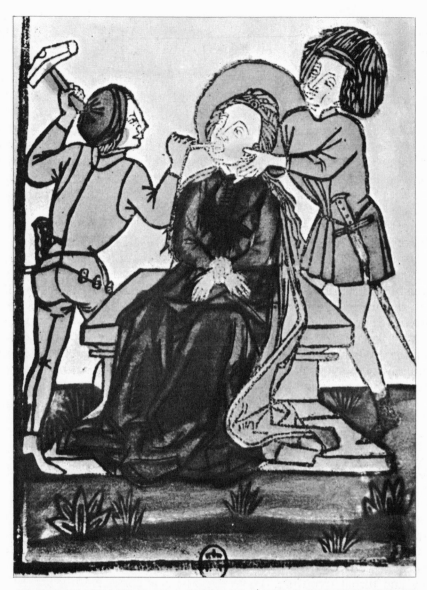

AN EARLY EXAMPLE OF A WOMANS DARING SPORTSMANSHIP

ST. APOLLONIA, PATRON SAINT OF DENTISTRY∾In the third century after Christ, Saint Apollonia lived in Alexandria. She embraced His faith. Some fanatic deniers confined her, knocked out her teeth with hammer and chisel. They threatened to throw her into flames should she not blaspheme her chosen religion. Tearing from her persecutors she cast herself into the fire. Many faithful learning of her sacrificial dental torture, began worshipping Apollonia as the Saint who would Help Head and Teeth Disorders.

TEETH TEETH TEETH

348

DENTISTRY IN SPORTS

Sports of sorts were probably played far back in time before man even knew of his own human existence. Puppies, tigers, and elephants play, competing with others of their kind. Dinosaurs probably did too. In early times man first grappled animals that attacked him, wrestling those and others for food. He fought men in play and probably less playfully for meat, and to prevent being eaten. He used his teeth to bite and fight as some wrestlers do today. Those knocked out had few dentists to replace them. As man civilized his mind found need for contest to display his strength, so that some could convince others of ability to conquer and lead. Certain of these efforts channeled into specialized refinements of war. Others turned in healthier directions towards organized competitive sports.

SPORTS ORIGIN

Something like wrestling was probably our original instinctive activity, combining blows of the fist as in boxing, plus any other actions of any muscles of any limbs or other body parts. As man exerted against others, seriously and in fun, he did all he could to win. There were no rules. Later details became important, skills developed, and ego and honor involved. Some preferred to stop rolling in dust and mud, and agreed to use their legs keeping bodies erect above ground. As they learned standing, springing limberly to deliver advantageous blows to opponents, or jump turning away to avoid them, pugilism later called boxing came. Some men wrestled, some preferred boxing, some both.

WRESTLING

Archaelogical excavation in Mesopotania, around old temple ruins at Kyafaje near Bagdad, unearthed two slabs of relief sculpture believed by experts to be 5000 years old. One carved in stone shows two pugilists. The other is bronze, of two wrestlers gripping each others hips. Both sports were popular in ancient Greece and Rome. Evidence is seen in old art and literature. Homer's Iliad tells of a famous wrestling match between Ulysses and Ajax. Early Greek wrestlers received high honors, and fought to musical flutes, under rules permitting breaking fingers, gouging eyes, biting and throat throttling. Tooth damage was considered minor. Slaves wrestled to death for amusement of noblemen and women. Ancient Jews were wrestling enthusiasts providing several famous champions. Rules differed with times and places. The Irish English and Scottish, each had individual brutal wrestling styles, while the French at one time only permitted holds above the waist.

In Japan where wrestling has always been a national sport, interest was so great that for twenty centuries, giant belly and sized Sumo wrestlers selected their finest sons and daughters for controlled intermarriage, so that mating would produce grapplers of desired immense mass, shape, strength and weight. During this period the Chinese practiced a different sort of sport also using selective breeding. They chose native carp fish, from which by controlled mating in small fish ponds, they developed unusual goldfish varieties. These of course were much smaller than Japanese wrestlers and more vividly colored. Species like calicos and other fantail types are most prized, when they have fat round abdomens like tiny Sumo wrestlers. They have fins of course rather than hands, which can't knock out each others teeth. At the same time Chinese practiced an athletic sport that included a form of wrestling and boxing combined. Today Japanese excel in jiujitsu wrestling. North American Indians wrestled before discovery by Columbus.

During early 1900's wrestling had popular professional prestige. Champion Frank Gotch fought 160 matches between 1905-13. Twenty a year. The Russian Lion and Terrible Turk also ruled. Later Strangler Lewis and Jim Londos were champions.

Scientific wrestling uses holds and muscle forces applied in such manner, that little of its important stresses are seen as action from outside. Wrestlers feel these high gripping exerted pressures, which though extreme often display little visible motion. Because of this, professional wrestling for audiences suffered boxing competition, where the action is all obvious. Watching real scientific wrestling is somewhat like watching chess. It can't be enjoyed unless its emotions are felt. Much of the energies are internally personal, best appreciated by those who play the game. For this reason professional scientific wrestling declined, but the sport's prestige continued in high schools colleges and athletic clubs. As boxing audiences grew while wrestlings declined, some sports promoters realized it was the intense visible actions that excited watchers and created a new wrestling style and era.

Wrestlers today perform squirming in misery, and appear to be rolling in pain, pounding mats with fists and palms, grunting, groaning, and gnashing teeth. They seem to despise each other. I've seen wrestlers spit in the others face. Audiences love such exhibition attending in great number. Today's top wrestlers are in the ring as often as six times a week. Some earn $100,000 a year. In some places women wrestle, sometimes in mud.

Even during today's wrestling exhibitions accidents happen. I spoke with Jules Strongbow, part Cherokee Indian, an old time professional, present wrestling matchmaker for Olympic Auditorium in Los Angeles. Jules says wrestlers still lose many teeth. They dislike wearing toothguards which become uncomfortable, since wrestling matches are continuous. There are no rest periods to remove guards, like boxers between rounds. During struggle, their heavy bodies hard knees and elbows, sometimes hit wrestlers teeth knocking them out. Jules himself lost two teeth twice that way. The first time many years ago wrestling Krippler Karl Davis. Primo Carnera the Italian, Heavyweight Boxing Champion of the World 1933, who later turned to wrestling, also told me of knocking out two more of Jules' teeth in Cleveland 1950.

BOXING

For a long time boxing has been the leading sport fought between individuals. The word boxer is from an old Pekin Chinese word meaning "righteous harmonious fists." Today's fight rings are rather boxlike. The sport is also called pugilism and prize fighting. Prizes are sometimes very high. In 1927 for the fight at which Jack Dempsey lost his world heavyweight crown to Gene Tunney, the gate was $2,638,660 of which Dempsey got $425,000 and Tunney the winner $990,445.

Pugilism derives from old latin words, pugnus which meant the fist, and pugil meaning one who fought with fists. Hands of such ancient pugil warriors were covered with cestus. Cestus was an old greek and roman word, describing a leather band worn as an enticing girdle by brides to excite love, and also used by fist fighters as a protective hand covering. Ancient Greeks fought man to man with such fat softened thin leather thongs, up to twelve feet long wrapped around fingers wrists and arms like bandages. These cestus, as early ancestors of modern boxing gloves helped fists faces and teeth. Museum art shows early Greeks using their teeth to tie these thongs, like boxers with glove lacing today. During the early Christian Roman Empire pugilistic gladiators were highly honored, often awarded a beautiful captive girl as winners prize. Such ultimate goal is rather similar for fighters today, though it is often the boxer won by the girl. Sometimes cestus were studded with lead, brass, and iron nuggets, for body and face and teeth smashing battles to death, between slaves in arenas entertaining Roman crowds.

There are few records of boxing for the intervening period until early 1700's. As the world flourished London became a large city, and for some reason the center for bare fisted, bare knuckled, fighting. James Figg was champion of the time. There were few rules. It was manly to kick a man that was down. Jaws were broken. Many teeth knocked out. Dentistry was mostly medicated trimming and patching of soft torn tissues. Few teeth were ever replaced. Fighters displayed spaces in their mouth proudly, as a badge of distinction. Bare fisted boxing was brutally bloody, with bleeding

TEETH TEETH TEETH

faces and fingers, though investigators feel fewer deaths occurred, since visual surface damages stopped bouts sooner.

Public objection arose and grew. In 1743 the then English champion Jack Broughton ennobled the sport with rules. These included marking the fighting area on the ground. Each boxer was entitled to a personal umpire and if both disagreed they selected a third. You could no longer hit a man down on the ground. There were still no rounds, fights were to finish or quit. Boxing was still fought bare fisted. Broughton also introduced "mufflers" another form of the old cestus, as a younger ancestor of present padded boxing gloves. Mufflers were thin coverings like ladies dress gloves. Even that little helped save some fingers, faces, fists and teeth. They were only used during sparring exhibitions and practice workouts. Mufflers were considered too effeminate for a real fight.

Pugilism popularity increased with respect for its participants. Jack Broughton is one of the few Englishmen not a member of the royal family buried in Westminster Abbey. Because of bloody brutality boxers were called bruisers, yet commanded a certain respect and admiration. Women publicly paraded crusading against fighting, as they have against alcohol and for their right to vote. Fighting for prizes was made illegal. Private clubs formed of which one had to be a member to attend bouts. To avoid the law, matches were held secretly in open fields out of town, inside barns and aboard barges at sea. Paid attendance and purses were poor. Sometimes winner took all, though a sympathetic crowd might pass a hat for donations to a loser that tried. Larger prizes were occasionally privately paid by sportsmen and professional gamblers. Sometimes to avoid the law medals were awarded as tokens, later secretly exchanged for cash.

There was little control. When a fighter was losing, his seconds might jump in attacking the opponent. Riots erupted and more than the puglists lost more than teeth. Matches were interrupted by police raids, stakeholders couldn't be found, winnings were hard to collect. Caught, charged with the crime of fighting for a prize, defendants claimed to be only sparring for sport. They were often released by a sympathetic judge who might have been one of the audience.

Bare fisted boxers couldn't fight often. Broken wrists knuckles and fingers ended many careers. Winners hand wounds often took longer healing than losers broken noses, teeth and split lips. All were occupational hazards of the sport, which to some extent exists today. Teeth lost by fighters was not as disturbing then, when dentistry was less advanced. Public opinion accepted tooth loss as natural and inevitable. Still boxing popularity increased while some enthusiasts crusaded for less brutality.

TEETH TEETH TEETH

CONTROLS APPEAR ∾ Communication was primitive. Travel and mail was by horseback and stagecoach. Roads were poor, passage depended on weather. Local groups started individual reforms. Gloves were required in some places. In some, fights stopped briefly when a man went down, separating bouts into irregular rounds. Wooden fences were placed around rings, to keep less honorable intruders and excited audiences out. Fighters were hurt against hard wood rails, sometimes intentionally, and stretched ropes were substituted. As the railroad invention spread man farther, and brought them together, the sport constantly increased and organized commercially. Audiences grew, rings were raised above ground so more standing could see. Choice front seats were sold at high prices. Prizes increased with respect and admiration for boxers. Yet objection continued, and in many places fighting for prizes was still against the law.

Between 1838 and 1853 in England, the London Prize Ring Rules were formulated. These increased the sports dignity and helped fighters, fists, faces and teeth. The ring was defined in size, and stakes provided for supporting ropes, to keep outsiders out. Only the fighters, their seconds, and the referee were permitted inside the ring. The referee had a watch for calling time. Rounds of indefinite length ended when a man went down, 30 seconds were allowed as a rest interval. Again, the floored fighter could not be struck. If a boxers seconds attacked his opponent the referee could declare the bout forfeit. Provision was made for use of gloves. They were usually thin, called skintights. Suspicious boxers seconds could demand the referee have the opponent open his fist, to see that no stones were held hidden. Rules included controls for the money stakeholder and defined pay off responsibilities. It is interesting that even these London Ring Rules of honorable agreement specified regulations for continuing the fight if police interrupted. The referee named the time and place for the bout to go on, the same day if possible, or as soon after at the nearest practical location.

As the independent United States grew and prospered so did pugilism. Irish immigrants appeared challenging English champions. Greatest was "The Great" John L. Sullivan, son of Michael of Tralee, County Kerry born near Boston 1858. Boisterous, loud, hard drinking, and pretty colleen chasing, John knocked out man after man. Popularity soared with his offer of $50 to anyone who could stand up with him for four rounds at Harry Mills Dance Hall Boxing Emporium near the Bowery, New York City. John L's teeth were beautiful. No one could touch them but himself, his dentist, or fingers and lips of lovely ladies. He knocked hundreds from mouths of others. Sullivan was reputed to have hit so hard, men's heads and shoulders struck the canvas before their following torso and buttocks.

He became famous in 1882 in a bare knuckled bout, taking the U.S. championship from Tipperary Ireland born Paddy Ryan, the Trojan Giant.

TEETH TEETH TEETH

Oscar Wilde described the fight for a British journal. John beat American and foreign challengers, in increasing number and popularity. Idol peaks were reached touring the country now offering a thousand dollars to anyone who could stand up to him for four full rounds. This offer was fought with gloves, protecting fingers faces and teeth, and helped popularize them. Other bouts were still fought without them. Sullivan's reputation spread touring Europe fighting to fame. Guest of the Prince of Wales, and King Edward VII, he also fought at Baron Rothschild's estate in Chantilly France. He was the pride of the boxing world.

PRIMITIVE PROTECTION ∾ Early fighters found protections of their own. From blows struck at the face most common damage was lips split against teeth, sometimes so severely seconds carried small scissors to snip off shredded strips. Boxers learned to place cotton padding and soft cloth underneath to protect them. Some held cloth, toothpicks, and twigs, between upper and lower teeth as a softer between the jaws absorber, for resistance against the shock of blows to the head.

Throughout John L's prominence he was a carousing hell bender. Though celebrated, many criticized him as a poor example of an idol. In 1889 Sullivan fought Jake Kilrain in what even then was an illegal bout, for heavyweight championship of the world. On July 7, to avoid police and state militia an entire chartered train with fighters and audience left New Orleans for a secret destination. At Richberg Mississippi, in a wood clearing, the ring surrounded by crowds of others waited. Some watched from trees. John Fitzpatrick later mayor of New Orleans, refereed. Bat Masterson famous sheriff of Dodge City, kept time. In seventy five rounds in two hours and sixteen minutes, Sullivan beat Kilrain in the last heavyweight bareknuckle championship bout, fought under otherwise London Prize Ring Rules.

A NEW ERA ∾ Before this in 1867, the eighth Marquis of Queensberry an English sportsman, as was custom in those times, gave his honored name to new boxing rules written by John Chambers. They lessened brutality even more, and made the sport more scientific. The Queensberry Rules established three minute rounds with one rest minute between. During the round if a man falls from a blow, weakness of any other reason, he is allowed ten seconds to rise unassisted, during which the standing boxer should return to his own corner. If the fallen fails to rise, the referee awards to the other. Larger gloves of best quality must be used. During the round only contestants and the single referee are permitted in the ring. Seconds must stay out. Queensberry rules were slowly adopted at first, but eventually spread being accepted for boxing around the world.

TEETH TEETH TEETH

Padded gloves save hands they cover, and teeth lips and other parts they hit. Yet teeth are knocked out and jaws broken with them. Some say boxing with gloves results in more serious inner body injury than before. Contest includes the dangers of damage. It wouldn't be much sport fighting with fists in large soft pillows, and then fighters could catch cold from the draft. One could just as well flip coins.

The Golden Nineties popularized variety vaudeville and a new boxing era. "Gentleman" Jim Corbett of San Francisco, another son of an Irishman, quiet, conservative, was universally respected as a more refined scientific pugilist. He was ridiculed by John L. as "That California Dude." In 1892 in New Orleans, Gentleman Jim with five ounce padded gloves under Queensberry Rules, beat Sullivan for a $25,000 prize to become the new world champion. John's public cried.

The new era also brought the first Negro world heavyweight champion. Jack Johnson born 1878 in Galveston Texas, only thirteen years after slavery's end. Johnson wasn't the first colored boxer. Before emancipation by Lincoln, black slaves were sometimes fought by their owners as financial pugilistic investments. Some humane less selfish sportsmen even shared prize money with boxer slaves, and after extended friendship might award them their grand prize of freedom. Negro boxers suffered prejudice by some and were kept from top sport echelons. John L. Sullivan wouldn't fight Peter Jackson, an Australian Negro. Gentleman Jim fought Jackson 61 rounds to a draw. Jack Johnson beat man after man, black and white. He was called the Galveston Giant. Fighting for pride, recognition for his people and victory, in 1908 Johnson beat white Canadian Tommy Burns, to win the championship and his new name Black Champion. He was a powerful puncher.

TWENTIETH CENTURY ∾ Nat Fleischer, editor publisher of The Ring considered boxing's world foremost authority, in his book "The Heavyweight Championship," G. Putnams Sons N.Y.C. 1944, described a bout at Colma California 1909, in which Johnson defended his title beating challenger Stan Ketchel. Nat Fleischer wrote, "A right uppercut with all the weight of Jack's massive shoulders behind it caught Stanley square on the mouth and shocked him into instant unconsciousness as if he had been hit by a hammer. Such was the fury of the blow that all of Ketchel's front teeth were broken off at the gums."

I've spoken with Nat Fleischer personally. He was there at Colma and saw the fight. "Doc" he said "the roots were left in Ketchel's jaws and a couple of the tooth crowns came off stuck in Johnson's glove." Nat got that very glove as one of his boxing trophies.

TEETH TEETH TEETH

Telegrams : "BRIDENTION, LONDON, W.1."

British Dental Association

Please address your reply to—
X̶T̶H̶E̶ ̶S̶E̶C̶R̶E̶T̶A̶R̶Y̶X̶X̶
Telephone: GROSVENOR 1592

13, HILL STREET,
BERKELEY SQUARE,
LONDON, W.1

11th. March, 1966

Sydney Garfield, Esq., D.D.S.,
415, North Camden Drive,
Beverly Hills,
California,
U.S.A."

Dear Dr. Garfield,

　　　　　Thank you for your letter of 1st. March relating to
mouthguards in boxing. After several enquiries I have found the following
information, which corroborates all you say in your letter.

　　　　　The mouthguard was introduced into British boxing in late
1913 or early 1914, Ted "Kid" Lewis being the first prominent boxer to
make use of it. Previously some boxers had used gutta-percha or some similar
substance to protect their teeth, but Jack Marks (really Jacob Marks) who
practised in the East End of London and had a great interest in boxing was the
inventor of a rubber guard. He first took an impression in gutta-percha and
then fabricated the rubber product. He went into production and his guard was
widely used. Another firm later made a "universal" guard which was supposed
to fit anybody; it did not, of course, do so, but sometimes by its lack of fit caused
bleeding and soreness, and was never popular.

　　　　　Lewis, the boxer, was first to introduce the guard to the United
States, as you have said, although at first there was opposition to his wearing
it in fights, until common-sense prevailed and other boxers there also adopted
it and it became as widely accepted as in Britain.

　　　　　　　Yours sincerely,
　　　　　　　E. Muriel Spencer
　　　　　　　(Librarian)

Johnson also beat Irish Victor McLaglen then fighting as "The Great Romano." McLaglen later left boxing to become a Motion Picture Academy Award winning star. From photographs I've seen, Johnson was successful at keeping his teeth from being knocked out. They were described by the London Times while Jack was on foreign tour as being "predominantly gold."

In early 1900's mouthguards also called toothguards, dentistry's greatest sport contribution appeared, though they were slow being adopted. Worn in the mouth around teeth like protective shock absorbers, they guard teeth lips and jaws from serious injury. Athletes sometimes wear mouthguards protecting both their upper and lower teeth. Most wear only upper guards.

I spoke with Howard Steindler at his Los Angeles Main Street Gym, where famous champions Archie Moore, Art Aragon, Carlos Ortiz, Joe Louis and others worked out. Howie is an old time trainer, manager, and boxing promoter. Howie said, "Doc, I've seen guys spit teeth out a hundred times." He followed with an interesting story. Howie had trained Mike Alfano, a New Jersey heavyweight. In 1941 at Lynn Mass. Mike was in the ring against Bill "Billie" Weinberg. Mike was wearing a mouthguard. Howie said, "Bill swung a heavy right and hit Mike's mouth. Billie's glove knocked Mike's lip right over the tops of his own teeth. I was in his corner, Doc, I saw it. His teeth went clear through a slit the punch cut in his lip." I asked, "You mean the punch actually got the teeth through the guard." "Oh no," Howie said. "It was Mike's lower lip. He only wore an upper guard. With lower protection it couldn't have happened."

I first met Lillian McLarnin by telephone. Clayton Frye of California's State Athletic Commission suggested I call Jim in Santa Monica. He was not at home. Since then we've become friends. Lillian and James McLarnin are examples of a long successful marriage. James "Jimmy" McLarnin was always greatly respected. He successfully fought flyweight, bantam, feather and welterweight while his own weight changed. Jim's been Welterweight Champion of the World. He took the crown from "Young" Corbett in 1933 and shared the championship with Barney Ross from thirty three to thirty five, when each took, lost, and regained the title from the other, back and forth. Since Jim was out I asked Lillian whether he'd ever suffered any fighter teeth damage. "Oh no Dr. Garfield," she said, "Jim never did. He always wore a good mouthguard. I took good care of it." Later I met Jim.

"Mouthguards are the greatest boxing invention ever," he said. "They've saved mine and many fighters teeth. The mouth is a target in a fight. It must be protected. Nobody," Jim said, "knows the importance of teeth better than I do. One time during my career my right arm and shoulder went bad. I didn't want to tell anyone. I couldn't throw a punch like I used to. Since my general health seemed O.K. I was afraid it could be my heart. Not wanting Lillian to worry I sneaked to Long Beach for examination by a specialist. Nothing was wrong. Later I discovered it was two ulcerated teeth. Two weeks after they were treated I was good as new. We always have our teeth checked regularly now.''

A chain is as strong as its weakest link and that's the link that fails first. A fighter with a weak jaw has what's called a glass jaw. Jack Dempsey had an iron jaw. At a bout promoted by Tex Rickard in Jersey City July 2 1921, well mannered Frenchman Georges Carpentier challenged Jack Dempsey for his world heavyweight crown. George Bernard Shaw predicted Dempsey would lose. Carpentier in the second round, delivered his right fist to strike hitting Dempsey's jaw with such force, Carpentier's thumb broke and his wrist wrenched. Shaw was wrong. Dempsey played with persistent George until bored, then knocked him out in the fourth.

I've always thought of Dempsey as the greatest since the era of John L. Sullivan. I discussed boxing and teeth with Jack Dempsey. He looked big, strong, virile. The first thing he said was, "You need good teeth for a firm solid jaw to be able to take a punch. With it you should have a good mouthpiece. It provides a feeling of protection and strength all around. Luckily, I've always had good teeth probably because I took care of them. I'm sorry for those that don't. You need teeth to enjoy a meal.''

I also spoke to Cassius Clay, Heavyweight Champion of the World when he knocked out Sonny Liston in Miami 1964. His bright shining teeth can be seen in his ready flashing smile. He asked that I address him by his new name Muhammad Ali, a name of his African ancestors as given by Muslim leader Elijah Muhammad. Muhammad Ali said he's had no fighting tooth problems. He has had three back teeth extracted, two on one side, one on the other, because of decay.

THE GOLDEN GLOVES ∾ Started 1926 by Arch Ward of the Chicago Tribune, then popularized by Paul Gallico with New York's Daily News, the Golden Gloves spread through our nation as a newspaper sponsored endeavor, helping boys through boxing as an amateur sport. Joe Louis, Rocky Graziano, Barney Ross, Floyd Patterson and others, came to fame through Golden Gloves. The boys fight for honor awarded as medals, and to the winner of each weight class a pair of small 14 carat boxing gloves of gold. Amateur bouts are less strenuous, only three rounds of only two minutes each, with one rest minute between. Golden Glovers must wear teeth protecting mouthguards. Padded gloves for professional fighters' fists usually weigh eight ounces each. Golden gloves are extra heavy padded, weigh sixteen ounces.

TEETH TEETH TEETH

Sebi Interlandi my friend and a former golden glover told me, "Syd, in a little while those gloves weigh a ton." Sebi stands for Sebastian. Sebi though big and powerful is clever sensitive and gentle. He is an intellectual, the type of athlete that carried a book under his arm. He described boxing to me as a symphony with muscles. Sebi fought heavyweight. He trained at Stillman's Gym, New York City, where he often worked out with Archie Moore, later light heavy champ of the world. The boys in the 1940's had little money. They wore inexpensive stock or standard mouthguards costing about 25 cents. They couldn't afford more expensive custom guards, fit exactly by a dentist. Stock guards come in small, medium, and large sizes, of which the closest is selected.

One day working out at Stillman's, Sebi took on a husky 18 year old. Workouts are supposed to be no more than that, but Sebi said, "This guy came at me like a tiger for the kill. He hit my lower jaw, first a left cross then a right, I felt it crack both right and left. It was horrible. My arms dropped." Sebi's lower jaw healed, but on each side he lost a tooth, where the fracture passed through the socket of its root. He had been wearing an upper stock mouthguard. I suggested dentist fit guards over both jaws might have prevented his fractures. "You may be right Syd," he said, "I've seen those custom guards, they cost more but do give better protection."

FOOTBALL

Football is the creation of invasion of a nation. About the year 1000 A.D. the Danes were trying to conquer Europe. They occupied England 1016 to 1042. After they were driven out, some Englishmen excavating a battlefield found a Dane's skull, and resentfully started kicking it around. If the Danish warriors teeth hadn't been lost by pyorrhea they were probably kicked out of his jaws by those first footballers. Today football players prefer kissing pretty teethed mouths of beautiful Danish blondes.

Between 1050 and 1075 skull kicking increased. Some may have kicked at the teeth first. When Danish skulls ran out, perhaps because of foot damages through inadequate shoes, inflated cow bladders were used. If the game had started in Holland wooden shoed Dutchmen would have finished the skulls even faster. The activity grew and for a long time was called "Kicking the Dane's Head" and later "Kicking the Bladder."

During the 12th century it spread widely. People of adjacent villages met halfway with a blown bladder, kicking it to the center of their opponent's town for victory. Many villagers joined, becoming rough mob teams. In addition to body head and teeth injury, crops were damaged, fences broken, livestock lost, and shops broken into. Authorities moved activities to open areas, and as the sport increased some started standardizing the game. Boundaries were marked for fields, with points awarded to opposite teams for kicking the bladder past opposite ends. Later in the twelfth century the name "Futballe" popularized, and bladders were to be activated only by feet. Probably less teeth and jaws were broken, though as in all life's games there must have been dirty players.

Futballe became so popular it interfered with bow and arrow archery, which was a military practice obligation of the time. King Henry II ordered a "cease playe" which stopped futballe for about 400 years. Early in the 16th century the Irish rebelled against English control and started a form of Gaelic football probably the roughest today. This encouraged Englishmen with renewed interest.

About this time firearms were invented, killing more enemies faster, needing less military slaughter production time. King James revoked Henry's rule, lifted futballe's ban, and blessed the game as honored sport. Other inventions gave man even more time. Football popularity grew with cities and towns supporting teams.

Added rules refined the game. Goal posts were erected at each end of fields, supporting cross bars, increasing needed skills. I don't know the influence on futballe players teethe at the time. Into the 1800's the ball could only be kicked. Picking it up and running was unthought of. In 1823 William Ellis of Rugby College did pick up a ball and ran, carrying it towards the goal. His captain apologized to the opposing team. The combined action of ball kicking, grabbing, carrying and running, soon captivated audiences. Every pioneer creates a path despite objection. A plaque has been placed at Rugby honoring Ellis for violating the rules.

Those were beginnings. The early game as played is more like today's soccer, popular through most of the world, though not played much in U.S. Rugby became the name of another game which found its place as an intermediate sport. The American version of football only changed the spelling slightly, while developing its own rules and skills. They're all rough, accident prone, and teeth, jaw, damaging.

RECENTLY ∾ Many professional football athletes lose teeth playing. Most do not wear mouthguards. Damage has been less severe since helmets and masks are worn. By telephone I made a date to visit the Los Angeles Rams at their San Fernando training field. George Menefee, Ram's trainer for more than twelve years, with Cincinatti U. before that, is a long time football man. George said, "Masks, especially those bird cages with steel bars around the face lessen mouth damage but can't stop all teeth, jaw, injury." Football forces are high, almost unbelievably. George introduced me to Bill Granholm, the Rams Equipment Manager for many years and another football veteran. Bill showed me masks and

TEETH TEETH TEETH

photos of others whose face protecting bars, almost 1/4 inch steel rod, had been bent during games. Bill said, "Manufacturers test this equipment to meet specification, and it seems you couldn't dent one with a sledge hammer, but these guys are tough, bend bars, break teeth, and sometimes more." Fullback Dick Bass told me, "Once in a scrimmage, a guy's foot got under my face bar, split it, and I lost four of my front teeth."

I met other Ram players, who like those of other pro teams had lost teeth yet don't wear guards. On the field and in the locker room I spoke with Deacon Jones. I could see missing teeth spaces, above and below in front, where his teeth used to be. Like most football players, the Deacon wears removable dentures while away from the game to replace them. He lost those teeth early in his football career. Jones is a powerful player, defensive left end for the Rams. Devoted to more than football he's greatly devoted to God, the minister of a Los Angeles church. I asked the Deacon if he wouldn't feel more secure with mouthguards, and admired his answer as a true sportsman. "When I play" Deacon said, "I just play football. I can't think of protecting anything. I play to win, that's all." There should be more of his kind. The health professions are there to protect people too busy to protect themselves.

I heard a story from several sources, dramatically demonstrating an attitude towards the fighting spirit of football prevalent in the past, before the realization that players could be protected. Joe Stydahar, All American at West Virginia, great linesman and tackle with the Chicago Bears in early 40's before protective mask days, later became coach for the Bears and Rams. During the fifties at Los Angeles Airport, on the way to San Antonio for an exhibition game with Baltimore, spirited coach Stydahar was heard telling his team to inspire their courage to battle, "Trouble with you guys - too many have your own teeth."

Across a dinner table, news commentator Bill Stout told me a similar story, of another coach of another famous team whose name Bill preferred I don't tell. This fellow, while interviewing prospective players for the new season asked, "Will everyone who wears dentures raise his hand." After hands were up, the coach said, "Everybody whose hands are down leave, and I'll talk with you other guys."

Clark Shaughnessy, among footballs greatest greats, with the game since 1914, told me a sentimentally touched toothless tale. Mr. Shaughnessy is a top football strategist. He's responsible for refining and perfecting the T Formation, a major scientific football technique advance. Clark, as coach in 1940, brought the T technique to Stanford U. revolutionizing the college game. As a pro-ball coach he's been called the "Brains" of the Chicago Bears. He also coached the L. A. Rams. Clark told me he'd always been touched regretfully in the past, though fortunately less with improving mouth protection in the last ten years, upon entering a football dressing room before the game. "The guys you knew would start coming in," Clark said, "and one by one, each changed their faces, taking out a part, left empty in their mouth, putting it on top of a locker shelf." Shaughnessy's a sensitive person. I loved the way he spoke. "Their street citizen faces became toothless game faces." After the game of course, their removable replaced dentures, recreated their people facing faces. Clark Shaughnessy said, "Helmets and masks help, mouthguards add good insurance."

Active participants in contact sports, find it practical to use removable dentures until retired from their active sports career. Then if they like, those who choose, sometimes replace them with teeth permanently attached in their mouth.

DENTAL SPORTS RESEARCH ∾ At Notre Dame University, a five year study of head related injuries suffered by college football players, was made by Drs. Stenger, Lawson, Wright and Ricketts, all Indiana dentists. Their conclusions appear in the Journal of the American Dental Association, Sept. 1964, titled "Mouthguards, protection against shock to head, neck and teeth." The project started during the 1958 football season, when a key player on the squad, as a result of concussion suffered during play, lost his control of equilibrium. His football days seemed ended. Earlier in high school, he had similarly suffered repeated concussion losses of consciousness in scrimmages on the field, yet despite this, because of ability, he was selected All American.

Treatment with experimental dental mouthguard apparatus, relieved the shock contacts between his teeth and temporomandibular jaw hinging skull joints. His equilibrium dramatically returned to normal. Wearing custom made mouthguards designed to accomplish the same result, he returned to his role on the team. From that time his head was clear and his concussions ended. He finished the season at Notre Dame, played in the North-South All Star game in Miami Florida, and continued with football for two years after graduation.

This stimulated interest in mouthguards, and their protection beyond the teeth to other parts of the body. Experiments were conducted with a mouthguard manufacturer. No commerical variety was found satisfactory under field conditions. Consulting with Notre Dame trainer Gene Paszkeit and football players, a custom design was developed during the early 1963 spring practice season, which protected teeth and permitted clear speech. Each member of the team was individually fit with such a custom model by the dentists in the study. Trainer Paszkeit said never before were there so few damages of all kinds as during that '63 spring season. There were no injuries to teeth or jaws, and a great reduction in concussions and neck

TEETH TEETH TEETH

injuries. Guards were continued through the entire '63 football season with similar results.

The study ended in 1963. Anxious to know the attitude after added mouthguard experience at Notre Dame, several years later from Los Angeles, I phoned trainer Gene Paszkeit long distance at South Bend, Indiana. We had an extended conversation. Gene was still as enthused with mouthguards as before but insisted, "They must be custom made. Stock guards aren't worth a darn. Dental made mouthguards are as important for protection as shoulder pads and helmets." Mr. Paszkeit felt the value of mouthguards went beyond that of saving teeth, which were well protected by face masks. "They cut down concussions and neck injury," he said. One boy expressing his feelings of mouthguard protection told him, "I feel I could run through a stone wall with them." Gene has spoken with football trainers of the Air Force Academy at Colorado Springs, the Naval Academy in Annapolis, and West Point in New York. They all seem to feel the same way.

For the professional point of view I spoke with Dr. John H. Stenger who conducted the original study, and is now team dentist at Notre Dame. He repeated the values of mouthpiece protection. In private practice Dr. Stenger devotes much time to problems of the bite-jaw-skull relationship, the source of many complex head and neck disorders. He stressed the importance of dentist taken impressions, and the critical jaw to skull bite relation measurements needed for mouthguard making.

MEDICAL SPORTS RESEARCH ∾ Paul C. Tricket M.D. a physician has been involved with athletics most of his life. He was sports active as a boy. His undergraduate athletic career included track, boxing, and football. He was flight surgeon in the U.S. Air Force. Since 1961 Dr. Tricket taught at Tulane University Medical School, New Orleans. As Director of Athletic Medicine he is also physician for Tulane's football team. Dr. Tricket's personal experience and interest led to him writing a book for trainers, coaches and physicians, "Prevention and Treatment of Athletic Injuries." Meredith Pub. Co. N.Y. 1965. An introduction by Morris Fishbein M.D. many year president of the American Medical Association is evidence of the book's value. Dr. Tricket being a medical doctor deals with injury to the athlete's entire body. He stresses importance of proper fit for all body protecting parts.

Discussing damages to the head Dr. Tricket wrote, "One of the most underrated pieces of equipment in football is the MOUTHPIECE. NO FOOTBALL PLAYER SHOULD BE ALLOWED TO STEP ONTO THE FIELD WITHOUT ONE! To be of maximum use it must be properly fitted by a dentist." Emphasis is copied from Dr. Tricket's book.

TEETH TEETH TEETH

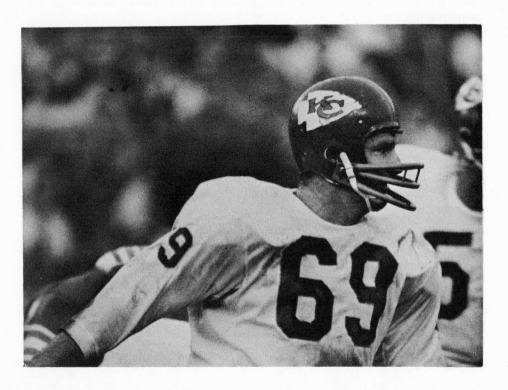

FACE MASK BARS & HELMET s.c.
worn by modern football warriors. Even such protective mouth armor in intensity of the games battle sometimes breaks. Cautious athletes also wear teeth protecting mouthguards. *photo-Life Magazine, N.Y., N.Y.*

ICE HOCKEY

Paying for a ticket, Admission; Walking aisles, Stepping stairs; Squeezing sideways to a seat; Looking, Talking, Waiting, Watching; Skaters swift over hard cold ice. Sticks raised Chasing, Searching Swinging, Dashing Crashing. Driving pucks through opponents goals. Ice hockey is Fast, Furious, Exciting, Dangerous. And accidents happen, injurying bodies, limbs, faces, jaws, teeth.

Towards the second half of the 1800's the game started somewhere over Canada's frozen lakes and ponds. Halifax, Kingston, and Montreal, make claim to the birth of its fame. In 1875 McGill University students started formal rules. Hockey grew, being first played professionally in 1900. In 1920 ice hockey was on the Winter Olympic program and has spread internationally. Because of tradition and the convenient availability of its natural long seasoned frozen facilities, Canada supplies most great players. Modern artificial ice rinks are improving the caliber of those in other countries. Hockey's prize of distinction is the Stanley Cup, awarded each year to the team that is world supreme.

Ice hockey is the most action packed, swiftest moving, skill demanding, roughest team game, causing more tooth damage than any other sport. Most of its athletes do not wear mouthguards. Very few seasoned hockey players have not lost several front teeth, usually of their upper jaw. Often of both. They're knocked out by elbows and hockey sticks, and sometimes struck by the hard rubber puck. Players wear cushioning protection over their lower bodies, and padded gloves cover their hands, but most do not protect their teeth. The alert fast action demands full vision that prohibits face masks, though goal defenders susceptible to extra heavy onslaught sometimes wear them.

Action is furious, demanding so much energy, that for peak efficiency players play only 1-1/2 to 2-1/2 minutes at a time, sometimes a little more. At a signal, a fresh player or group of two or three, leave a long bench along the rink side, entering to replace an equal number of two minute used exhaused perspiring men, leaving the ice for rest on the bench to recharge their body batteries. Hockey players do lots of gum chewing as tension release mechanism. Most smoke few cigarettes. Each team has six men on the ice, five and a goal guarder. Two or three times that number sit along the side recuperating, resting wounds, and waiting for their next chance to play.

Lynn Patrick, Manager Coach for the Los Angeles Blades Ice Hockey Team, lost several teeth playing hockey himself. Lynn used to be with the New York Rangers. During the 1936-37 season Patrick shared a two bedroom apartment in Flushing Long Island with Mac Colville. While practicing at the Madison Square Garden Mac left for the dentist. When Lynn got home Mac was seated reading by a lamp. Lynn asked, "Well Mac, how are you." Mac answered without words, merely lifting his head, looking up open mouthed, showing torn red, stitched, toothless gums.

Thursday evening March 17, 1966, I attended a game at the Los Angeles Sports Arena between the Blades and the Portland Buckaroos, with coach Lynn Patrick, J. H. Winer M.D. team physician, and Aldin Young D.D.S. team dentist. Professional hockey rules require that the home team have a physician at each game. Dr. Winer told me, "It's a rare hockey game at which no blood is shed and stitched flesh patching is not needed." Most damages are to faces and eyebrows, often split scalps need sewing. Dr. Winer said, "There are lots of oral lacerations, split lips and cheeks." The presence of a dentist is not required though Dr. Young attends most Blade games. From Canada, Aldin Young was himself a hockey player when younger. Still involved with the game, Aldin seated at my left near the Blades goal, yelled excited with every intense action.

Dr. Young is a pioneer, introducing mouthguards to ice hockey. Objection to tooth protection from the past carries over, based largely on unsuccessful results with inadequate, stock sized, store counter sold, low priced appliances. They cannot fit properly, loosen and distract the player, interfere with talking and mouthbreathing. Hockey players in action gasp for needing great gulps of air. Experimenting for over a year Dr. Young developed a satisfactory design for ice hockey. It must be custom made by a dentist.

Mark Boileau, a French Canadian, is captain of the Blades. He plays the forward line in the center position. Mark lost four upper central teeth at hockey. Hockey players do not generally get fixed bridgework to replace their missing teeth, that could easily be broken again. They must remove their removable dentures during games, since they could come off, even causing choking to death. The vacated spaces of missing teeth, present their remaining adjacent existing teeth more prominently sharp, to damage the soft cheeks and lips. Several times in the past, hit in action, Mark's canines or eye teeth at each side of his lost teeth area, penetrated cutting through his upper lip to the outside. Scars show the sites. About two months ago Dr. Young made a guard for Mark that I could detect in his mouth on the rink. He's suffered no lip or teeth damage since. Mark Boileau told me, "I wouldn't play without it, and I can chew gum. I forget I'm wearing it. It's great for confidence, helps you play better."

Three weeks later by request Dr. Young made a guard for Willie O'Ree. Willie is a forward right winger. He's played the game for a long time, with the Quebec Aces in Quebec Canada, and the Kingston Frontenacs before the L.A. Blades. Willie too, lost lots of teeth. He took out his denture, removing part of himself to show me. Willie said, "Dr. Garfield, I wish I had this guard ten years ago. I'd still have my own teeth."

Hockey games consist of three twenty minutes play periods, with ten minute intermission rest intervals between, in which the ice surface is cleaned and flushed. During the second interval Dr. Young took from his pocket a plastic envelope, containing a new toothguard he made for Bob Wilson, defense player who came to the Blades from Buffalo last year. Bob also lost teeth at hockey. After the second period he gave Wilson the guard while he rushed by to the locker room. After the game won by the Portland Buckaroos, Doc Young and I joined the players. We asked Bob how he liked his guard. He answered, "Great, it felt strange at first, but I was hit in the mouth and didn't bleed. I know my lip would have split without it. Thanks Doc, it's great." In the dressing room two other players approached Dr. Young asking he make mouthguards for them.

BASKETBALL

Basketball is an American invention created by intention. In 1891 Dr. James A. Naismith, instructor at the International Y.M.C.A. Training School, Springfield Mass., now Springfield College, originated the game. Dr. Naismith felt gymnasium activities like Indian club twirling, bar bell swinging, weight lifting, and chinning, provided limited interest, were not stimulating enough participation. He felt a competitive team game was needed for mature individuals, which didn't present the strenuous dangers of sports like football. He reasoned accidents resulted from rushing towards goals at opposite ends of playing fields. Dr. Naismith thought that if goals were made horizontal, balls would have to be thrown gently up, so as to follow the path of a loop falling down to get in. He invented the game with peach baskets. It was soon apparent their bottoms should be cut out. At first no backboards were used, balls were lost from the court and interfered with by audiences. Wood, then wire mesh, were later adapted as barriers. Now backboards are often strong clear glass for better vision from behind. As basketball popularity grew, it was evident speed, skill, dexterity, and coordinated teamwork were needed.

In 1927 Abe Saperstein became the greatest Basketball Ambassador of International Good Will when he organized the "Harlem Globetrotters." His Negro team covered millions of miles touring the world, Alaska, Egypt, Cuba, Spain, Russia, China, Africa, Sweden, others and on. There were not many countries they didn't play. All these tall athletes leaping gracefully like ballerinas, skillfully dancing with basketballs they bounced and threw, tossed to drop through loops, spread good will for the United States throughout the world.

TEETH TEETH TEETH

Basketball isn't as gentle as originally intended. It is not considered a contact sport. According to rules the only thing a player may touch for is the ball, in fact intentional body contact between opponents is declared foul, and the offending team suffers a penalty.

Players wear no outer protective padding or face masks and hardly need them. They do not use mouthguards. Teeth are accidently damaged but not often. Basketballing teeth themselves however sometimes damage other parts. While leaping high, hand or hands stretched, reaching with the ball to drop it through the goal, or for a ball bouncing rebounding from the round steel ring it hit missing entrance, excited players are sometimes wide open mouthed, with their stretched tensed tongue tip extending through. It has happened at such time, that an opponent striving with an upward stroke to block the shot, or retrieve the ball for himself hit the players chin, snapping its teeth to snip off the tip of their own tongue. Frank O'Neill trainer for Fred Schaus' Los Angeles Lakers Basketball Team, told me Rudy La Russo an outstanding rebounder, one of the best defensive players in the game, bit his own tongue several times, once almost completely through.

I do not recommend basketball athletes wear mouthguards, but for those few with long tensed tongues that stick out to sometimes be bitten, a dentist if asked to, could design a guard that would help. It would more properly be called a tongue guard.

THE SPORT OF KINGS

Royalty is on the way out, but the thrill of racing horses makes every man a king, and riders of racing horses sometimes lose teeth. Johnny Longden was all time king of jockeys, winning more races than any other. Longden retired from his racing career on Saturday, Mar. 12, '66 when he brought George Royal in first, at his own last race, for his 6032nd victory in the San Juan Capistrano Handicap at Santa Anita. Johnny Longden told me, that several years ago at Del Mar Race Track, the horse he rode took him through the rail into the center field for a fall, where he hit a water sprinkler, causing dental damages that cost $4000 to restore.

Horses restrained, excited, frightened at the gate, have thrown their heads back hitting the jockeys huddled over them, striking their jaws together fracturing teeth.

As horses race ahead down the track, their torsos rock in responsive rhythm with their legs thrusting back against the turf. Skilled jockeys lean huddling close forward to lessen their envelope outline of resistance to the air. They are a united union as the jockey alert peers ahead, guiding his living power animal with words and touches and tugs at the neck, with pressures and beats of his arms and legs. As he looks forward to the sides and above, pounding hooves of horses before him have thrown clods of turf up bruising into his face. Goggles protect the eyes, in some cases embedded stones have injured jockeys' teeth.

Racing horses sometime fall, breaking their own teeth and jaws, more often those of those who ride them, especially in steeplechasing. Steeplechase racing supposedly evolved from groups of horsemen galloping, jumping over hedge and wall obstacles of the countryside, towards prominent goals like church steeples. Steeplechasing is popular in Europe.

Raymond Robaire is a Parisian, Frenchman, American sportsman, restauranteur, my friend and patient. Raymond lived, owned and raced horses in Maisons Laffitte for about ten years. In the Los Angeles area Raymond has owned and raced horses for five years. His horses have been ridden by Johnny Longden and Willie Shoemaker at Santa Anita and Hollywood Park. Maison Laffitte is a world famous European horse racing community along the border of the Seine River six miles from Paris. Eighty percent of its residents earn their livelihood with race horses. Raymond told me, "Steeplechasing is very popular in France and very dangerous." In Europe the same men that train horses often ride them. Thoroughbred horses are high strung, sometimes referred to as fickle, and nervous. They are sensitive, easily frightened. They're usually trained to jump hurdles alongside a familiar more experienced horse. While learning to jump, running towards the hurdle, the horse may frighten even by a shadow, suddenly stopping throwing the jockey over his head.

Horse and rider numbers are not limited in steeplechase racing. There may be as many as twenty five. As they race down the turf close, fighting for first, one fall could pile up all, like automobiles on crowded freeway. Raymond told me, "Very few veteran steeplechase trainers and jockeys have not lost teeth. I believe, Sydney," he suggested, "mouthguards should be used in steeplechasing. If properly introduced they'd be welcomed."

MOUTHGUARDS

Mouthguards, also called Toothguards and Mouthpieces originated in boxing, probably because the sport presents the face and mouth as a prime object of attack. I met with dentists and dental technicians who design, prescribe and make mouthguards; fighters, football and hockey players who wear them; athletic trainers, coaches, managers, promoters, and members of governmental athletic agencies controlling their use. Mouthguards are probably the principal dental contribution of athletic significance. Since their value to athletics is interwoven with the progress of each sport described, some details may be repeated.

HISTORY OF MOUTHGUARDS ∾ In early pugilism days, smashed lips, broken noses teeth and jaws, from blows to the face, were expected and accepted like thunder and rain after lightning. Little was done for protection. Most common injury was to the soft inner lip lining, where it crushed tearing over hard tooth fronts, and split over their sharp biting edges. Some clever boxers put soft cotton padding and other substances under their lips, over the teeth and gums, cushioning the blows for lip portection. This was done for a long time. Some boxers still do during practice. Loose cotton under lips is unstable, and in action of battle distractingly difficult to manage.

In the early 1900's Jacob "Jack" Marks, a dentist practicing in the East End of London, was greatly interested in boxing. He took impressions and made models of fighters teeth and jaws, around which he molded a rubber strip that fit over the outer front teeth and gum surfaces, as a protective shield under the lips. They were held in place by fitting accurately into between each tooth space. They were called "gum shields" at the time, and served primarily to protect lips from internal damages. Dr. Marks is considered the inventor of the mouthguard. Ted "Kid" Lewis a clever London boxer, was also interested in mouthguards. He helped Dr. Marks develop the guard and did much to popularize them.

Shields were used mostly around upper teeth, since those stick out further, and are closer to the target for a blow to the nose. Handling separate upper and lower shields would be difficult during a fight. Gum shields were very helpful.

As the United States expanded to lead the world industrially it also provided the largest paying audiences pugilistically. Kid Lewis came to the New York - Boston area to fight, and demonstrated the value of his gum shield mouth piece. He used it in gyms but was prohibited from wearing it in official fights on the grounds that shields were considered foreign bodies, prohibited by London Prize Ring and Queensberry Rules. Proving his ability as a scientific boxer the Kid became Champion Welterweight of the World between 1915 and 1919. During this period he fought Jack Britton twenty-six times throughout the states, losing his title to Jack and recapturing it. Convinced of his teeth protection apparatus' value, Lewis persisted and is responsible for introducing mouthguards to America.

From Los Angeles, I spoke with Mr. Lewis by telephone, where as an old boxing veteran he lives among friends in a hotel outside London. We've had several cross-country trans-Atlantic conversations. "Doc," he said, "They wouldn't let me use shields in the beginning. After the first

TEETH TEETH TEETH

round I'd sneak it in when they weren't looking. It stopped those bloody cuts. I'd hit Jack in the mouth and he'd bleed every time. He'd hit me without much damage. After a few fights Britton wanted one and I helped him get it. Then other guys got shields and they started letting us use 'em. Those they have now are even much better.''

While it was obvious guards shielded lips it was also noticed their rubber resiliency helped save teeth. Improvements were made extending them completely over the teeths biting edges, and continuing a layer around behind more completely surrounding the teeth, front and back, holding on gripping better, distributing the forces as support in back against blows. This is essentially the design of upper mouthguards today.

In the 1920's Jim Farley, later to become Postmaster General of the United States, became New York State's Athletic Commissioner. New York City and its Madison Square Garden were becoming the boxing center of the world. Alert Mr. Farley saw the value of mouthpieces and worked to popularize their use in New York's boxing rings. The use of mouthguards by boxers continually though slowly spread, and has become mandatory in numbers of states for official fights. In 1962 California law demanded their use.

Boxing prominence is primarily professional. Its organized control is independent within each state. Some make no mouthguard provision though their value is being increasingly realized, spreading to other sports.

UNIVERSAL USE ∾ Since 1962 all U.S. high school football teams must provide mouthpieces for players. In some schools because of cost, less expensive ready made or self fit guards are used. The American Dental Association sponsors a program through which dentists donate their services towards providing custom fit guards for high school players. In the Los Angeles area every year hundreds of dentists donate their skills free, making thousands of mouthguards for high school football players.

University football attitude differs. Some feel helmets and face masks are enough protection, that tooth guards interfere with play. Some teams use face masks and toothguards. Some coaches let each individual athlete decide. It seems the use of custom made guards may be more popular in public institutions because of the cost. Around professional football locker rooms it's obvious many players have lost teeth and few wear mouthguards.

It's hard to teach an old dog new tricks, or an athlete who developed his skills without dentist custom made toothguards to use them. It's not easy to convince football players of mouthguard value, when they already have some protection from masks and helmets. Especially if they've had poor past experience with cheap poorly fit mouthpieces, and talked with others

TEETH TEETH TEETH

that also did, and are hardly aware of the important differences between dentist custom fit guards and the store variety. It's as logical as expecting to buy fillings, dental bridges, and dentures that could fit, across a counter.

Professional football players usually get there from college, and college men get there from high school. It's likely the 1962 and later, enforced mouthguard using generation of high school football athletes, as they reach professional status will prefer guards with their games. Gene Paszkeit, Notre Dame trainer, and Dr. Stenger, Notre Dame football team dentist, told me the high school boys coming through with toothguards take personal pride caring for their guards and won't play without them. Dr. Maurice Tyler, a dentist with the Los Angeles School System, especially interested in the high school football program told me, "Syd, we've been perfecting these mouthguards every year. Soon these boys learning to use them in high school will feel naked on the field without them."

THE MOUTHGUARD ∾ Mouthguards are molded of soft resilient, strong rubber or rubber like plastic. Plate 20-1, THE MOUTHGUARD - ATHLETIC TEETH JAW PROTECTOR, illustrates a variety of guards and their values. Drawings A, B, C, D, E, F, G are all of dentist fitted custom made mouthguards. Each is molded over an individual model of its particular athletes jaw, and is adjusted by a dentist if necessary for that athlete's mouth. It will fit only that athlete's mouth. Like fingerprints, no two are ever exactly alike. Drawings A & B are of a modern popular upper mouthguard, as used by most athletes, providing satisfactory protective service. It contacts teeth of the lower jaw equally distributing blows, efficiently absorbing shocks to the head. Around the outside and inside it protects and supports the teeth and other tissues it covers. Its inside view shows the individually molded shapes of each tooth it intimately fits.

Drawings C, D, E, F, G are all shown as cross-sections through the front teeth, jaws, and lips, Each also continues around back, on both right and left sides, closely fitting and protecting the back teeth. Drawing C is of the early 1900 invented "gum shield" which primarily protected the lip. Drawing D is a section of the popular modern upper guard as shown in A & B. It is popularly used in boxing, football, and other sports. The combination of its intimately fitting inner and outer flanges, connected by its tooth edge channel layer, greatly reinforces the entire guard, just as in building construction a steel structural U shaped channel is far superior to a flat strip. Forces delivered at a local spot that could ordinarily knock out teeth, is absorbed by the intimate fit to all the teeth, transferring and distributing the blow along the entire jaw for better resistance.

It has also been found that as the athlete closes his opposite jaw into the resilient material of the tooth edge layer, his jaw muscles automatically

TEETH TEETH TEETH

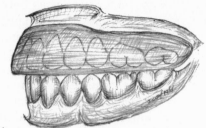

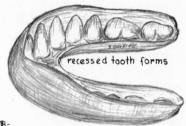

A- SIDE VIEW OF UPPER GUARD IN USE

B- SIDE-INSIDE VIEW OF UPPER GUARD

recessed tooth forms

DENTAL CUSTOM MADE UPPER MOUTHGUARD

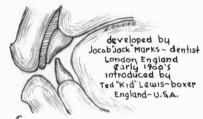

developed by
Jacob "Jack" Marks ~ dentist
London, England
early 1900's
introduced by
Ted "Kid" Lewis ~ boxer
England ~ U.S.A.

C- *the early* GUM SHIELD OR GUARD

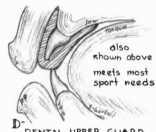

also
shown above

meets most
sport needs

D- DENTAL UPPER GUARD

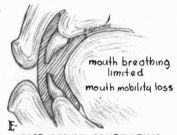

mouth breathing
limited

mouth mobility loss

E- UPPER-LOWER COMBINATION

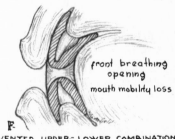

front breathing
opening

mouth mobility loss

F- VENTED UPPER-LOWER COMBINATION

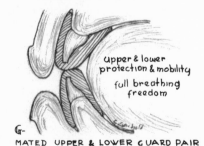

upper & lower
protection & mobility

full breathing
freedom

G- MATED UPPER & LOWER GUARD PAIR

least teeth-jaw
protection

factory molded
edges irritate
lips, gums, tongue

H- STOCK GUARD ~ sold in standard sizes

DESIGN DETAIL VARIETIES
ALL GUARDS SHOWN CROSS-SECTIONED AT FRONT TEETH ~ ALL CONTINUE BACK BOTH SIDES
ALL EXCEPT -H- ARE DENTIST FITTED & INDIVIDUALLY MOLDED FOR EACH ATHLETES TEETH & JAWS

PLATE 20-1 THE MOUTHGUARD ~ ATHLETIC, TEETH, JAW, PROTECTOR S.Garfield

TEETH TEETH TEETH

combine with his jaw hinging joints back on each side of the head, to unify his lower face block into a compact unit, better able to withstand blows to the jaws and skull. Athletes wearing such guards, greatly lessen dangers of concussion loss of consciousness, and more serious injury to the brain. Boxers wearing these guards can better withstand knockout punches, delivered to the jaw. For maximum efficiency, after fabrication in the laboratory, mouthguards may require trial fit and adjustment by the dentist. Such guards are also made for the lower jaw. Individual guards, both upper and lower, as in drawing G worn together, would be even more valuable.

Drawing E shows a combination upper and lower one piece mouthguard. These provide better protection to jaws closed together. Some boxers like them. They may obstruct mouth breathing. Punches to noses often cause bleeding which blocks needed nose breathing. Drawing F shows a one piece, upper and lower air-vented-in-front combination, which helps this problem. Athletes who've lost their teeth and can't control single jaw mouthguards, find combination guards will work.

STOCK — READY MADE MOUTHGUARDS ∾ Someone always tries to make things cheaper, they should if they keep the quality. There are lower costing, less satisfactory, ready made mouthguards available in a few standard sizes in sporting goods stores. They're sometimes sold in drug stores near gymnasiums. Drawing H shows such a mouthguard. It is not dental custom made. It is also shown in cross section through the front teeth jaws and lips. It also continues around back on both sides. It is available in a few mass production standard molded sizes. Even the closest fit is a poor fit. They do not embrace and support the individual teeth. They must be made flexibly flimsy, to adapt to the almost infinite variety of human jaw and teeth arch sizes and forms. It would be extremely rare coincidence that their factory molded constant teeth edge thickness, provided the proper bite relation. Their outer surfaces contain ridge edges, from the factory molds they're made in, that bruise the lips and annoy the tongue. They're often distractingly difficult to keep in place and interfere with speech.

There are higher priced still inexpensive varieties that provide for some individual custom adoption by the athlete himself. They are better than the store standard or stock variety, but less satisfactory than the dentist made product. Mouthguards for protecting jaws and teeth must be as personally individual as dentures for eating that replace missing teeth. They both involve similar dental mouth details. For maximum efficiency they must be made by a dentist.

TEETH TEETH TEETH

A PERSONAL TEST PROGRAM

As part of my mouthguard research I tried mouthguards for myself. In a sports supply store I bought an inexpensive standard mouthguard, marked medium size, which seemed closest for me. I couldn't try first without buying. It seemed a trifle too small, but the next size large was way too big. The same guard is designed for both upper and lower use. It was rubberlike. I put it to place and could feel it forced to spread, fitting over my upper teeth. I am a gagger. It annoyed me to keep it in my mouth. It slipped from position constantly. I had to keep biting together to stabilize it. Enclosed instructions suggested cutting off excesses with a scissor. The overall size was a little too small, but some places were too big and I cut those away. It seemed to stay in place better at times, but often slipped from position. I could feel its irregularities along my gums and under my lips. I could speak with it, though not clearly, and talking made it fall faster. It was generally uncomfortable to feel and use and still caused gagging.

I took an impression of my upper jaw and made a model. According to my prescribed instruction, a dental laboratory cured a rubberlike mouthguard to exactly fit my own mouth model. When delivered to my office, I could see inside the mouthguard each individual tooth as it fit my model and mouth. I placed it to position over my upper teeth. I'm a terrible gagger, it's even hard to take my X-rays. It fit snugly to place but induced gagging. I couldn't speak well. In my office laboratory I ground bulk from the palatal surface. It was more tolerable, my speech improved. There was too much bulk under my lips. I ground that off, was more comfortable, and could talk better. As I closed together the bite wasn't right. Biting on ink marking paper, I ground off the excess to fit my lower teeth. The guard was becoming rather acceptable, but its surface was annoying rough from grinding. Polishing substances in my lab used for grinding conventional denture materials didn't work right. I got the proper supplies, refined and polished the mouthguard, and soon hardly knew I was wearing it. I could speak well and felt a sense of security with the mouthguard in my mouth. I like it.

TEST LIMITS ∾ I did not submit myself to blows on the jaw for test resistance to my teeth being knocked out.

MOUTHGUARDS CAN TREAT TEETH ∾ Sometimes blows to the mouth are especially heavy. The mouthpiece may be strong enough to prevent the loss of teeth, but the force so severe the guard deflects and teeth loosen. In such cases the same dental guard that prevent their loss can

TEETH TEETH TEETH

also help them heal. After examination and treatment, the dentist may recommend wearing the accurate fitting mouthpiece, to keep the loose teeth stabilized as a supporting splint in the mouth, which can also hold medications, keep the area clean, and help the surrounding bone retighten.

A MOUTHPIECE STORY ∾ On Mar. 3, 1966 in Los Angeles, I attended a ten round heavyweight bout that went all the way, between local Amos "Big Train" Lincoln and Billy Daniels from New York City. Coincidentally sitting near me at ringside, also watching the match, was singer Billy "Ole Black Magic" Daniels, unrelated to the fighter. It soon became apparent to me watching closely, as each heavyweight's mouthpiece was removed after every round, that Big Train Lincoln was wearing a dental custom made combination upper and lower air vented guard. Daniels used an upper store bought stock guard. Though both fighters hit each other's mouths, in a short time Daniels bled profusely yet Lincoln's mouth was clean. He did lose a little blood from over one eye. Twice Daniels' non-dentist-fit, stock mouthpiece, fell from his mouth, and the bout was stopped according to California rules, until washed by his seconds and replaced. The rest may have been welcomed by Billy, who wasn't doing well, and lost the match by unanimous decision.

EVEN BILLIARDS

Accidents happen in every sort of sport, don't blame a particular game. Billiards also called pool, uses skill and a long thin leather tipped stick called a cue or cue stick, to hit a small white ivory ball called a cue ball, directed at another ball hit into holes called pockets, along the borders of a table top. Billiards can damage teeth.

While writing this chapter concerning sports, I asked patient, dancer, actress Eleanor Powell who originally encouraged me to write the book, whether she would care to read my manuscript. She read and said she enjoyed it, and, "Well you know Syd, those porcelain jackets you made for Peter were caused by a sport accident." Peter Ford is the son of actors Glenn Ford and Eleanor Powell. "About thirteen years ago," Eleanor said, "Glenn was doing a picture in Brazil called "Americana." The story was woven around Brahman cattle. Some of the filming was in deep jungle. I remember seeing an old bull sacrificed, torn bloodily apart and devoured in a few minutes by schools of small piranha fish, in a river where the animal was led to divert attack from a large herd crossing downstream. Pete was eight at the time. We both joined Glenn near Rio de Janeiro as guests of a wealthy rancher.

TEETH TEETH TEETH

One day Glenn and the Brazilian rancher were playing billiards. Pete watched closely, resting his head on his palms over the billiard table edge, keenly interested, eyes widely opened, following every play. The Brazilian measured a critical shot, drawing his cue stick back and forth, the tip end slowly sliding, supported guided between adjacent fingers close behind a ball. Peter watched alerted, parting his lips, exposing his teeth. The Brazilians right hand drove hard, the tip of the stick miscued, improperly striking the ball, to jump from the table, hitting between Peter's upper left central and lateral incisors, fracturing each adjacent tooth crown corner off."

I do not prescribe wearing toothguards, while resting your head on your palms at the edge of a billiard table while watching the game played in Brazil.

I do not prescribe wearing mouthguards with safety belts while driving, though for those who care to it might save their teeth. I do not recommend mouthguard protection against the dangers of love. Even the most expert dentally adjusted equipment could lessen the thrill of a kiss.

Life Throughout involves with Contest
Imperfection Correction delivers our Best

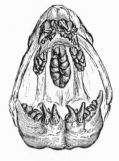

WOLF FISH
Anarrhichas lupus
showing great variety
of tooth forms. Front
pointed grasping &
biting teeth. Inner
blunt crushing teeth
also called SEA CAT
fair food value

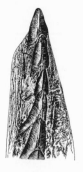

SECTION cut through
JAW of *Pseudoscarus*
or PARROT FISH
shows a succession
of six teeth forming
beneath following
to erupt
little food value

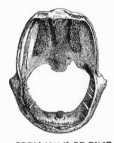

OPEN JAWS OF PIKE
ESOX lucius
Myriads of hinged
teeth along upper
palate back into throat
& some under tongue
Pointed short and long
individual teeth
around lower jaw
borders~ a food fish

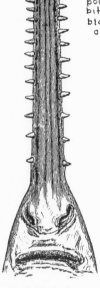

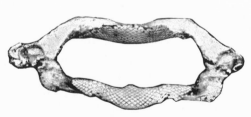

S H A R K
with some attached spine

A YOUNG SAWFISH
Pristis
seen from beneath
Rostral teeth projecting
along both sides of
its long rostrum beak
Pavement teeth inside
its bottom side mouth

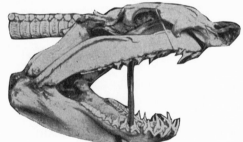

Myliobates or BAT RAY
Pavement teeth shown covering
open jaws like tiles over a floor
skates ~ rays ~ sawfish

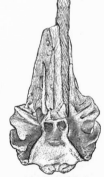

NARWHAL
from beneath
Long tusk &
unerupted tooth

TEETH ~ JAWS ~ SKULLS of WATER ANIMALS S.G.
ONLY A FEW OF A GREAT VARIETY

TEETH TEETH TEETH

TEETH BENEATH THE WATERS

Little more than a quarter of Earth's surface is land. This from deep below, spreading, rising, penetrates, exposing to us through the face of water, waters drawn down filling the voids, covering almost three quarters of our planet. Reaching to depth of six and a half miles. These waters fresh and salt, envelope what amounts to another world, a liquid environment of water. A world we enter but briefly, to dive and swim in, sometimes explore. Sometimes reach into for food. Some waters are cold arctic, some hot springs.

Many creatures live in these waters, abundantly towards the top, diminishing with depth. Animals have been found three and a half miles down. Varieties include worms, corals, snails, starfish that are really not fish, jellyfish that aren't fish either, octopus, sharks called cartilagenous fish, real fish, whales, animals growing inside shells, animals that grow around outside their shells, others probably not yet even discovered. Most of these creatures have teeth, or primitive types of teeth.

FISH TEETH TYPES

Tiny marine sea horses, and giant fresh water sturgeon reaching 24 feet at 3200 pounds, have no teeth at all. Myxine hagfishes or slime eels, not true eels, are long, slimy, slender like snakes. They have no bones, scales, or side fins. Their eyes are under the skin. They have no jaws. They have a single sharp pointed tooth, centered projecting forward from their mouth roof, and hardened toothlike edges along each tongue side. Their mouth is small round, with lips diverging to tiny tentacles. Sucking they attach to other fish, and use their centered tooth as a surgical lancet, to penetrate the flesh for blood food. Their toothlike tongue edges actively follow boring into the body, which they enter devouring their victim from the inside. Though they like to become very intimate they should not be considered friendly. Myxines are found along coasts of large parts of the world. Myxine Bdellostoma of Chile has a bright yellow tooth. Myxine Glutinosa of Europe reaches 3 feet long. We're not anxious to meet them, they could eat your heart out.

Parrot fish teeth like parrot bird beaks, function forward in front without lips over them. They seem completely solid around each jaw. Divided by a front centered vertical line they look like broad teeth, one right one left, both top and bottom. They really consist of smaller individual hard enameled teeth, intimately fused to each other, blending with their inner supporting bone. Parrot fish use them to bite, crush and eat barnacles, crustaceans like crabs, and corals. Their strong enamel teeth grind hard coral to sand, which they swallow eating, to digest the small amount of soft inner live content. A single parrot fish's teeth grind consuming thirty pounds of coral a day, converting to over five tons, or ten thousand pounds of sand in a year. Some fish have several teeth, some many more. Certain bony fishes have thousands of teeth, lining the jaws, roof, and floor of their mouth, attaching to the tongue down into the throat.

Few fish chew. They swallow torn off pieces, or entire prey, usually smaller fish whole. Their teeth, sharp pointed, back directed, holding, prevent escape of their slippery subjects. Cod and pike have a hinged type of tooth. Not rigidly fixed at the base, they attach with flexible elastic fibers to the jaws, swingable rearward towards the throat. It may seem to some curious victims comfortable relaxing in the dark back inside. The teeth yielding gently deflect, permitting easy passage one way only. Instantly erected, sharply aggressively pointed against retreat, escape is impossible.

Fish teeth vary. Some large mouthed Siluroid catfish, of fresh river waters in Europe and Asia, within their long flexible sensory perception barbels, encircling their lips like cats whiskers, have strong hard, inch and a half and longer teeth, rigidly fixed to their jaws. Tiny mouthed Chaetodonts from tropical salt seas, gorgeously patterned, vari-colored and irridescent bright, have fine short flexible wavy teeth, like soft little hairs.

Fish don't drink. Anyone who "drinks like a fish" won't get much at all. The only water entering fish stomachs is that swallowed with food. Constant, opening mouth closing fish procedure, only pumps water through their gills. Dissolved oxygen in the water is extracted for breathing, as it passes through the fine capillary blooded gill network on each side of the fish head. That water doesn't enter fish throats. Fish have nostrils, not for breathing, on each side of their snout. These connect with olfactory sacs, for smell sensation of substances in the water.

SHARKS

Sharks are vertebrates of the scientific Class: Chondrichthyes or cartilagenous fishes. Vertebrates are animals with a structural framework, like a spinal column or backbone. Vertebrates include man. Sharks vertebral column and other body structures are of cartilage or gristle, not bone. In Greek chondros means cartilage, ichthyes means fish. Ichthyology is the study of fish. The word fish is from the Latin "pisces." Fish that have bone structures, like sardines, salmon, common eels, tuna and others are of the Class: Osteichythes. Osteo means bone. Sharks entire skeletons are of cartilage, sometimes reinforced with deposits of harder lime. Their jaws are movable with the cranium or skull. They have hard enamel covered teeth. Most sharks live in open waters, more numerous towards the tropics. Some leave the salted seas, entering narrowing rivers invading the land. Some sharks live permanently in fresh water. Certain sharks on rare occastions even enter polar regions. They are all predacious, living preying on other animals appropriate to their size. Some largest capture seals and sea lions. Harmless whale sharks up to 50 feet long feed on tiny plankton.

I've always loved adventure, traveling far primitive and foreign lands, fascinated with life, plant, animal, human, wild, land and sea. In native canoe I've penetrated dense Mexican jungle, on camelback crossed Egyptian desert. In Casablanca and Marakesh, Morrocan North Africa, I've experienced intrigue. Alaskan waters encircled me with schools of whales. Diving into waters underworlds found other creatures of such seas. I seek the unusual and though danger frightens, it is excitement unequalled. Such living gives life many lives for me, stimulating, educational, pleasured, romantic.

During search for authentic informative material for this chapter, I once unexpectedly found myself closely surrounded by large numbers of the open jaws of sharks, each and all studded with sharp pointed protruding teeth. Sharks of all kinds, of many sizes, menacing, from the small three foot dog shark, to large vicious tiger sharks, and great white sharks that reach thirty one feet long, man eaters. Jaws open, aggressively gaping. Such variety could rarely if ever be found assembled in common waters. Probably never. They were skeletal specimens around the office of Dr. Sheldon Applegate, Associate Curator of Paleontology, where I met him at the Los Angeles County Museum in Exposition Park. I examined these specimens small and large, jaws, tissues, teeth. Some shark teeth were broken, some were missing, none showed decay. Shark teeth vary. Some are pointed and sharp. Most are triangular and sharp. A few are like knives and little saws and sharp. They're always very sharp.

Like other fish, sharks have many teeth, lose many teeth, grow many teeth, often swallow their own detached and embedded in their victims. They've been found in sharks dissected stomachs. Around the entire forward edge of sharks upper and lower jaws, prominent functional teeth are studded abreast, pointed sharp, next to each other in line, presenting a

TEETH TEETH TEETH

continuous advancing front of teeth. Behind each individual tooth inside, there is another tooth growing. Behind that another, behind that another, behind that another and another behind that. It's best to examine unalive sharks. A skeletal specimen hangs in my home, in which I counted six teeth behind each other in every row. Like soldiers ready to take the place of those lost in battle.

Shark and other fish teeth die and fall at early fish teeth ages. They don't live long enough to decay. Continuously Erupting teeth, Using teeth, Losing teeth, Replacing teeth, fish especially sharks are sort of teeth factories. Teeth; Teeth; Teeth; Teeth; Teeth; Teeth; Teeth; The bottom of the ocean is covered with teeth. In some places this is actually so. They accumulate in crevices. As fish die they fall, partly eaten, their remains decompose. Harder resistant tooth material survives, collects, increases in quantity, where they have been found over large areas by investigators of the ocean floor.

Most shark teeth lead the lives described. There are exceptions. Dave Powell, Curator of Fishes at Sea World San Diego, told me of a small free swimming copepod crustacean, that attacks the teeth of blue colored Bonita Sharks. The copepod has a body about one half inch long, usually followed by two filamentous egg sacs each an inch long. They sometimes attach to the outer shark skin seemingly harmlessly. They often enter the sharks mouth to attack their teeth attachments. They project grasping extensions, deep into the flesh surrounding bonita shark teeth, and boring in consume and destroy the soft adjacent tissues, often causing severe tooth loss. Bonita shark tooth tissue is apparently copepod delicacy. The teeth themselves too hard to damage fall away. Dave told me, "Doctor I've seen as many as fifteen in a shark's mouth. It looked a mess."

Sharks feed a way of their own. Humans feed their way. They can cut off a piece on a plate. Their hands help hold, delivering food to front teeth which bite into cutting off. Human jaws closing together are also adapted to perform sideways slicing actions. Try it. The hand helps tear, separating the outer piece away. People with teeth can bite off well.

Shark jaws can only open and close directly as a hinge. No side action is possible. Luckily they have no hands to hold while biting off particular pieces. The shark darts in at his victim, may turn to present his undersided mouth, then bites in holding on. He starts to roll and twists and shakes his body one way and another. His exerted torso oscillations, against the inertia of his struggling victims body mass in the water, helps his closing teeth quickly saw through, severing the engaged part as a bite. Then he swallows. So whenever you are bitten by a shark I will tell you what to do.

TEETH TEETH TEETH

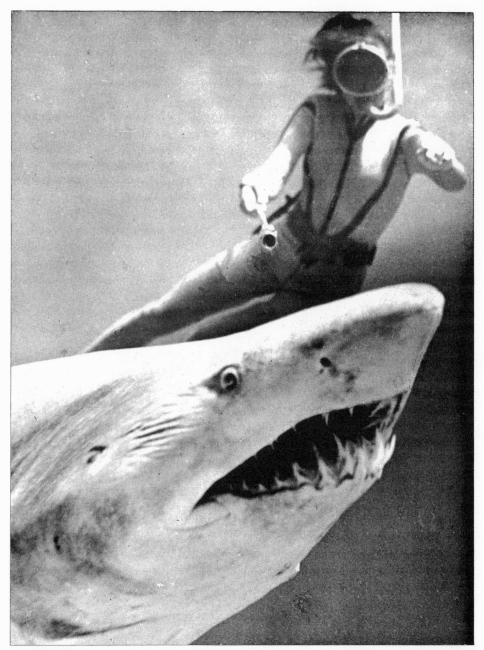

Photographer~ Ben Cropp, Sydney, Australia ~ Ben must have been quite close. The sharks teeth can be seen, one behind another, continually erupting succeeding replacing those lost in use. Powerful jaw muscles are evident around the angle of its mouth.

TEETH TEETH TEETH

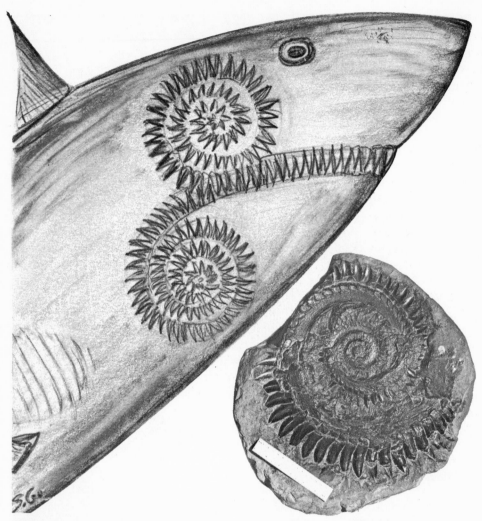

COILING ROWS OF SPIRAL ROLLS OF SUCCESSIVE REPLACEABLE TEETH

Helicoprion an extinct shark lived in the Permian Period 225 million years ago. No relatives of Helicoprion are known to live today. The lower right circular photo is of one of it's Teeth Roll Fossil Specimens found near Montpelier, Idaho, now at the Los Angeles County Museum of Natural History. The drawing above shows an internal view of the probable relation of its upper and lower rolls of spiraling teeth, forming at the centers, enlarging while coiling around and erupting forward for use in the mouth, followed by eventual loss and continual successive replacement. Existing few specimens do not definitely determine whether Helicoprion had a single row of teeth above and below centered in its head, or like todays sharks and most other teeth on both sides of the mouth. Size of Helicoprion can be estimated from the 6 inch rule on the photo indicating the single specimens 17 inch diameter. Teeth of some extinct animals are the only remaining evidence of their early existence, because teeth though subject to decay, are the hardest substance of bodies.

TEETH TEETH TEETH

Do not fight back resisting. You will only be bitten off faster. If you relax and calmly lie back it might take a little longer. The best thing to do in trying to remain wholesome, and stop yourself from being separated from yourself, is not to lose your head. Try to coordinate with the shark. Act as a good dancing partner, blend with him as a unit in movement. Jig with the shark when he jigs. Jag when he jags. Don't jag when he jigs or jig when he jags, and PRAY.

CETACEANS ∾ WHALES, DOLPHINS, PORPOISES

The largest living creature in or out of water is the whale. Blue whales have been found 105 feet long weighing 130 tons, well over a quarter of a million pounds. That's a whale of a whale. Whales are of the highest zoological class Mammals, like man. The class name mammal derives from the mammary glands or teats that its female members use to suckle, feeding their milk to dependent young. Whales are of the mammalian order Cetacea comprising whales, dolphins, porpoises. Cetus is Latin for whale.

Distinction between whales, porpoises and dolphins has not been definitely established, though particular creatures through time have become identified with particular names. In some areas certain animals are called one, while in other places similar appearing may be named another. It is interesting that the creature called the Killer Whale, which reaches thirty feet long, is considered by some marine zoologists to be the largest dolphinoid or dolphin cetacean. That's a whale of a dolphin. The name whale is most usually applied to the larger cetaceans. Porpoises are often those with dorsal fins, or fins on top, that are triangular in shape. They have blunt snouts and chisel shaped teeth. Dolphins often have dorsal fins which curve pointed backwards, longer snouts and pointed teeth. Some cetaceans have no dorsal fins at all.

Cetaceans vary in size and form, though they're always stoutish, heavy rounded of body. Greatest variation is in head design. Some are blunt, round in front, even somewhat square. Some are pointed in front, extended or shortened. Some have mouths that split their heads, halfway between top and bottom. Some have jaws thick or thin, either on top or bottom. Some cetacean mouths are close to the top, so that the upper jaw, which could be long or short is shallow, while its lower is massive. Some mouths lie close to the bottom of the head, as ours do, leaving a thin lower jaw mating well with a tremendous above. Strangest mates combine as compatible couples.

Whales and other cetaceans look like blunted fish and live swimming in water like fish, but are not fish. They are mammals like man. They breathe air, which they must rise to the water surface for periodically, every several

TEETH TEETH TEETH

or more minutes of their lives, twenty four hours of every day of their lives. If they fail to breathe this way they drown. Seriously sick cetaceans are sometimes supported by others to keep them from drowning. Through blowhole nostrils at the top of their head, inhaled air enters going down for use in whale lungs. The sighting sign of the old whalers "thar she blows" is the whale's exhaled body warmed used air, clearing from its nostrils, dragging surface sea water with it, and condensing moisture from cooler ocean air, to form the picturesque fountain like spout. Fish breathe, gulping water as they swim along in it, forced through their gills which extract dissolved oxygen. They have no lungs. Fish tails are vertical for directional guidance like a rudder. Whale and other cetacean tails are horizontal, for frequent up and down going control needed to breathe.

Whales have skin like man, thick like some, sometimes several hairs like some, not scales like fish. Fish pectoral or chest fins, have fine rays of varied numbers. The fore or chest limbs of a whale called fins and flippers, are covered with flesh and skin, shaped looking like fins. They help whales swim like fish. Inside these finlike appendages, from the body structure out, there is a humerus bone like in man's arm, going to radius and ulna bones as in man's forearm, connecting with inner wristlike carple bones then four or five finger bones. They never hold toothbrushes like some people don't. Whales have large brains. They communicate with each other using a system of sonarlike high frequency sound, which they emit by vibrations in their blowholes, and also use for navigation like radar. The Susu, a river dolphin of India, seems to be normally blind maneuvering entirely by its sound system.

The cetacean sex drive can be strong. Captive dolphins and whales, male and female in large tanks, sometimes attempt masturbation and homosexual intercourse. Whale courtship is somethat like man's. I've seen whales chase, nip, playfully bite and kiss lips to lips, before sexual intercourse. Reproduction is viviparous like man's, meaning the female delivers her young alive at birth. Whales don't lay eggs. Whale males have a penis, females a vagina. After a whaling intercourse and eleven months or more depending on the species, the whalet developing within the uterus is born alive, usually one at a birth, up to twenty three feet long. That's a whale of a baby whale. Diaper service would be very expensive. Cetacean pregnant females suffering difficulty delivering their young, are sometimes helped by other whales, who gently assist passage of the new born whalet from the birth canal. That's a whale of an obstretician or midwife. Though whale teeth sometimes decay, I've never heard of whale dentists. Mother whales in the water nurse their young with milk from their breasts, as fewer human mothers are doing. They're very protective watching their whalets well.

TEETH TEETH TEETH

TEETH BENEATH THE WATERS

Most fish are oviparous. Females have no uterus for developing their young. Eggs produced in ovaries are released through oviducts, layed in great numbers into the water. Brook trout according to size lay 80 to 5600 eggs, ocean sunfish 300 million eggs at a time. The male fish near its female, from his testes ejaculates tremendous numbers of free swimming microscopic sperm into the water. Most waste. Some manage their own personal microscopic intercourse with individual eggs they encounter, penetrate and fertilize, outside the parent fish bodies. Certain marine varieties hatch in a few hours. Temperature is a factor. Brook trout eggs below 40°F take 90 days or more. Hatchlings of most fish fend for themselves, soon being eaten by others, including their own parents.

The zoological order Cetacea which includes Whales contains two sub-orders or groups, classified according to their teeth, Toothless Whales and Toothed Whales. Toothless whales do not have teeth, toothed whales do have teeth.

WHALES WITHOUT TEETH

Toothless whales are of the zoological suborder Mysticeti. Mystax in ancient Greece meant mustache. Instead of teeth the toothless whale has mustache-like dental apparatus. Whale information is limited though increasing. At the rate we are killing them we may never know much about them. Man killed, and other discovered dead specimens, of pregnant female whales of both toothed and toothless varieties, reveal embryonic or fetal young whales developing in the uterus, with rudimentary primary or baby teeth like those of humans forming their first set. In the pregnant toothless whale, these primary teeth are then naturally lost while the young are still developing in the uterus. As the uterus nourished unborn toothless whale continues to grow, nature then replaces its lost primary teeth, with a dental structure of developing whalebone, also called baleen.

Baleen is not bone. It is plastic like, of a dense horny fingernail like quality. Baleen attaches to inside the whale's upper jaw, parallel to its cheeks on each side, as a series of large sheets hanging down from the top. As the baleen extends down inside the mouth towards the bottom, the sheets thin, separating, fraying, and spreading wide into long fine close hairs like of a broom. With the whale's mouth closed they fold up, in, and back, lining the mouth roof, laying over the whale's tongue. Somewhat like an inner mouth roof, long haired, nearly arranged, mustache. Ancient editions of Aristotle called such whales Mystakoketos, meaning whale with a mustache.

The feeding toothless whale swims ahead, jaws apart wide, through dense schools of small marine animals, taking mouthfuls, past its raised

TEETH TEETH TEETH

baleen. When he's gotten enough, the whale's mouth partially closes. The baleen drops towards the lower jaw edges, sealing along the lips as a sieve. The whale closes closer, forcefully expelling the water, as his living seafood collects in masses inside along the baleen edges. Some children squirt water out between teeth, like their toothless whale relatives do. With a sweep of his tongue wiping them off, the whale collects his food and swallows, as some men do with their mustache. That's a whale of a meal. I don't think Jonah got in that way. Baleen or whalebone or toothless whales, are among the larger cetaceans of the oceans. Smallest is the Pigmy Fin Whale also called the Minke which grows to twenty eight feet.

TOOTHLESS WHALE DENTAL DIFFICULTY ∾ The most valued whalebone whale was the Bowhead or Greenland Whale or Right Whale. They reach about fifty feet. Their mouths are tremendous occupying the middle of their heads, which take the entire forward third of their body. Such a whale of a mouth, had whale like amounts, of whale sized sheets of whalebone. They have tiny eyes at the mouth intersecting ends of their jaws, on each side above, just in front of their small chest fins. They have no dorsal fin. Not much is known of baleen or whalebone diseases of today. Mysticeti whales especially the Right Whale have suffered severely from a terrible mouth problem large parasite. In fact they were almost completely exterminated by it. They were called Right Whales since their whalebone dental sheets were up to twelve feet, even longer, making them the most desirable or right variety for pursuit, by cruel selfish mammal animals that chased them in ships, killed them, invaded their mouths, and took their whalebone to make women's corset stays. The development of modern plastics and other materials, has completely eliminated the need for whalebone, unfortunately rather late for the whale.

CETACEANS WITH TEETH

Through the long continuing past lower animal forms developed to higher. Some progressed evolving to dominant mammals and founded the Age of Mammals. Among them there were the whales. Some of these whales became the toothless Mysticeti whales of today. From the Eocene Epoch, ranging vaguely perhaps 50 million years ago, we've found fossils of Odontoceti whales, whales with teeth. Squalodon had about 60 teeth. Zeuglodon three hundred and sixty, a whale of a collection of whale teeth. Like man today, their teeth were Heterodont. That means teeth in different parts of the jaw have different shapes, better suiting them to more ideally do different types of tooth work, needed at their locations. Sharp front teeth bite off better. Pointed teeth seize and hold. Blunt backers grind. Those

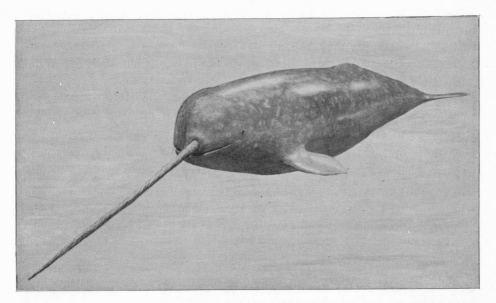

NARWHAL- *Monodon monoceros* - A TOOTHED WHALE OF THE ARCTIC

The Narwhal attains a body length of over twenty feet. From the left side of the males head a tooth projects growing as a left twisting spiral hollow ivory tusk sometimes reaching to nine feet, even more. Inside the skulls opposite side a small tooth exists invisible unerupted. Rare males grow two projecting tusks, one left, one right. Female narwhal tusk teeth both remain underdeveloped, small unseen unerupted never coming through. Narwhals are born with several other smaller teeth soon lost.

TEETH TEETH TEETH

early toothed whales may have had different ways of securing food, and preparing it for digestion. Our toothy cetaceans today or Odontoceti include whales porpoises and dolphins. All have somewhat Homodont teeth. That means their teeth are mostly rather alike, similarly formed along their jaws. There is great difference however between the teeth of some cetaceans and others.

The Sperm whale also called Cachalot grows to 60 feet. Very active they can leap completely from the water, falling back with sound like a shot. Its head is blunt massive on top to the front. Its lower shallow jaw can open down almost to ninety degrees. It is the only whale with a throat large enough to pass a man. The lower jaw has numerous teeth held tightly by their tough gums, which when stripped away often take the teeth with it. They are not firmly rooted in bone. The upper jaw has only a few stunted teeth. Sperm whale teeth have little value. The whale feeds on fish and large squid or cuttlefish, which they swim into wide mouthed and swallow whole. Sperm whales are hunted for their blubber and spermaceti, a white oily wax used in ointments, contained in cell spaces of its large upper head. I've been told whale meat tastes good, though most in our part of the world is canned to cat and dog food. Sperm whales are the prime source of ambergris, a waxy substance sought as a scent holding base for perfume. It is created in the whale's alimentary canal, as a pathological product reacting against an irritant in its cuttlefish food. Ambergris is found in sperm whale stomachs, and sometimes thrown up as a valuable whale vomit which floats, and is searched for in tropical oceans.

Ziphoid whales grow to thirty feet. Their front head is pointed long like a beak. They have no teeth in their upper jaw. The lower has two single thin strong straplike teeth or tusks, rising on each side, outside around the upper jaw to ten inches long. They have tooth tips on top sometimes curving inwards toward each other, which could act as jaw opening stop limits. These teeth seem of little value. The larger teeth of males may be used in sexual pursuit and attack. Female ziphoids have been found with series of double parallel healed scarred lines around their vaginal slits.

The mythical unicorn horse had a horn from the center of its head. The unicorn of the sea is a real whale, with a real tooth projecting like a horn, from the left near the center of its head. The longest, straightest, strongest, tooth of time is the Narwhals. Supported attached in the upper front skull, with a three or four inch diameter round ivory like base, the tooth extends ahead, narrowing twisting tapered, to a thin pointed tip, in exceptional specimens up to twelve feet long away. That's a narwhale of a tooth. There

TEETH TEETH TEETH

is only one like it to a family of four, two father teeth and two mothers. Both male and female narwhals have only two teeth each in their upper jaw, with none below. Only one of all these can be seen. Through the evolution of time, for reasons we'll probably never know, the male narwhals left tooth kept to its own territorial side, yet evolved migrating up, to penetrate above through its lip outside the mouth, directed straight ahead, twisting to the left on its axis like a spiraling sword. The twist helps its structural properties. In a narwhal body up to twenty feet that left tooth could extend seven to ten feet ahead. Most narwhals are torsoed and tusked shorter. The opposite right male tooth is small, unerupted invisible beneath the flesh. Rare narwhal males have been found with two long tusks. Female tusks are always more modest, entirely out of sight. They're both short, perhaps eight inches long, unerupted inside the bone. The nar of narwhal is from an old Norse word meaning corpse or dead body, because of its whitish grey color. Differently from other whales that travel spanning oceans, narwhals range only the Arctic.

The Common Dolphin, Delphinus Delphis, of world wide warm waters, grows to six or more feet and has 200 teeth, probably more than any other living mammal. The Bottlenose Dolphin is friendly and clever, some perform in sea circuses. They have about 100 teeth.

TEETHED CETACEAN TEETH PROBLEMS ∾ For information concerning cetacean dental disease I inspected a limited number of dead and live specimens, read numerous scientific papers, and consulted marine scientists and caretakers that worked with such animals. At the Los Angeles County Museum of Natural History I met Dr. David K. Caldwell, Curator of Ichthyology and Marine Zoology. Dr. Caldwell showed me the diseased skull of a fresh water dolphin from the Amazon River, Colombia, South America. The animal died within two weeks after capture. I examined the specimen, some of its teeth were darkly stained and covered with deposits. Between stains, some tooth parts were a dullish slightly yellow white, similar in appearance to soft human teeth. I probed with an instrument finding they were soft. All were severely worn along the jaws, almost to the gums in some places. There were areas of bone degeneration similar to human peridontal disease. A few teeth were decayed. In the lower left jaw rear molar region, between two decayed teeth towards the root tips, there was an abscess loss of bone from the tooth ridge down which spread inside, extensively undermining a large part of that side and perforating through the outer jaw surface eroding into almost an inch opening. The disease of long duration, could have caused the dolphin's death. Before antibiotics similar jaw infections killed humans. Dr.

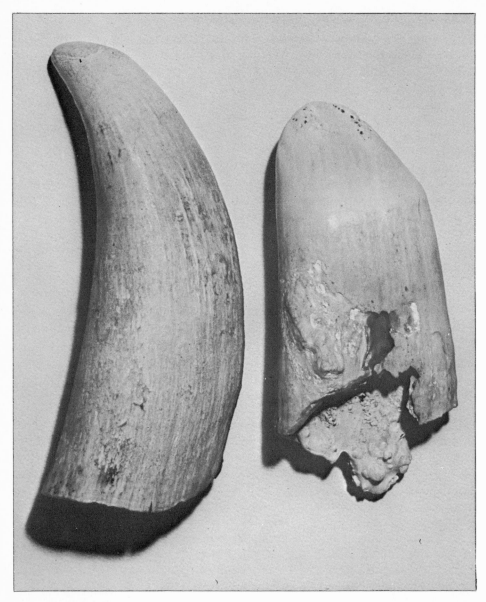

TWO SPERM WHALE TEETH

The sperm whale up to 60 feet long, is the only whale with a throat large enough to pass a person. Its lower jaw has long conical curved tapering teeth. Shown actual size one is slightly worn at the tip. The other even bigger originally shows severe wear, extensive decay and peridontal degeneration. close examination discloses a natural attempt at repair with secondary dentin as occasionally occurs with humans.   photo-Leland Auslender   S.G.

TEETH TEETH TEETH

Caldwell had seen even more pathological dental cases, in the same and other species. Several other dolphin specimens also had severely worn teeth though otherwise undiseased. The Museum also had whale teeth with heavy wear. Some of these also had large pyorrhetic deposits, root degeneration and decay. Most museum whale skull specimens showed healthy teeth and jaws.

I corresponded and spoke several times by trans-Pacific telephone with Dr. Masaharu Nishiwaki of the Whaling Research Institute, Tokyo, Japan. Despite difficulty understanding Dr. Nishiwaki's spoken English, which far surpassed my complete inability to speak Japanese, our communications were valuable. Dr. Nishiwaki also told me of severe whale tooth wear, peridontal disease and tooth decay, though again many whale teeth were worn though otherwise healthy. He never said any whales ate candy. The doctor sent me a large sperm whale tooth, containing a two inch cavity, showing formation of secondary dentin. This is an attempt at natural self tooth repair sometimes also occurring in human teeth.

The Killer Whale of Atlantic and Pacific Oceans, also called the Grampus, reaches twenty to thirty feet long. It is black with yellow white patches beneath going up its sides. They're fast, travel in packs. Their mouth opens wide to bite and seize. Their strong sharp pointed canine like teeth several inches long, interdigitate deeply from their upper and lower jaws. They attack to kill, devouring big fish and seals, and even join ganging in numbers to slay other whales many times their own size. They tear and strip victims tails, tongues, flippers, fins, and lips, then wait for death from loss of blood to devour the carcass. Killer whales have been found beached, with severe unevenly worn teeth and dislocated jaw-bite relation problems, similar though worse than that of man. It is felt killer whales' jaw misalignment could be caused by their violent feeding action of grasping large victim bodies, and tear twisting parts of their prey. Specimens have been found with broken infected jaws. Tomes' "Dental Anatomy" 1914 describes one, in Britain's Oxford Museum found 1873, whose improper lower jaw bite relation caused such excessive teeth wear that their internal pulp was exposed, infecting through those teeth to abscess and destroy the supporting jawbone around them. More recently Dr. Caldwell of Los Angeles Museum, Brown of Marineland Pacific, Palos Verdes, and other investigators report similar findings.

CETACEAN PSYCHOLOGY ∾ At the University of California Los Angeles, I met Dr. Kenneth Norris, Professor of Zoology. Dr. Norris a former Curator of Marineland of the Pacific, has also been design consultant for several large oceanariums of the world. He edited "Whales, Dolphins and Porpoises," Univ. of Calif. Press 1966, a thorough treatise

TEETH TEETH TEETH

by numerous specialists. Dr. Norris' findings of these water mammals' physical and dental disease seemed similar to those described. He introduced additional psychological factors. Among his researches Dr. Norris studied cetaceans of the Hawaiian area. A young Pacific Bottlenose Dolphin caught in ocean waters, was kept and trained in a netted lagoon at Coconut Island, Kaneohe Bay, Oahu. The dolphin adapted, soon befriending other sea animals and humans of the project. He learned to love his keeper and depended on him. After six months the dolphin was taken one half mile from shore, where in its former natural water home it was released for observation.

Dr. Norris told me, "The dolphin left alone seemed instantly terrorized. Flapping his flippers, rolling his eyes nervously, he chattered his jaws and teeth. You could hear them." Dr. Norris said such teeth jaw chattering often occurred when dolphins felt threatened in nature. The behavior is recognized by others as a warning, at the approach of sharks and killer whales.

Dr. David K. Caldwell of the Los Angeles County Museum described a similar, even more significant incident, seen during an accidentally caused cetacean psychological behavior experience in Florida 1957. A group of Atlantic Bottlenose Dolphins in apparent good health were at the Gulfarium, Fort Walton Beach, Florida, on the Gulf of Mexico. At one time their observation tank needed extensive replumbing of the water exchange system. The banging noises of metal piping and structural supports being cut and assembled for their multi-gallon aquaria disturbed the animals. From the first, typical dolphin fright behavior was seen. Sound transfers through water far more effectively than through air. Human divers in the tanks said the sounds were deafening. The dolphins were under extreme psychological stress. The construction took a long time. Dolphin knowledge is new. The supervisors did not sense the serious situation. After several weeks, one by one, in a short time, six of the animals died.

Autopsy by a three man team, of veterinary surgeon, medical doctor, and Gulfarium biologist, revealed all the dolphins had severe duodenal ulcers considered the probable cause of death. More recent studies, confirm these intelligent nervous animals respond like man to stress and disease situations. Dolphins and other cetaceans occasionally become emotionally involved, refusing to feed even on to death, with the loss of a close companion. Autopsy of such sensitive water mammals also revealed perforated gastric ulcers. Many of their teeth were worn.

I suggest excessive wear of dolphin, porpoise, and whale teeth, could be caused by the nervous stress of life in the modern world of water they're

TEETH TEETH TEETH

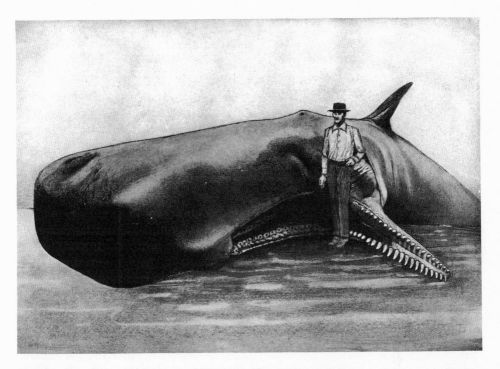

SPERM WHALE∾AN ODONTOCETI OR TOOTHED WHALE. The sperm whale grows to sixty or more feet long. Teeth in the long narrow mouths of their massive bulk upper head, grow to ten inches long. They help seize giant squid for food. Sperm whales are sometimes found with decayed teeth, and often with a pyorrhetic degeneration and loss of their upper teeth. Healthier lower teeth could result from their long lower jaws opened wide swimming into prey, deriving some beneficial cleaning from the water forced passing through.

TEETH TEETH TEETH

subjected to. Some people in the tense trials of our times, wear their teeth in a grinding called bruxism. It is reasonable to believe these intelligent mammals of the sea, whales being hunted and decimated and other cetaceans in strained life situations, could be sea bruxing their teeth away. Cetaceans also seem to be losing their teeth with evolutionary time. Many with teeth hardly use them. Some have a few teeth with no apparent functional value at all, like man's appendix. Many cetacean teeth have no enamel. The teeth of whales and others may be disappearing, as it is thought man's third molar or wisdom tooth is leaving him.

AQUARIUMS

Few can explore waters of the world. A few that do, bring numerous creatures from far spread spaces to populated places, where aquaria try to provide natural habitats, so sea animals can be seen closely, through glass and from the surface. Marineland of the Pacific at Palos Verdes California, has large fresh and salt water tanks, where water animals of the world, those that live on the bottom, free swimming fish, sharks, whales and others, are kept for scientific study and public observation. There are many tanks of many sizes. Some are immense, several stories high deep, each surrounded by viewing platforms, from which swimming water creatures can be watched at different levels through windows, looking up from below, straight ahead alongside, down through glass, and directly in from up above.

Dave Brown an old friend, was Curator of Mammals at Marineland. I phoned Dave, told him of my fishy writing, and asked if there were dental problems with the captive creatures in his care. "We certainly do have them," Dave said, "It's been a long time since I've seen you Syd, come on down, let's talk about it." This started a series of Marineland visits.

Captive animals of aquaria, come from different distant aquatic areas, often hotter or colder than their new home. There may also be differences in the waters. Most creatures arrive healthy, some are diseased. Bacterial pathogens may exist in aquariums, unknown in the natural habitat. Animals away from home, like humans, may be more susceptible. They sometimes get sick. Sea animals, fishes, sharks, porpoises, others, suffer disease of their outer skin and inner organs as humans do. Treating captive water creatures isn't easy. Sharks and whales won't say it hurts or where. Unfortunately disease when it can be seen has often become severe. The animals in pain may be irritable and such patients don't lie down for treatment. The doctor may need a sea diving suit. Several men, nets, gun for shooting tranquilizers and anesthetics, may be needed to capture restrain and control the sea patient. Some seem to understand and try being

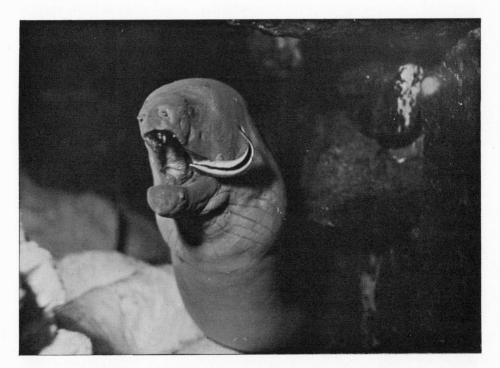

THE CLEANERFISH TEETHCLEANER SERVING A MORAY EEL

The tiny cleanerfish *Labroides dimidiatus* of Philippine waters scavenges cleaning debris from the teeth, mouth & gills of other fish. At the steinhart Aquarium, San Francisco some were introduced to tanks containing large voracious varieties from foreign waters over 10,000 miles from cleanerfish regions. The bigger fish calmly opened their mouths for cleanerfish treatment where at times one or several at a time darted picking particles from teeth & adjacent oral areas. They explored the throat & occasionally left the widened mouth pecking through gill slit side exit openings. *photo~* steinhart Aquar., Calif. Acad. of Sciences   S.G.

TEETH TEETH TEETH

cooperatively responsive. Institutions like Marineland are also scientific sea laboratories, cooperating with government fishery bureaus, museums, and universities. They may have several hospital tanks where temperatures and chemical conditions are carefully controlled. The patients get better than their natural care, some live longer than in the wild.

Fish in nature and captivity suffer bacterial infections and larger parasite worms. Some constipated are given castor oil. They get eye, liver, kidney, and heart diseases. Some get air bladder troubles which disturbs their ability to keep positioned in the water. This blows them up like people with dropsy, though people do not have air bladders. Some fish get ulcers, that turn to tumors of the lips, which surround their teeth and spread through the head, even becoming cancerous, from persistent pounding swimming into glass tank windows. All these usually unknown to their owners, even happen to tiny fish in home aquariums. Whales, porpoises, dolphins, seals, walruses all mammals like man suffer similar diseases to man. They never get cancer from smoking.

The Los Angeles County Museum publication, Contributions in Science, No 95 April 4, 1966 Brown, Caldwell and Caldwell, reports the psychotic behavior of a large male pilot whale at Marineland. The animal captured Jan 1, 1959 participated in normal social and sex play with female whales and appeared intelligent. After ten months, he was trained to perform in a whale show that included feeding exhibition. In time his behavior became erratic. He stopped play and sex activity. Several reports were made of his unusual conduct. He alternated periods of depression with failure to feed, and aggressive vicious attacks on smaller females that previously were his friends. The attacks became increasingly psychotic and dangerous. On Aug. 9, 1962 tranquilizers were administered by mouth. He seemed to improve immediately. They were continued for seven days when on Aug. 16, he suddenly attacked killing a small 780 pound female. Her autopsy revealed a broken lower right jaw and severe damages through the chest region, including a large tear through the right ventricle of her heart. The male was confined.

During summer of 1963 he again stopped feeding. Appetite stimulating drugs didn't help and he lost over 500 pounds. No infection or disease could be detected. On Oct. 10, 1963, antidepressant psychotherapeutic drugs were administered by tube deep into the throat. He improved dramatically and started feeding. Treatment was continued for three months and he resumed normal behavior. No longer a show performer he renewed social and sex play with whale friends.

Most sea mammals and other water creatures are healthy, though disease occasionally occurs. They are sometimes given blood chemistry, blood pressure, fecal and other medical tests. Dental x-rays have been taken of

TEETH TEETH TEETH

dead specimens. Microscopic diagnosis is used. Constipation is helped by mineral oil. Hernias occur. Liver, kidney, heart and lung problems appear. Pneumonia is common. Erysipelas until recently fatal to dolphins, is now prevented and successfully controlled by periodic vaccine injections. Warm blooded sea creatures when infected get fevers. Their temperatures are often taken by rectal thermometer. Penicillin, multi-spectrum antibiotics, vitamins and other drugs help. Many with dental diseases, either captured that way or aquarium acquired have been cured.

SEALS   SEA LIONS   WALRUSES

Seals, Sea Lions, and Walruses, live in water and on land. They feed from the sea. They form a group of mammals called Pinnipedia. They're pinnipeds. Pinni is from Latin meaning fin and feather, pedis is foot. They're fin footed. Their feet used to walk waddling, are also developed webbed as fins or paddles for swimming. Modern man uses plastic foot fins, feet attachable, to help him swim like pinnipeds. Both seals and sea lions look similar to each other, and both lose their first set of teeth at about the time they're born. Their ears make the difference.

SEALS also called True Seals have no outer ears. Their ear canal is flush with their seal skin, hidden by surrounding fur. Their scientific name is Phocidae. Phoca is Latin for seal, idae means of the group. Their pinniped hind feet are rather confined towards the center of their body, less maneuverable on land.

SEA LIONS are scientifically designated Otaridae. Otos in Greek means ear. They have small well developed visible outer ears, leading like ours to the inner canal. They're also called Eared Seals. Their hind feet are more separate, spreading to each side, giving the animal more agility on land. Sea lions are more usually circus performers. Both seals and sea lions sometimes have tooth troubles.

Dave Brown of Marineland told me of a valuable trained California Sea Lion that was not performing properly. It stopped responding to its keeper and wouldn't take the trainer's acting cues. It stopped feeding. Examination revealed pus had penetrated bone and skin, draining through the fur, beneath its lower left jaw. Examination inside the mouth disclosed severe peridontal disease, and decay abscessed teeth. Those teeth were extracted and the area cleaned and drained. Deposits were scaled from surrounding teeth. Antibiotics and other medicants were applied. Healing was routine. The seal was soon happy, eating, actively performing again. The same thing happens to human actors though pus doesn't come through their fur.

TEETH TEETH TEETH

TEETH BENEATH THE WATERS

WALRUS are pinnipeds scientifically classified by their teeth. They're Odobaenidae. Odo in Greek means tooth, bainen to walk. They're a group that walks, sometimes climbing, with their teeth. Walrus' two upper canine teeth form downward hooked tusks, up to 3 inch diameter and 36 inches long on exceptional specimens. They often hook those strong tusks above over blocks of ice, pulling with their powerful neck muscles, their monstrous fat soft blubber covered bodies which may weight almost two tons, clambering up shimmering, like large globs of shaking jelly, slithering over crags of ice and rocks. That could be called tooth walking. It could become the name of a dance.

The walrus, native to northern Arctic oceans, big, awkward, clumsy, is sometimes dangerous, especially large male bulls, aggressively possessive in the mating season. Sometimes they're sociable and gentle. May 1961, Dave Brown as part of a collecting party rescued four young orphaned baby pups, two males, two females, from an ice pack in the Bering Sea, beneath the Chukchi Sea, within sight of Soviet mainland, between Siberia and Nome, Alaska. They were less than two weeks old, still carrying attached remnants of umbilical cords. The largest a male weighed 154 pounds.

Walrus lose their first or milk teeth at about birth. Their canine tusks are not seen yet. While normally nursing mother walrus milk to the age of 16 to 24 months, their permanent teeth and tusks are coming through. Too young to feed themselves, Dave in Alaska started with a stomach tube fed baby walrus formula, of cooked chopped clams, peanut oil and vitamins. Baby walruses fall to many diseases. Preventative antibiotic injections were given daily. Taken to Marineland, they learned to feed from nippled bottles, were tendered more care than many human infants, and cured of several baby walrus sicknesses similar to humans. Under such conditions walrus infant survival is probably better than in nature. In 1965 that 154 pound boy, by then had been named Farouk, and grown to 1600 pounds. He may reach 3500. Their Marineland keeper and friend Eddie Asper introduced me personally.

I was delighted with the warmth they slobbered their large masses along the cage floor towards me, and gently raised large wide bright brown eyed heads, nuzzling up awkwardly close to be scratched petted. Though gentle and friendly those heavy hulks were potentially dangerous. Their weighty movements could fracture limbs. Male walrus canine tusks are larger especially thicker than females. All have internal live pulp along their length nourishing the tooth. They pass down from under thick upper lips, extending below over lower, small walrus receded chins. Above those tusks on out, from their broad upper lip skin surfaces, both male and female walruses, have large thick semitransparent yellowish, whiskery,

TEETH TEETH TEETH

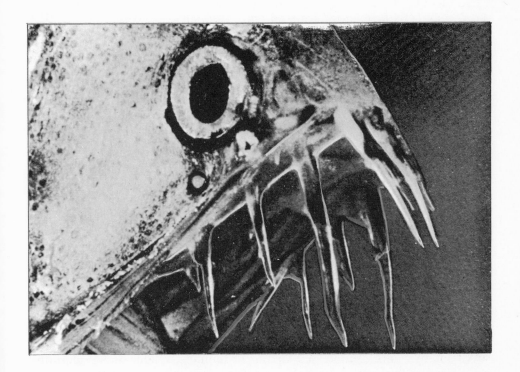

LONG CURVED THIN STRONG, TO TWO MILES DEEP SEA, TEETH OF THE VIPERFISH

Viperfish are of the Family Chauliodontidae. Chauliodus in latin means Exserted or Outward Tooth. When viperfish jaws normally close their upper and lower teeth extend meeting outside their mouths. The upper jaw photo shown is enlarged. Viperfish reach a maximum of one ounce weight at nine inch length. Viperfish Chauliodus macouni of California Pacific Coasts are found at depths of 5000 feet. Viperfish Chauliodus sloani of Eastern Atlantic Waters reach to 10000 feet deep and more.

long drooping mustache hairs, sweeping right and left, just like Uncle Charlie's mustaches. Uncle Charlie who lives in Detroit, has big thick tobacco yellowed mustaches sweeping down just like walruses. Aunt Mamie's mustache is shorter.

Walrus mustache hairs are called vibrissae. Each hair has muscles at its attached base, by which the walrus can activate moving it, individually and in groups. Uncle Charlie can't do that though he can wiggle his ears. Vibrissae are valuable to walrus as sensory perceptors searching for food. In Alaskan and Siberian waters, walrus may eat some seaweeds, mostly crustaceans like crabs, and mollusks like clams. They swim head down closely along the ocean bottom, feeling sensing with vibrissae for food. Tusks may be useful digging through sand and soil. Some walrus even attack large seals for food, and use their molars to crush the bones.

Through Marineland's windows beneath the water I saw walrus immersed gliding through head first, with few fin motions, like a small soft silent, sinuous submarine under the sea. They twist with grace as their masses rotate, and turn smoothly gliding ahead, often back down, coasting with torso inert at rest, submerged moving forward, seemingly weightless. Only one of the four had tusks. Walrus in captivity also swim with their heads down, close along the bottoms of pools usually made of concrete. They seem to be searching for something. Their tusks though hard, rubbing against the floors stony structures, wear off through to the inner live pulp, down level with their lips. Looking closer I could see stumps of the tusks worn away flush, and to even below the soft lip surfaces, at both corners of their mouths. The worn end of each tusk that could hardly be seen, was a stained ring of ivory, dirty black at their soft pulp central inner core. This could be an entry for infection.

Outside the pool around the surface of their enclosure, as the walruses among other friendly gestures opened their mouths, I could see inside within the front muzzles of their jaws, their teeth. The lowers near the front were obvious, stained and worn. Their uppers were hardly discernible. Bending a bit to look up under, I could then see them close beneath, also stained and worn, inside behind their downward curving upper jaw, supported blending with their massive emerging tusk foundation. Where the canine tusks came from the skull, under the upper lip and all around into the mouth, the tissues were tenderest soft pink, delicate stretchy, pulling as the lips moved, more delicate than any around human teeth. This too could be a vulnerable entry for infection. It is.

In zoos and aquaria, infections starting in around walrus tusks invade the skull, often causing death. I've seen photographs of the skull of a walrus killed by such disease at the New York City Aquarium. A large part of the bone was destroyed, from the tusk socket around in towards the brain case.

TEETH TEETH TEETH

TEETH BENEATH THE WATERS

For a long time, such dental disease has been a constant threat to the maintenance of these valuable animals.

Modern veterinary, medical, dental, methods and drugs, are increasingly beneficial though limited. It isn't easy treating live massive beasts. Ideal x-ray and surgical facilities aren't available. I once asked Ken Curgess, Curator of Mammals at Sea World San Diego, whether their recently acquired elephant seals had any dental problems. Elephant seals are also called sea elephants. Males may grow to twenty feet long and have an extended trunk or probosis like an elephants. "I don't know doctor," he said, "you can't get close enough to tell. With big ones like those you have to wait till the animal's in trouble."

One March 1963 day at Marineland, Farouk their large male walrus, one year ten months old weighing 850 pounds was irritable, looked sick, and wouldn't eat. His upper left jaw swelled massive along its tusk prominence towards the front, with a bloody discharge from the left nostril. Touching the tusks soft surrounding tissue caused instant painful withdrawal, suggesting an acute dento-alveolar abscess into the head. This could be fatal. The animal was isolated.

Though difficult to control, broad spectrum antibiotics were given, a specimen of nasal pus was taken for culture identification of the infectious organisms, and the area was cleaned and drained. Later specific antibiotics were used against the identified germs. Surgical cleaning and drainage was continued as possible. Within a week improving, Farouk slowly started taking special fortified foods. Chemo-antibiotic therapy was continued, and in less than a month his appetite returned to the normal fifty pounds of fish and clams a day. He resumed loves with his female companions. In mid-1966 weighing over 2000 pounds, Farouk still a lover, eats 100 pounds a day. Sometimes infected tusks, in captive walrus that recover, fall out, and the socket heals unlikely to reinfect again, just like the sites where teeth are lost from human mouths. Walrus without tusks are less normally attractive, and less feared by competitive lovers, just like their human counterparts.

It isn't practical to provide relatively small deep exhibition pools, with natural environment of thick sandy soil bottoms, growing clams and other natural food for walrus. Cleaning and water exchange supply would be impossible. Recently walrus pools are heavily coated with new soft tenacious plastic linings, to lessen the abrasion of their tusks and adjacent tissues. The walrus tear the plastic coatings. In Coney Island, Dr. Ross Nigrelli, Pathologist and Director of the New York City Aquarium, told me of their attempts of protect worn walrus tusk ends from infection with protective tip-covering metal jackets.

I had several phone conversations with Dr. Francis H. Fay, biologist

TEETH TEETH TEETH

with the Zoonotic Disease Section, Arctic Research Center, Anchorage Alaska. In their far native north, walrus also break tusks climbing rocks and ice. Their dental disease is similar to that of temperate captive climates, though far less common, being limited to perhaps one or two percent of the walrus population. High incidence in zoos and aquaria is probably due to walrus wearing their tusks on pool floors, the greater virility of germs in warmer parts of the world, and increased animal susceptibility in their foreign environment.

SWORDFISH & SAWFISH

Swordfish and sawfish, both big, have unique dental apparatus and names mistaken by some for the other. Both describe the beaks of the fish that bear them. Swordfish beaks are long, narrow like a sword. Sawfishes long beaks or snouts are flat, wide like a saw blade, with teeth along both edges.

SWORDFISH ∾ The swordfish, sleek, streamlined, swift, of temperate and tropical seas, averaging 8 feet, purplish blue above, turning lighter sides to silvery belly beneath, is excellent food. A record catch 14 feet 11 1/2 inches long weighed 1182 pounds. Its sword was 4 1/2 feet long. Broadbill swordfish is considered the world's greatest gamefish. Extremely difficult to hook, only five hundred are recorded caught by rod and reel. Most get to market harpooned.

It has a bony skeleton. The intermaxillary and maxillary bones of its upper head consolidate, projecting tapered forward, narrowing extended to a long hard thin pointed rigid swordlike beak. Its lower movable jaw when closed blends into behind the beak, forming the front pointed narrow mouth, spreading back wider joining the head as a whole. Swordfish have no significant teeth. Their sword on the lower surface has villiform teeth. These are small emerging rudimentary, regular rough projections, probably survivors of larger functional teeth, from an earlier evolutionary form of the fish. Its young hatched from tiny eggs laid in the water, have no swords. After a few months at about 8 inches, their sword starts developing.

Swordfish are considered part of a group called Spearfish which includes swordfish, sailfish, marlin and other particular fish named spearfish. They all have forward projecting pointed spears. They're flatted vertically side to side with tall dorsal fins above. The sailfishes dorsal fin, especially large, runs almost the length of its back, can be erected widespread like a sail, and folds down the side like a sail. Sailfish have teeth. All have widespread caudal or tailfins with narrow extensions pointed up and down.

TEETH TEETH TEETH

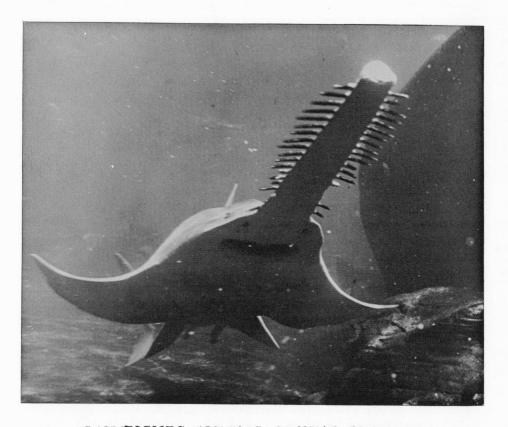

SAWFISHES SPECIAL DENTAL DISEASE s.g.

Suffered by some captive SAWFISH *Pristis*. Rostral teeth of long rostrum beak normally projecting along both sides, evenly spaced, equally lengthed sometimes disease & degenerate irregularly even falling off. Inside the fishes underside mouth its eating pavement teeth being continually replaced as worn away are healthy during their shorter life. *photo*-Marineland of the Pacific, Palos Verdes, Calif.

TEETH TEETH TEETH

Using their spear like a club, they sometimes strike through schools of mackeral and herring as prey, slashing from the side. Swordfish have been said to attack whales, which is doubtful. They do strike direct, penetrating into wooden boats with their sword, which they sometimes snap off to get free. They could be caught that way. London's Natural History Museum has a small piece of timber with three broken protruding swordfish spears.

SAWFISH ∾ The sawfish, ugly, grotesque, awkward, slow, is not a bone backbone fish, but a more primitive form with a skeleton of cartilage, scientifically grouped with sharks, skates, rays. They live along coasts of subtropical and tropical waters, entering rivers of the Americas, Africa and India. Many inhabit the Gulf of Mexico. Though not choice food, young sawfish are sometimes eaten. Sawfish look somewhat like squat shark, with wide flappy sidefins like a ray, with a long flat double tooth edged snout, sticking out far in front. They are depressed downward, wide from side to side, flat along their bottom and spend most of their time on the bottom. They are sharky grey brown, whitish on their bottom. Usually reaching ten to twenty feet, one, thirty one feet long weighed 5700 pounds.

The hard structures of their upper head, flatten and prolong forward, to a rigid spatula like leather surface looking snout, called the rostrum. This forms the blade of its saw, taking about the forward fourth of its length. It is a double saw. Along each blade edge, right and left, large teeth called rostral teeth, grow from the sockets with inner nutritive pulp. These teeth, a single permanent set, are irreplaceable. I measured the sawed off saw of a sixteen foot sawfish. It was eight inches wide one inch thick, at the cut from the head end, forty inches long tapered to its thin three inch wide rounded front end. Along each edge, equidivided, there were two inch long sharp teeth. Twenty along one side, nineteen on the other. Sawfish have been found with rostrums six feet long, one foot wide.

The fish has two distinctly different types of teeth, located in different places. Beneath, back from the rostrum, separate and unconnected is its mouth. The mouth is a thin movable narrow lipped slit, within the flat underhead, running across wide from side to side. The inner lips and jaws are covered with tiny massed teeth called pavement teeth. These are many many miniature teeth close together, lining the sawfish mouths surface, like short hard little groups of tiny tiles. They form opposing pavements or pads of teeth, up and down, which work against each other like grindstones, crushing grinding sawfish food. Pavement dentition are common to mouths of many rays and skates. They are continually being grown, used, worn, lost and replaced, like teeth of other fish. They have little time to sicken.

TEETH TEETH TEETH

21
TEETH BENEATH THE WATERS

Sawfish bear young alive, intact in proper proportion, saw, teeth, everything. Large mothers give birth to fully formed sawfishlets, two even three feet long. Luckily for her delicate insides and birth canal, her infants saws and teeth are soft at birth. They soon harden in the water. Charles Grover, assistant to the curator at Marineland Pacific, showed me a dried newborn specimen in his office. It was 33 inches long of which the saw took 8 1/2. It saw teeth were sharply pointed up to 3/16 of an inch long.

Sawfish don't use their saws like people use saws. They never swim back and forth, sawing pieces off victims that would never stay still. They strike their long head extended toothedged blades sideways, through schools of fish to kill. As their victims fall, they follow to grasp and grind them with their mouth teeth. They sometimes just swallow.

When tired of fishing upper waters, they often enjoy slithering in stops and spurts, bellies against the bottom. They sometimes use their saws to find foods of the ocean floor. Moving slowly along, they rake, swinging their long tooth snout side to side, through the sandy soil. Some of their underswings sift snails, sea cucumbers, crabs, clams, and other seafoods sawfish enjoy. While raking for food or fun, the sands also clean their saw teeth, they may even clean their teeth intentionally that way. One would have to study sawfish talk, no course of which I know is given, to find out.

John Prescott, Curator at Marineland Palos Verdes, collected many sawfish in southern waters. He told me, "No, I've never seen any specimens caught with other than clean healthy saw teeth." When sawfish are kept captive some suffer dental disease. In large aquarium collections, duplicating the natural environment, of all its diverse creatures from far different places is impossible. Perfect provision for some might be harmful to others. Compromise must be made. Most large tanks have big bare concrete floors, with occasional rocks and sunken boat hulls for underwater decoration. This permits easier cleaning. It's probably better for many inhabitants, but doesn't have sand for bottoming sawfish. Ideal conditions, unattainable for all, would include valuable specimens eating each other as in nature. Many fish are hand fed by human divers. Through glass at Marineland Pacific I could see smaller fish being placed by divers directly into mouths of sluggish sawfish for feeding. Over the years and many visits I would wait to see them swim close for detailed study. New arrival sawfish had clean sharply defined healthy rostral teeth, along their long snout saws. Some that had been around longer, had teeth with unattractive irregular deposits, much like that of human peridontal disease. Older inhabitants had areas eroded from some teeth, adjacent to deposits, and places where lost teeth were missing.

TEETH TEETH TEETH

John Prescott Marineland Curator, and Charles Grover his assistant, took me behind the scenes to their marine laboratory tanks. Most sawfish after a year or several, suffer internally and dentally and die. Prescott in his office showed me the saw of a deceased sawfish. There were pyorrhetic deposits among many eroded teeth, and degenerative invasion of the sockets of some that were lost. I was reminded of pyorrhetic human jaw specimens. Mr. Prescott told me he kept one sawfish alive for four years, considered a long time by some aquarium keepers.

Marine Studios, at Marineland Florida near St. Augustine, has had a group of five sawfish living in their tanks from seventeen to twenty years. Probably a record. All are from local Florida waters. I phoned Cliff Townsend curator at Marine Studios and asked about their teeth. "Perfect," he said, "they look as good as when caught from the ocean." I asked whether their tank had a bare concrete floor, anxiously awaiting his answer. "No," he said, "we keep a covering layer four or five inches thick, of broken shell fragments. Sawfish seem to like browsing in it. They occasionally rake their saw teeth through. Sometimes they completely bury themselves."

There is a brightly colored tropical fish called Surgeon Fish. They grow to two feet long. Just forward of their tail, surgeon fish can snap out scalpel like sharp bony knives, used for attack and defense. I don't think they are ever paid to perform professional dental surgery. Unwary fishermen lifting them by the tail, have had their hands seriously slashed. They are also called Doctor Fish and Medicos. Though Cuttlefish manufacture an ink, I never heard of an Author or Writer Fish and know nothing of any of their teeth.

Beneath Deep Seas are Teeth of Fish
Some Sleepers leave theirs Immersed in a Dish

TEETH BENEATH THE WATERS

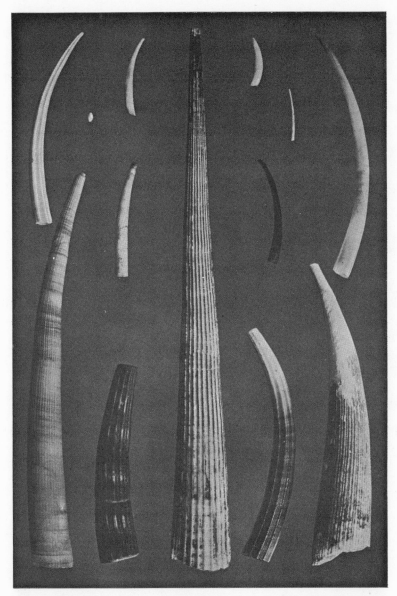

TOOTHSHELLS   **MOLLUSKS**   **class SCAPHOPODA**

Toothshells are not teeth or tusks. These hollow skeletal shells only use the name Tooth. Their inner space houses soft creatures that live in the sea. Their larger end half embedded in sand, has a mouth containing numerous tiny Radula Teeth. These grind food which passes through digesting and wastes, evacuating from their water exposed narrow end.

TEETH TEETH TEETH

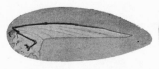
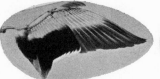
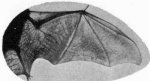

PTERODACTYL ~ Reptiles
toothed & toothless

BIRD
none have teeth

BAT ~ Mammals
have teeth

COMPARATIVE WING STRUCTURES

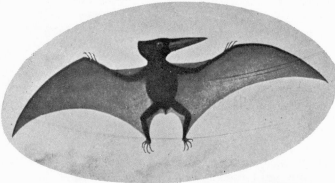

Pterodactyl
PTERANODON

wingspan to 25 ft.
had no teeth

Pterodactyl
RHAMPHORHYNCHUS
had teeth

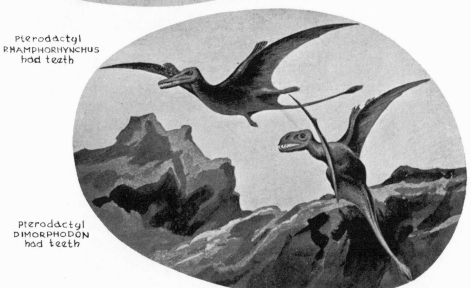

Pterodactyl
DIMORPHODON
had teeth

excavated from exposed land layers of approx. 5000 feet depth
from Jurassic Mesozoic Earth stratas of 150 million years ago

TOOTHED & TOOTHLESS EXTINCT FLYING REPTILES
Portrayed from fossil skeletal specimens

TEETH TEETH TEETH

22

ANIMAL TEETH

Animals have always fascinated man, though some are repulsed by certain of them. Perhaps through evolution, the enthused sense their ancestral relation, while those who dislike animals resent that hereditary affiliation. Animals on land and beneath the sea do have teeth to serve them. Most that fly into the sky, do not, though they do deserve them. There just isn't justice. Birds do not have teeth. Anything as rare as the teeth of any existing bird doesn't exist at all. Once there were toothed birds.

Skeletal bird fossils from the Mezoic Era of the Cretacious Epoch, of the Age of Reptiles 120 million years ago, have been found with teeth in their jawbones. Hesperornis was an aquatic bird about six feel long. Ichthyornis was a smaller bird of flight similar to some today. Both, now extinct, had teeth. Birds kept their teeth until the Tertiary Epoch, about 70 million years ago, when after 50 million years of toothy experience they abandoned them, some may think like wise old birds.

Modern birds have a bony beak, often with notched edges, which fulfill some tooth function. These help seize, pick, and tear food. Birds do not really chew. They pass tossing their food, sometimes with a few closing controlling grasps, through the mouth back into their throat and gizzard. Gizzard walls have strong muscles, lined inside with hard projecting shallow ridges of corny epithelium or skin, like little-teeth-lined stomachs. Their gizzard muscle activated ridges, grind birds' food. Birds are also sort of subsconscious dentists, though they have no professional education or license to practice. They select bits of gravel and pebbles, swallowed into their gizzard for added food grinding, like with lots of little false teeth.

There are animals that look like birds and fly like birds and do have teeth. They are not birds. They are mammals called bats. Their young like those of humans develop in the uterus to be born alive. While still unborn, growing in the uterus, the young of certain bats erupt a first set of teeth, shed and lose them there, and grow their permanent second set while still inside, with which they are born to the outside.

DAY WITH A VET ∞ Victor Tierstein an animal doctor, has been my friend since we met as members of the Los Angeles Zoological Society. Vic's degree is D.V.M. doctor of veterinary medicine. From 1939 through

TEETH TEETH TEETH

411

1955, except for a few military service years, Dr. Tierstein treated animals of the world at the Los Angeles Zoo, in addition to his private practice. At present Vic limits his field to horses, and on special occasion treats other beasts. Dr. Tierstein has rendered veterinary medical and dental services, for major motion picture studios like Paramount, MGM, Twentieth Century Fox, and Columbia. He's been veterinary physician, surgeon and dentist to animal motion picture stars. I asked Vic to discuss animal dentistry. He answered, "Sure Syd, why don't you join me on one of my regular practice days." Saturday Jan 9, 1965 I did and loved it.

With me Dr. Tierstein made six separate calls around Los Angeles County. He treated over a dozen horses, some, very valuable prize Arabians. None of his treatment that day was dental, though Dr. Tierstein told me of such previous experiences with horses and wild animals. He treated horses for worms, back and hide fungus, body and leg wounds. He thoroughly examined one horse for a prospective purchaser. He explored three expensive horses internally, inserting his rubber gloved hand into the rectum, and feeling along through the intestinal wall for the uterus filled embryonic fetus. Two horses were pregnant, one wasn't. We visited and Vic treated, a two and a half hour old colt and its mother mare. He surgically cut her attached, dragging long along the ground, afterbirth tissues. Dr. Tierstein also removed a lost thermometer, from deep inside the intestines of a sick valuable race horse, where it had been inserted too deep through the rectum by a caretaker trainer. It was a day I will never forget.

LION ∾ During the 1940's Dr. Victor Tierstein was called by the Paul Getty estate, saying a female African lion suffered an accident, that might have broken her back. J. Paul Getty the multimillionaire oil man had a museum near Malibu, and a private zoo in the area. Dr. Tierstein arrived to be met by Tom Flemming an old man, the animals keeper for years. The lioness was in a large tall cage with a growing tree near its center. Somehow she had fallen from high and was in agony with a paralyzed back. She pawed viciously, reaching menacing dangerously, when Vic approached. Since Tom was her friend, Dr. Tierstein asked that he stay in close sight, between him and the lion. The animal in pain, fearfully clawed to attack the doctor as he tried to touch her. Somehow Tom didn't cooperate completely. Vic repeatedly had to ask that he keep between him and his wild patient. At a particular moment Tom turned away, and the lion lunged at Dr. Tierstein, grasping his left leg between her jaws. Vic wore heavy leather cowboy boots. He could feel her fangs penetrate the leather, enter his flesh into the muscles of his leg. He felt the blood flow hot, filling his boot. He screamed in pained horror, at the old man for help, who only awkwardly jumped in to grab the lion's tail. After tugging, during Dr. Tierstein's terror, the lion let loose. Vic very tenderly, removing his own boot, was amazed to see the old man laughing, hunched bent over hands on his knees, shaking. He thought him crazy. Vic looked at his leg. It was untouched. Tom laughing, explained the lioness had no teeth. They were removed when she was a cub. Yet Dr. Tierstein said, "I could feel her teeth, penetrating my leather boot, entering my leg, and could feel the blood running down." Extreme fear can unreasonably affect anyone's imagination.

TIGER ∾ One 1950 day Victor Tierstein D.V.M. in Los Angeles, was telephoned by Clyde Beatty the wild animal trainer, from his winter quarters in El Monte, California. Mr. Beatty had a dental problem with a Bengal Indian Roll-Over Tiger. The roll-over tiger is especially valuable, prized for circus performance. Not all are intelligent enough for such training, which takes a long time.

Dr. Tierstein agreed to come the next day. He asked Mr. Beatty to save some of his professional time, and weigh the tiger before he got there. Beatty said he would. Doctors need their patient's weight to determine the quantity of anesthetic for surgery. Weighing a wild dangerous animal is often difficult. Sometimes a squeeze cage is needed. The empty squeeze cage is moved, with its sliding door end adjacent and contacting the door of the caged animal. While in complete contact both doors are opened. If the animal doesn't itself enter the squeeze cage, it is driven there with poles, reaching through the bars, and the squeeze cage door is closed confining it. The weight of cage and doors are known, and subtracted from the total weight with the animal inside. The squeeze cage door is so designed, that it can then be moved inwards, pushed with rods or pulled with cables, towards its opposite cage wall, safely squeezing confining and holding the animal securely between them. Controlled this way anesthesia is administered, usually by injection to the caged animal. When the animal is anesthetized immobilized, surgery or other procedures can be safely performed in or out of the cage.

The next day Dr. Tierstein arrived finding the tiger sick, emaciated, with a seriously infected lower right canine tusk. Beatty said it weighed about 250 pounds. It looked rather thin to Dr. Tierstein who asked if it had actually been weighed. Clyde said he'd been too busy, but from personal knowledge of tigers, felt sure 250 was a good estimate, and Tierstein could proceed on that basis. Vic had also been around tigers, some weigh 250, others up to 350. Their long luxurious fur misleadingly makes them seem larger. Wild they can't be touched. He thought this animal had lost a lot of weight. If it were much lighter the anesthetic dose could kill. Too little

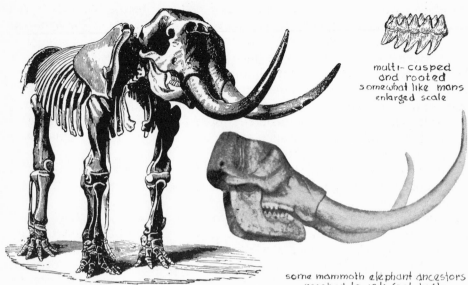

multi-cusped
and rooted
somewhat like mans
enlarged scale

some mammoth elephant ancestors
reached to 13½ feet high

AMERICAN MASTODON~Appeared in Pleistocene Period with primitive man about 1 million years ago

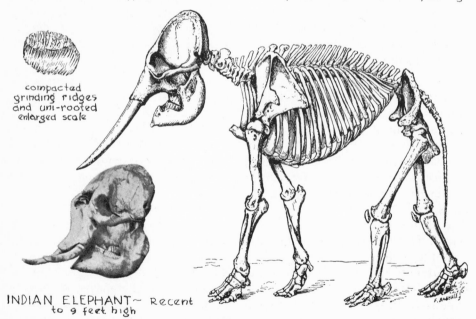

compacted
grinding ridges
and uni-rooted
enlarged scale

INDIAN ELEPHANT~ Recent
to 9 feet high

AN ELEPHANT AND AN ANCESTOR s.c.

Each specimen shows an entire skeleton and molar tooth drawing and a skull photograph
The long incisor tusks are seen related to the mouths inner food grinding molars
skeletal & skull material from the British Natural History Museum~ London, England

TEETH TEETH TEETH

anesthesia would leave him dangerously difficult to operate. Clyde felt sure of his estimate, and had no available weighing facilities. The tiger was very sick. Additional delay might weaken him too much.

Mr. Beatty was anxious to go ahead. Dr. Tierstein feeling 250 pounds too high, told Beatty he would administer Nembutal as an anesthetic for a 150 pound animal. He felt time was important, and Clyde reassured him that from his own experience with tigers and that particular one, even 250 was safe. Dr. Tierstein administered a dose for 150 pounds and operated successfully. He left with detailed instructions for care as the animal came out of anesthesia. That's routine practice.

The next day Dr. Tierstein returned. The tiger never reviving died anesthetized. Vic weighed him at only 75 pounds. His large skeletal, deep fur covered frame was misleading.

Clyde Beatty knowing Dr. Tierstein was returning to Los Angeles, asked if he would deliver the dead tiger to a taxidermist in Hollywood, directly along the way. He wanted it stuffed and mounted. Vic was glad to help. Beatty had a man tie the tiger on the flat back of an open trailer without rails. The trailer was hitched to Doc's car. He was to leave it with the taxidermist. Vic left for Hollywood and unexpected experience. Along the streets, on the Hollywood freeway, then back on the bumpy streets again, the old trailer with poor shock absorbers bumped up and down. People stared, cars slowed closer to look following. The tiger loosely tied bounced lifelike, as though fighting for freedom.

ELEPHANT ∾ In 1961 Paramount Studios produced "Hatari" starring John Wayne and Elsa Martinelli. The story started in Tanganyika, along the east central coast of Africa. Elsa protraying "Dallas" loved animals, and was followed everywhere by three pet baby elephants, two females and a male. After all African filming was finished, the cast returned to California, for more convenient less expensive completion of several scenes. For realism some native set materials, monkeys, cheetahs, hyenas, birds, and the three elephants, with native animal trainers were also taken. The elephants were stars. As filming resumed in the Los Angeles area, Dr. Victor Tierstein was engaged to insure their health.

As the picture filming proceeded, Tembo the smallest, Dallas' favorite, important to the story, became hard to control. Tembo is the Swahili word for elephant. Interruption of such motion picture making can be extremely expensive, involving stars high salaries, many less high salaries, and the useless wasted use of expensive equipment. Dr. Tierstein's examination of Tembo, a young male bull, showed swelling of his lower right jaw in the first and second molar teeth region. Elephants aren't as easy to treat as humans, though they may seem easier than some. Dr. Tierstein with controlling help, drained the area and applied antibiotics. The swelling subsided. Movie making could continue. After several days Tembo's jaw expanded again, renewing the trouble. Filming couldn't continue without the elephant's important written role. A trainer felt he had first seen the swelling appear and go in Tanganyika. Dr. Tierstein asked to see rushes of the African shots.

Studying the animals behavior in the early film, and examining Tembo as close as he could, Dr. Tierstein diagnosed the disease malacia, similar to human osteomyelitis, an infection inflammation of an animals bone marrow that sometimes starts with teeth. Malacia is generally incurable in elephants. Radical surgery was impractical. Vic kept Tembo comfortable with repeated minor surgeries, antibiotic and other therapy. The animal seemed to understand. After "Hatari" was finished Tembo was transferred to a zoo, where despite care he died in a short time.

SNAKE ∾ In jungles and zoos snakes sometimes suffer disease called Canker Mouth. Snake canker mouth is similar to human pyorrhea. Dirt deep between the snakes long pointed teeth, causes infectious inflammation around the base of the teeth, destroying the gums and supporting bone. The teeth loosen and are lost. The snake in pain can't feed, sickens, sometimes dies.

In zoos, boa constrictors are especially susceptible to canker mouth. Boas like pythons, have strong massive muscles along their length. They are not poisonous. They often drop from above upon their prey, wrapping around, encircling and grasping. Like a self closing thick steel cable, their powerful coils tighten, strongly crushing body and bones. Sometimes they strike to seize their victim between sharp pointed teeth, folded hooked back, holding against escape. Their upper and lower jaws disengage, separating open behind from their skull attachment, like disconnecting hinges, stretching wide apart to swallow, engorging kill even far larger than themselves.

Snakes are cold blooded. Their body temperature is not kept constant like mammal humans, but varies with that of their environment. Slow, sluggish, less alert when cold, snakes breed better, eat more, are more active and dangerous when warm. Snakes in zoos are exhibited under warming electric lights to interest zoo visitors. They are safer handled when cool.

At one time at the Los Angeles Zoo reptiles were the charge of William Lasky, son of Jesse Lasky, motion picture producer. Bill before then and now is in the motion picture and T.V. field. His love of nature, zoology, and all animals, motivated his work at the zoo. I've visited Bill's home in Malibu Canyon, where he has a large private collection of birds, many he

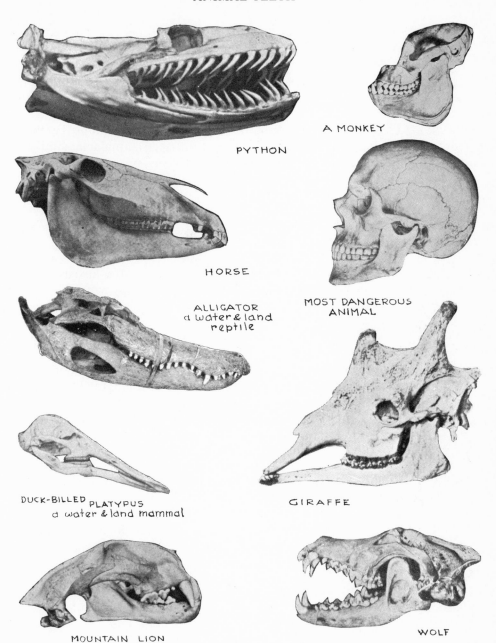

A MONKEY

PYTHON

HORSE

MOST DANGEROUS
ANIMAL

ALLIGATOR
a water & land
reptile

DUCK-BILLED PLATYPUS
a water & land mammal

GIRAFFE

MOUNTAIN LION

WOLF

TEETH ~ JAWS ~ SKULLS of LAND ANIMALS s.G.
ONLY A FEW OF MANY VARIETIES

TEETH TEETH TEETH

gathered himself around the world. Some are very rare.

Bill also called Lasky at the zoo, had in his care a twelve foot long boa constrictor with a body several inches thick. The snake had canker mouth, was irritably disturbed by its disease. Bill had handled the boa before, felt he knew it well. He lifted the snake from its exhibit cage, then carrying it, was joined by Victor Tierstein the zoo veterinarian. They walked up a hill towards the animal hospital.

Suddenly the draped hanging snake coiled, tightening up powerfully around Bill's arm. He screamed afraid it would snap. Vic grabbed to pull the snake away with little success. He was afraid to leave Bill for help. Such a snake could kill a man, some have. He pounded at its' head. The snake darting evasively snapped, biting into the doctor's hand. As he pulled held by its teeth, he bled slippery and pounded with his other. For reasons perhaps only known to snakes, for no cause Bill or Doc could see, it suddenly relaxed and let go. Both Bill and Vic sighed relief. Carefully they delivered the boa into a box at the hospital to cool.

Later the snake was treated, with veterinary dental surgery procedure, like humans with similar problems. Anesthesia was applied. The area was carefully cleaned and medicated. Some gum tissue was trimmed for corrective hygiene. Some teeth were extracted. Recovery was uneventfully successful. After healing dentures were not made to replace the missing teeth. They could be swallowed with another victim.

Serpent is from the Latin word, to creep. Serpent tongues are long, narrow thin flexible ribbonlike, forked double to two pointed tips. They can be protruded darting, through a notch in the lower jaw when closed, and move back and forth, activated by tiny sensitive muscles to wave vibrating enchantingly, like an evasive delicate flame. Their tongues help snakes smell. Serpent or snake teeth, both words really mean the same, stick from both jaws and from bones in the roof of the mouth. Their teeth have a backward slant to seize and hold their prey. Snakes do not tear or chew or bite off pieces. They swallow whole. Most snakes are not poisonous. Poisonous snakes have a pair of specialized teeth called fangs, hinging back down from bones of the upper jaw. They are grooved or tubular to carry their toxins. These passages conduct the poisons from glands close in the snake's upper head, into its victim. Like other snake teeth, there are fangs behind them, developing continually, available for use to replace those lost. They are sometimes left in the victim. There are small snakes called Toothless Snakes. They have teeth only temporarily, while developing inside the egg. They use these teeth to help break through their shell hatching, then lose them for life. There is a type of treacherous

TEETH TEETH TEETH

scoundrel human called low down snake, that deceives like a serpent. Most are born without visible teeth, though they soon grow them, and sometimes also lose them in later life.

CHIMPANZEE ∾ Like people in jungles and zoos, chimpanzees in jungles and zoos have trouble with their teeth. Chimpanzees are mammals of the order Primate, which includes Man, Lemurs, Marmosets, Monkeys and Apes. Primate means prime, first in quality, rank, authority. Chimpanzees are Anthropoid Apes. Anthropoid means resembling man. Apes are the larger tailless monkeys most closely related to man. Chimpanzees among men often ape or mimic them, many of whom ape or mimic apes. Many members of each group act like each other. Both, living in natural primitive and modern civilized environments, have similar dental diseases. Chimpanzees, of the equatorial forest and bush of Africa, have been found with tooth decay or caries and other diseases of the mouth. Some of those animals in their native habitat, suffer more dental problems than chimpanzees with controlled diets and proper treatment in animal laboratories and zoos. Like man some have teeth better than others, perhaps for similar unknown reasons.

Skippy was a motion picture star. In the "The Jungle Princess" he played with Dorothy Lamour. He did a jungle series with Johnny Weismuller and Maureen O'Sullivan. Johnny played Tarzan. Skippy portrayed a wild chimpanzee pet named "Cheetah." Like some other actors and actresses Skippy's teeth were neglected. In 1942 at about twenty years of age, middle aged for a chimp, Skippy left show business to retire at the Los Angeles Zoo. He was given a cage apartment of his own among other country neighbors. It isn't pleasant confined in a small enclosure. It's not the freedom of swinging through trees. Most who resent being growled, clawed, snapped and sometimes spit at, fail to understand the position of caged animals. Few would be content, caught and kept, supplied food, tender words, and cautious strokes through bars. It would be unusual experience being kept by wild animals. Perhaps given mates of our choice we'd like the small cage from which they couldn't get away. Some animals are supplied with two or three. Divorce wouldn't work. Would we wear clothes. Close quarters can cause frustrated resentment. Men in enforced confinement, sometimes become as wild as caged beasts and kill. They may be aping apes.

Charles Allen was Chief Animal Keeper. An expert, Charlie knew and loved animals. Charlie welcomed the caged former star chimpanzee, who like other stars temperamentally unpredictable, sometimes scratched, and once bit tearing his hand badly. Charlie was disappointed and hurt emotionally, though many casually accept the human behavior of developing machines used to maim and kill many of their own kind. Charlie understood and wouldn't hold a grudge. He extended his bandaged hand which Skippy first avoided, then shamefacedly accepted. Hugging they established permanent friendship.

Earl Chumley, Skippy's personal keeper, became the chimp's favorite friend. Earl who is also my friend told me, "Doc, you should have seen that chimp. He loved baloney sandwiches, especially with lots of mustard. After he saw me having mine for lunch, he held those I gave him just like a person, taking bites like anyone else. And he'd wipe the mustard off his lips. Sundays he'd jump up and down, screaming till I'd give him an ice cream cone, which he held licking like anyone else for dessert." Skippy was fed and enjoyed cooked meat three times a week. Contrary to earlier belief, it's been found primates in their natural habitat eat insects and meat when they can get it, though there are no ice cream cones. At the zoo Skippy was still a showman. Assistant Chief Animal Keeper Aaron Krieger, told me of skits he'd perform at request. Asked to "Make like Bob Hope," Skippy promptly responded with chimpanzee gesture, turning his head grinning widely, showing his teeth together. Each fist clenched and opening, and each arm to its side, he'd chomp those teeth clacking up and down, spreading waving his limbs widely apart. He did best for biggest audiences.

Skippy's teeth were bad when he first moved to the zoo. They'd been long neglected and were severely pyorrhetic. Chimpanzee pyorrhea is very much like man's. Earl Chumley said, "When Skippy's teeth hurt he'd pound screeching, calling me to his cage. He'd open his mouth and pointing touched the bad ones. His infected teeth harmed his health." The zoo veterinarian scaled and cleaned them, occasionally extracted one or two. His dental disease degenerated until Skippy's teeth became so loose he pulled several himself. He'd proudly hold them between his fingers and show them to zoo personnel. Van Yrineo an old faithful animal keeper said, "Skippy was his own dentist." Many captive chimps have been known to pull their own pyorrhetic teeth. On september 26, 1962 at about forty years of age Skippy died. Veterinary diagnosis was circulatory disease and heart failure.

OUR ANIMAL RELATIONS ∾ Visiting zoos and public parks was more popular pastime, when they were harder to get to. Since passing trolleys have been replaced by high speed autos, and other things making life easier, man has been losing his contacts with natural environment. We are in a rush to nowhere. Many are running from themselves. A trip to the zoo is advised for friends, and may renew old associations. In addition to the romantic imagery, involved with each animal's adventurous original location, some will find and recognize, more than one familiar affiliated relation. No matter where we come from we're really all quite alike.

There are lowly worms, toads and rats, though we needn't visit zoos to find them. Man's closest relations are considered gorillas. We may recognize an ape, like that boar of a baboon, that looks like the monkey that lives down the street. There are slick sloths, sneaky snakes, sly foxes weasels and wolves, as dangerous to cute innocent chicks as any others in town. Most zoos have big dark wide eyed, cute, honey bears. Many are from South America. I once had one at home myself. On outer sides of the bars, some visitors detect honeys as cute as a bee, that seem especially desirable bared. Some of the darlings are deers. Being clever animals, experience has taught them to flee from most men that approach them. There are swine of all kinds, greedy hogs and fat pigs that love to wallow in filth.

Most zoos like other areas of Earth have stubborn mules and asses. Asses of Asia and North Africa, like local domestic ass, are quadrupeds of genus Equus Asinus. They're smaller than horses, with short manes and long ears. Domesticated ass are easy to influence and useful to man, they like being petted and fondled. Wild ass like the Kiang of Tibet, are attractive large and small, yet hate to be touched. They are haughty, independent, hard to control, will bite if irritated. In nature asses take good care of themselves, keep clean and healthy. Sometimes closely confined and neglected in zoos, even young active attractive asses get dirty and smell. Like their close relative the horse, ass molars in back are wide and flat for grinding. All types of horse and ass teeth sometimes suffer dental disease.

PREHISTORIC ∞ For a hundred million years between 200 and 100 million years ago, the predominant animals of Earth were reptiles. It was the Age of Reptiles. They occupied most available area. It wasn't a man's world yet. Most Primitive Man and Woman hadn't even appeared until perhaps a million years ago. Some reptiles were small. Some could fly. Wing bones of Pterodactyls supported a flight membrane somewhat like that of bats. Some Pterodactyls had teeth. One variety Pteranodon, had a wingspan of twenty five feet and no teeth. Some reptiles like dinosaurs were bigger than elephants. Many walked on four feet. Others like Ceratosaurus, stood kangaroo like on their two hind feet, with a muscular tail for their third triangular support. Their two shorter front fingered appendages, which they also sometimes dropped down on, had value as hands for grasping and guiding food into their mouths. They had teeth.

Reptiles, Dinosaur, Brontosaurus, Brachiosaurus, and Diplodactus, were the largest land animals known. Up to ninety feet long weighing forty tons.

Their heads and mouths were very small. Some had brains hardly larger than that of a cat. They too had teeth. The hadrosaur Duck Bill dinosaur Anatosaurus, a grass and plant eater, had jaws with close dental collections containing over a thousand teeth. Some dinosaurs consumed up to one thousand pounds of food a day. Their small toothed mouth needed constant grinding, to keep that enormous girth alive. Their teeth were subjected to continuous abuse. Fossils of such teeth have been found severely worn decayed. It seems that even that multitude of millions of years ago, germs had evolved to create dental infection. Diseased dinosaur mouths could have caused death by starvation.

CROCODILE & ALLIGATOR ∾ The zoological Class: Reptilia or reptiles includes lizards, snakes, turtles, tortoises, crocodiles and alligators. Crocodiles and alligators are of the Order: Loricata. Lorica is an old Latin word for cloth of mail, like the protective metal plates sometimes attached over leather, as was worn by old knights of shining armor. Reptilia loricata, crocodiles and alligators, have bodies covered especially on top, with knobby hard protective bonelike scales or plates, attached to their own body leather. Some small alligators are stuffed for souvenirs. Softer outer edge parts, and underbody sections of large animals, are used for shoes, ladies handbags, and in narrow strips to help hold men's pants up.

The distinction between crocodiles and alligators is not definitely defined. Some similar creatures are called one or the other in different parts of the world. All are found in regions of sub and tropical temperatures, and zoos of any other area that gets them. Very small ones have been found in bathtubs.

A primary distinctive characteristic involves their jaws and teeth. Crocodile snouts are longer and narrower than alligators. The crocodiles lower jaw, irregular along its edges, is wider than the upper. Crocodile lips are thin. When crocodile mouths are closed, the lower teeth along their borders are seen sticking upright all around, like little pointed spears surrounding their upper jaws confined within them.

Alligators have large thick upper lips, distributed too far around for a fully contacting kiss. When alligator jaws are closed, their lower teeth stick up into sockets along the outer edge of their upper jaw, and into fleshy pockets of those upper large lips that lap over and hide them. The lower fourth canine tooth of certain alligators, on each side grow especially long. In some older specimens such long lower pointed up canines perforate their upper lips, which heal as circles of flesh around their protruding tusks. They can be seen coming through, with the mouth closed. This may be a symbol of distinctive alligator dignity, unappreciated by modern young gators.

TEETH TEETH TEETH

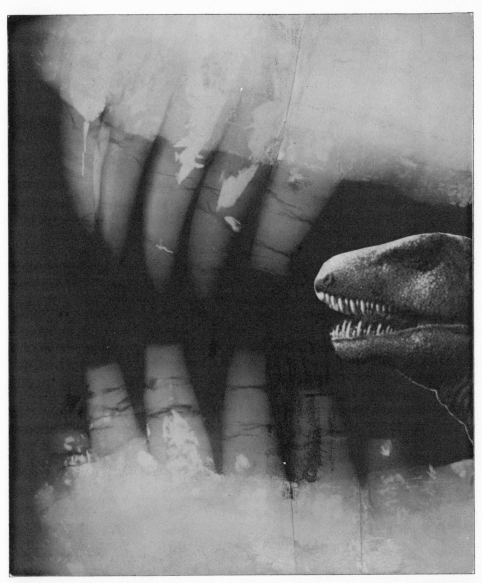

Life size x-rays assembled from several taken of fossil fragments of Dinosaur Allosaurus found in Utah. Allosaurus lived in the Jurassic Period 175 million years ago, reached 35 feet long standing 10 feet high. Pictured superimposed is the head of Dinosaur Tyrannosaurus a related similar larger successor. Tyrannosaurus lived during the Cretaceous Period 100 million years ago, reached 50 feet long at 19 feet high. Both were carnivorous or meat eaters.

X-RAY OF DINOSAUR TEETH 175 MILLION YEARS OLD

Fossil fragment x-rays from Los Angeles County Museum of Natural History, L.A. calif. Dinosaur head from a mural by R.F. Zallinger at Peabody Museum Yale Univ., New Haven, Conn.

TEETH TEETH TEETH

Alligators inhabit warmer regions of the Americas and China. Most rarely reach ten feet in length, though specimens have been found over sixteen. Crocodiles are also found in the Americas, and tropical waters of Australia, Asia and Africa. Many populate the Nile River. Ancient Egyptians worshipped crocodiles, adorning some with gold. Some were mummified. Exceptional crocodiles have been found up to thirty three feet long.

Crocodile and alligator temporomandibular joints, the jaw hinging system are uniquely different from man's. Human lower jaws move down to open, hinging about a socket in the upper skull. Croc-gator sockets are in their lower jaws. Their upper opens going up from their skull, so that alligators and crocodiles can conveniently open their mouths up, while flat prostrate on the ground. No record can be found of the original patent.

There are little flying dental hygienists that enter wide open crocodile mouths, to hop around cleaning their teeth. The Nile Bird also called Crocodile Bird, a small black and white stilt legged plover, picks food debris from croc tooth crevices, as food for itself. It's a mutually satisfactory relationship. Crocodiles seize and pull large animals into rivers to kill and devour, yet never harm the little bird. Crocodiles are not very sensitive. The plover also renders a warning of danger service. At approach of potential crocodile enemies, its screech and flapping wings flying away, alert the croc who slithers into the river.

Crocodiles are dangerous to man, perhaps more to women. Every year many females washing along riverbanks are seized by crocodiles and eaten. Natives feel most damage is done by old male crocodillia who prefer young girls. That's understandable. It is not a mutually satisfactory relationship. The natives enjoy crocodile meat, though I don't know whether they practice sex discrimination.

Among cultures that suffer from crocodiles an ancient fable persists. A boy was seized by a crocodile. His father begged the beast to spare him. The crocodile said, "I will return your son unharmed if you can answer my question correctly." The question was, "Will I return your son." If the father says "yes" the crocodile keeps the boy and his answer is wrong. If the father says "no" and he is returned, the answer is still incorrect.

ANATOMICAL EXAMINATION ∾ It would be extremely difficult to closely examine teeth of live alligators or crocodiles. I obtained the skull of a large American alligator from south Florida waters. The beast had probably been about eleven or more feet long. Such animals are fast disappearing, being displaced from their swamp and bayou homes, by man's advancing concrete steel roads, spreading to provide more human houses. The alligator skull measured two feet, from the tip of its snout to

TEETH TEETH TEETH

the back of its lower jaws mouth hinging joint, from which I could lift swinging the upper jaw up. Both jaws, upper and lower, were excellent examples of ideal engineering size and shape design, efficiently using their bone and teeth material, to best do the alligator grasping biting eating job they were intended for. The skull was also a beautiful specimen of nature formed sculpture. It was an art object, created by the many millions of years of all the elements and forces that made it. The upper mandible or jaws bright white bone surface was mottled with an irregularly distributed pattern of blackish shallow pits, more profusely prominent towards the front. This is an aging change that occurs to older gators, from the smoother surfaces of younger skulls.

From the snout far back along the long cranium on each side, close to the skull center, were the eye sockets, and shortly behind that it had a small double lobed brain case or think chamber, no larger than my thumb. Man's brain being far too big, squeezed way back behind his eyes, to spread filling most of the head. This alligator skull specimen when closed, presented no tusks of its lower jaw prominently sticking up. Its upper teeth were most obvious, pointed down around outside its lower jaw, which was narrower and lay inside between them. Opening and closing the jaws, I could see that most upper and lower teeth did not substantially interdigitate, meeting with each other, as in the mouth of man. As I opened and closed the jaws experimentally, several times the upper skull slipped, into a pathological crossbite improper bite relation. I've seen crocodiles and alligators in tropical jungle, but had little opportunity to study them closely. From the way they snap and grab and twist their victims in water, it would not surprise me to find these animals suffer crossbite and jaw joint problems in nature.

Seen from the front, the alligators upper closed jaw protrudes around forward of the lower, and shows its upper front teeth passing down long as tusks, pointed menacing aggressive around in front, and part way back on each side. Towards the back of each side, its shorter upper teeth tips end over a bone ledge, along the lower jaw sides. The lower jaws teeth pointing up had sockets provided in the upper jawbone, into which they neatly fit.

I counted the teeth. There were eighty. Forty in each jaw. Twenty on each side, right and left of each jaw. Several were missing from their sockets. Peering into those sockets, I could see new tooth tips deep, arising to replace them. All the teeth, though different in size along their ridges, were rather similarly shaped. They were conically pointed, slightly curved, many turned back like a Turkish simitar or sword. Held tight between it would be hard to escape them. Their tips seemed enamel covered. Except for brown yellow encrusted stains around some of the teeth tips I saw no evidence of disease. The bone surrounding the teeth had rather substantial

TEETH TEETH TEETH

integrity, though there was some slight hint of degeneration between several far back teeth.

The skull tusks came from bone sockets, slightly larger than themselves, surrounded by thin channels of space around them. Most were held tight by some remnant shreds of dried organic tooth attaching tissues. Some were loose. Their attachments probably eaten away by bacteria, that eventually consume all death succumbed animals, converting every live being back to the soils of earth. One tooth pulled away easily. I pried several carefully with long narrow thin sharp instruments. The largest measured two and a half inches long, three quarter inch diameter at the base. The alligator's teeth were completely hollow inside, almost paper thin in some places, thickening towards their hard enamel point tips. These vacant spaces, probably had contained large soft vital tooth feeding live biological substances, that grow reptilian teeth faster, continually replacing lost ones. Inside the sockets of those I had removed, I could see at their deep bottoms, little new tooth tips arising. Teeth, teeth, teeth, ALLIGATOR TEETH TEETH.

FIGHTING BULLS ∾ I left for Mexico with William Deanyer a hypnotist, anxious to try his technique to increase bravery in bullfighters, and Lyn Sherwood who publishes the Clarin, an English language periodical devoted to bullfighting. Lyn's wife Virginia came along. I had interesting experience with bullfighting teeth near Tecate Mexico. Toro is Spanish for bull. Teeth of toreros, who are any of those engaged in bullfighting, and include matadors those more closely involved who kill the bull, are like teeth of any other people, some better some worse. Matadors may grind their teeth together, wearing them away and perhaps loosening them more than most, in the intensity of personal danger and the kill. Teeth of black fighting bulls or toros, are somewhat similar to other bulls, with similar added bullfight considerations.

Dr. Jose Velasco a medical doctor, studied his profession in Mexico City and Barcelona Spain. We've become friends. Dr. Velasco practices surgery in Tijuana Mexico, and is Surgeon for Tijuana's Monumental Bull Ring, one of the biggest in Mexico and the world. He's repaired many torero and matador bullfight horn gored wounds. Jose tried to discourage me, but when I insisted, helped me achieve my Debutante or fight my first bull. Though young and small it was active and brave, and charged with fury directed at my red cape, hand held hanging close, brushing my body as it passed, thrill frightening me while I stood still, seeming brave though scared in the sun. I will never forget the day.

Tecate, south along the border about twenty five miles east of Tijuana, has near it Ganaderia Las Juntas. Ganaderia means Cattle Ranch. Las

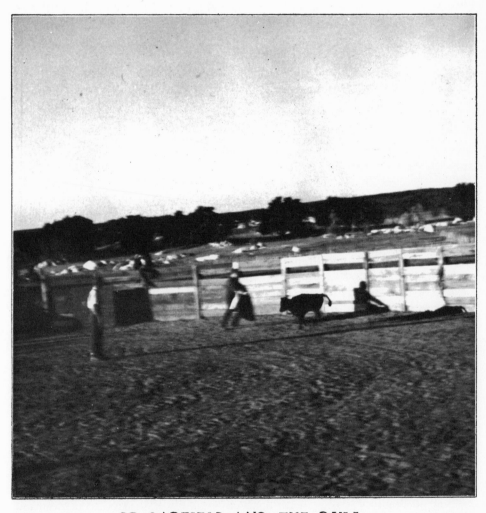

DR. GARFIELD AND THE BULL

MATADOR "EL CHARRO" ELISIO GOMES, WATCHES FROM THE LEFT
enlarged from a photo by Wm. Deanyer

TEETH TEETH TEETH

Juntas its identifying name means Togetherness. Ganaderia Las Juntas raises black fighting bulls in addition to other cattle. The ranch also has a small bull ring, perhaps 90 feet in diameter, used for teaching bullfighting. The ranch is managed by Elisio Gomez, a former active matador called El Charro, who raises the bulls and also teaches bullfighting. Elisio speaks only Spanish. I speak only English. Dr. Jose Velasco interpreting for me, asked Elisio whether he knew of any diseases of fighting bull teeth. Matador Gomez replied, "The Dentista had better examine such bulls teeth himself." He could recall no particular problems.

In preparation for battle, bulls are kept in a roofed dark enclosure for several hours. Released, they leave between close high parallel double walled strong fences, to enter sunlight rushing into the ring. Smaller younger, less dangerous bulls and cows of fight bred stock, are used to teach. Most are not fought to the death. Students ready for the kill pay for their fight victim. If especially talented it may be provided by a sponsor.

In Las Juntas ring, Matador El Charro always waited ready for his bullfight beginner to enter, challenge and taunt the black animal, into close body charges. At times of serious danger to undergraduates, El Charro skillfully intervened to divert the beast. I could see between charges the exhausted bull rest, panting chest heaving heavily, saliva drooling stringy, sometimes with blood from its lips. While alert and taut towards my small four footed horned black opponent, I felt the pride of cheering OLE's from the side. I've never killed a bull. Returning to outside the bull rings high fence and safety, I felt myself panting chest heaving heavily, though no stringy bloody saliva drooled from my lips.

Outside the ring I approached a bull that had fought and lost like most, being debellied skinned and butchered for market. Its horns pointed sharp ten inches long. With a steel rod I pried forcing its jaws apart. Fighting bulls like other cattle are ruminants, along with sheep, goats, deer, giraffes and camels. They have no front upper teeth. Their lower front teeth are a small, sharp, single edged, separate group. Above their lower front teeth the upper jaw is bare, surrounded with a ridge that looks like ridges of humans that have lost their teeth. The ruminants upper front toothless ridge is called a Dental Pad. It is covered with hard corny tough epithelium or skin. Ruminants will nip, tearing soft grass with their lips, and grasp long grasses and leaves, wrapping around with their long curling muscular prehensile tongue. Monkeys have prehensile tails. Ruminants use their lower front teeth as knives, to shear those grasses against their upper hard dental pad, separating from its outside rooted connection to swallow.

The dead black four footed fighter's mouth, had eight severely worn sharp lower incisors, close around in front. I could see each tooth edge crowns exposed inner yellow dentin, surrounded by its narrow outer

TEETH TEETH TEETH

enamel ring. I was amazed to find its upper jaws dental pad marked with deep matching fresh teeth edge cuts, bleeding where the bull apparently in its fright like a man in fright, bit into his own mouth flesh.

Later in Los Angeles, I consulted with two veterinary doctor friends that work with domestic cattle. They were both surprised. One emphasized, "Really Syd are you sure those cuts were fresh, that the bull bit through that hard upper pad."

Far further back in the bull's open mouth, separated from the front by a long stretch of toothless jaw, I could see individual island collections of large sharp cusp pointed molar teeth, both above and below, along its upper and lower jaws, each side right and left. Though light was poor, it was evident they were darkly stained, covered with heavy brownish black deposits. It was interesting that though these back molar teeth existed above and below, acting as jaw closure stops, the bull in its tense fright situation managed to bite itself. Human jaws can be similarly manipulated.

Anxious to examine bull teeth more closely, I borrowed a thin narrow pointed sharp knife, from the man that had been butchering the animal. I inserted the tip carefully around the root, hard deep into the lower front jawbone, to sever the tissues and remove a tooth entirely whole, for detailed inspection. As I pulled it from place, I was disappointed to see the root partly gone, apparently broken from its attaching bone beneath. Wanting a perfect specimen, with the knife I cut even more precisely, and deeper around the next incisor tooth, not knowing how long a bulls tooth root might be, cutting carefully deep away to avoid any root damage. Pulling this one out, I was again disappointed with the second incomplete root, annoyed at what I thought might have been less than ideal care, or possibly inadequate instruments. I consider myself a competent surgeon though I had never operated bulls before. Using the knife again as the only tool available, I cut in even more carefully and deeper, avoiding the root so as to embrace surrounding tissues and protect it. At great depth I scooped in the dead bulls lower jaw from beneath, lifting the knife point like a ladle, to raise the root unharmed from below. I was amazed this time to see coming out, more than the single incisor I was after. Included coming up from far inside, was a much wider larger crowned permanent bull tooth, which also had only a partly developed root. I scooped deep again, and got another permanent or adult bull tooth with an incomplete root. I noticed both larger teeth were in their developing teeth sacs.

The facts were evident. All the previous erupted teeth I had removed were baby fighting bull teeth, like the baby or primary teeth of humans. I had not broken their roots. The roots had been naturally biologically partly

TEETH TEETH TEETH

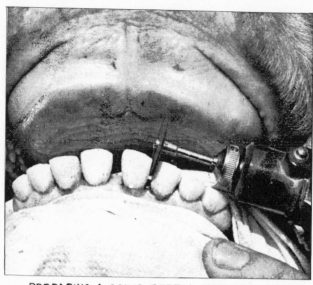

PREPARING A COWS TEETH FOR CROWNS
cattle are ruminants. They have both upper & lower rear
food grinding molars. In front of the mouth they have only
lower teeth used to nip & tear grasses clamping against
their bare upper front hard ridge called the Dental Pad

cattle grazing in sandy soils wear their teeth severly, cant
feed, may even die of starvation. Stainless steel bovine crowns
developed by Dr. Ward Newcomb a Chapell Nebraska dentist help
cattle health, extend life, increase milk and beef production

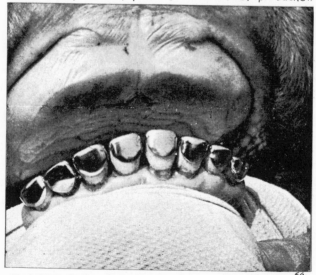

CATTLE DENTAL CROWNS
PRESERVE TEETH, HEALTH & PROLONG THE LIFE OF COWS & BULLS

TEETH TEETH TEETH

resorbed, destroyed by their invisible permanent or adult bull teeth, following from far beneath to succeed them. The deep unerupted larger permanent teeth, were themselves not yet fully formed, still having only partial roots. Teeth, teeth, teeth, BULL TEETH. Later in the afternoon passing the killed bull again, I could see flowers had been put in its mouth.

FRIENDLY ANIMAL TEETH

Pets in homes have problems like masters though they don't pay taxes. Dental related diseases of cats and dogs consist of about five to ten percent of such veterinary medicine. Animal bad breath is caused by dental disease and from further inside the body. Some suffer a pyorrhetic type of gum recession and jawbone infection, with teeth loosening and loss, increasing as in man with age. Teeth dirt and other deposits cause infections and abscess. Extractions are often necessary.

Animal teeth scaling like similar human treatment helps. There are cat and dog veterinary specialists that even fill teeth. Problems seem to increase with softer varieties of inferior canned foods containing excess starches. Veterinary study indicates hard food chewing helps.

Some love any mongrel, mutt or alleycat. Others with particular snobbish sensitivities discriminate. Selective mating of cats and dogs, created upper classes of pet aristocracy, who proudly boast and display written proof of their ancestral lineage. Some such beautiful dogs are big. Some people who prefer certain parts of women big, and live in particular types of modern homes and apartments, favor dogs small. So dogs were grown smaller. They didn't tie, growing the entire animal down, as Japanese once did with baby girls' feet. Possibly this could have been done, but tying an entire animal would have resulted in expanded distorted bumps, between adjacent cords. They selected particular small males and females, whose breeding gave great reduction in size, yet retained desired body proportions properly. These miniature toy dog varieties, look good and are good, are much wanted and valuable. For some unknown reason, their entire body reduces in perfect comfirmation except the teeth. It seems the new smaller jaws develop and grow the same old bigger teeth, which crowd orthodontically disfigured, in their animals faces. For some of these valued dogs, certain teeth are extracted. Veterinary dentists sometimes use wires to straighten such teeth, as dental orthodontists do for children. As with children, the better looking straightened teeth also helps the dog's health.

Rin Tin Tin a German Shepherd dog, was a world famous animal motion picture star. Shortly after World War I, Rin was introduced to silent films at Warner Bros. Studios by Lee Duncan. The dog's fame grew. Rin shorter lived than his human continuing audience retired in time, and was replaced by successors honored to continue using his name. Frank Barnes, considered by some the best dog trainer in the business, coached animal actors for hundreds of motion picture and television productions since 1927. Frank's dog prodigies appeared with Jackie Coogan, Henry Fonda, George Raft, Joan Bennett, Dick Powell, Jerry Lewis, Dean Martin, many others. Barnes was owner trainer of the German Shepherd JR, who played Rin Tin Tin, in "The Adventures of Rin Tin Tin" television series.

I asked Frank about Rin Tin Tin's dental problems. "He never had any Doc," Frank said. "I always took good care of my dogs teeth. I prepared the mother even before breeding, with calcium and cod liver oil. And I fed the pups well, nothing but the best balanced food. I cleaned my dogs teeth regularly, just like a dentist does. Cleaner than many actors and directors teeth. I scraped them and used dental floss. Rin Tin Tin had good teeth. They had to look good for close ups when he snarled." Frank Barnes also demanded other special considerations for his dog heroes. "I never let Rinny grab a real gun from a heavy." Heavy is movie terminology for the villain. "The studio had to provide a prop of soft wood or rubber, which was switched at the right time. I couldn't afford to let him bite on anything hard like steel. JR's teeth had to keep sharp, so that he could release good girls and guys by biting through rope."

Many scenes of the long series involved playing with children. Since filming was continuous and heavy, Frank stipulated that JR not be engaged in intimate fighting, as a child's careless movement could provoke the dog dangerously. Just as with human stars for such action shots, a dog actor double was used.

My friend and patient Hugh Hooker was among Hollywood's greatest stunt men. Hugh dared dangers of all kinds. He's fought as many a good and bad cowboy, and also taken high falls dressed as heroines. He's encountered intimate hazardous situations with galloping horses and grappled ferocious dogs. Hugh loved animals.

Hugh was a stunt man in the Rin Tin Tin series and acted in many of the man fighting dog shots. At lunch Hugh told me, "Syd we used a vicious less valuable dog, for those Rin Tin Tin against the villain battles. Fighting I got real close to that dog. I'm not a dentist but his teeth looked bad to me, and his breath was terrible."

Wild and Tame Creatures with Fangs Strong White
Better Love and Mate and Face Lifes Fight

TEETH TEETH TEETH

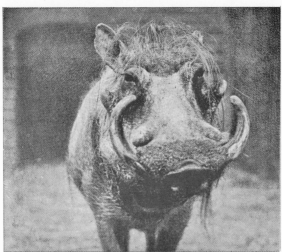

This normal warthog may look attractive to others.
Rarely a wrong turned tusk grows back into an eye & blinds.
Other wild swine varieties like Babirusa sometimes suffer similarly.
Such tusky tooth trouble also occurs among certain rodents
even growing to penetrate into the brain causing death.

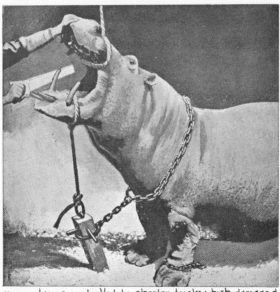

Hippopotamus controlled to shorten tusks which damaged
its upper jaw, made feeding difficult, harming its health.

TOO LONG TUSK TOOTH TROUBLE

LIKE MAN, ANIMALS EVEN IN NATURE BECAUSE OF BAD TEETH
& BITE RELATIONS SOMETIMES SUFFER SERIOUSLY ~ S.G.

TEETH TEETH TEETH

23

THE FUTURE

The future of dentistry will be its eventual disappearance as a profession. The same fate awaits the medical profession. Hand in hand, these curers of bodies ills will be left behind in distance to disappear. They and allied healing scientists, parasitologists, microbiologists and virologists, biological physicists and chemists, and biological atom experts who are yet about to appear, will no longer be needed. All these united as a conquering army, will find the subtle causes of the constant aging changing breakdown of our bodies. These detected factors will be eliminated, disease will no longer exist, and doctors of health like the ice man will no longer be needed. Science and knowledge will be the fountain of youth and man may even live forever. At one time there were no men at all, then they did come to be. Perhaps some day man will never die, living on and between this and other earths.

Already dentistry has changed things. Far fewer teeth need to be extracted. Less removable dentures are being made. Great progress has been accomplished in restorative technique. Teeth decays cause is being found, and its ills will be eliminated. Peridontal disease, pyorrhea, is being controlled and cured. Eventually the intimate nature of dental defects will be known and eradicated. We'll have no more trouble with our teeth than with our toenails.

In early times man's foremost enemies aside from other men and the elements were those that visibly attacked him. Wolves and tigers and crocodiles, and in imaginary days of Sinbad the Sailor, the giant legendary bird the roc, that swooped down carrying him away. Later man detected other personal assailants. Worms that he saw in his evacuated stools, and worms he saw in bodies of fish and land animals he ate. Smaller parasites like germs were harder to see and conquer. The microscope helped, antiseptics and antibiotics too. It's still quite a war. Our medical army is well equipped, improving its battle strategies with experience, and we are winning, though many are still being lost in the fight for life.

Man is gaining substantial control of parasitic disease, and probably will soon eradicate these body invaders who eat our tissues as we consume foods that nurture us. It's a battle for survival of the fittest. We will win.

Every progressing era looks back upon their past as ages of ignorance. Man is egotistical, and whatever the time of his existence, feels modern, all

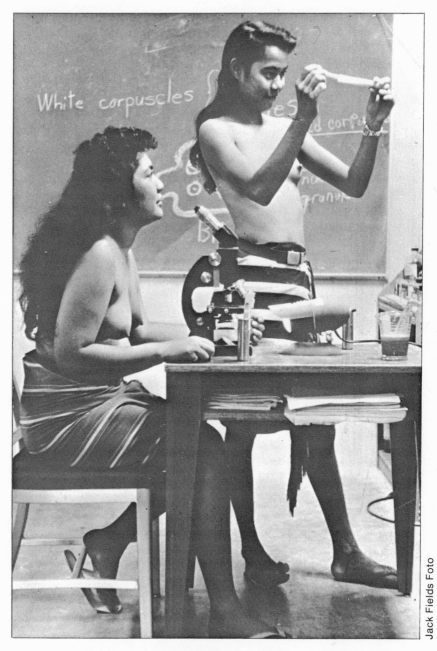

Jack Fields Foto

MODERN HEALTH EDUCATION REACHES TO REMOTE MICRONESIA ISLANDERS.

TEETH TEETH TEETH

wise, intelligently informed. Things he believes, he establishes as fact, while other attitudes are labeled heretic, not to be tolerated. Yet led by creative dissenters of perseverance, we forge ahead.

Really we are only now first entering transition, from not knowing, to a time of awareness with knowledge and science. All that has been accomplished and delights us, is little compared to what is to be. The canoe amazed the cave man. Sailing vessels' use of newly captured wind power intrigued the oarsman. Steam pushing pistons, to turn wheels and propellers, fascinated the world. Only a hundred years ago, any who seriously described jet transport and color television would have been ridiculed, and if persistent perhaps incarcerated. And this time of moon missiles is only the beginning. Changes are about to take place we can hardly imagine. Just as we find specimen curiosity in prehistoric man, the new beings that will live and move through space, may look back upon our era as one of elemental beginning.

Possibilities for man in this future excite the imagination. Let me present one. The human animal body, even that of a grasshopper, is multi millions of times more intricately coordinated than any space missile or electronic brain. And we within these of our bodies, who've designed those missiles and brains, have developed a scientific concept more advanced than any within our own selves. This is the phenomenon of nuclear fission or atomic transmutation. With this technique tiny bits of matter are converted to tremendous quantities of energy. The matter itself becomes energy itself. Neat and efficient. At present we mostly use things like uranium. In time any substance may be convertible to energy, and eventually energy converitible to any material at all. Precious stuff, platinum gold oils, won't be sought any longer. They'll be makeable from anything, like any other thing desired. The potentialities are limitless.

These bodies, mans, grasshoppers, earthworms, and elephants, all wonderful as they are, grow and derive energy in an old fashioned way. By simple chemical combustion, like a burning smoking candle. We consume enormous amounts of food through our mouths and air through noses. All this requires a lung pump system, and other complicated internal organic equipment, that frequently breaks down, just to produce a relatively small amount of energy. And all this stuff we consume is hardly used, inefficiently leaving us as tremendous amounts of waste, so great, it should have at least one full daily, we hope, evacuation as a foul stinking mess. The liquids as urine through urethral openings, and solids as fecal material through the rectum. A smelly procedure and quite inconvenient. Sometimes of course, this complex material moving ejection equipment

TEETH TEETH TEETH

breaks down, and we cannot even force the darn stuff out. Disease, pain, and bloody distress may be suffered, to the delight of medical proctologists, who earn an especially good living from patching rectal exit valves. What is not sauce for the gander, is sauce for the goose.

If man's body had evolved beyond on, to function by nuclear fission, and who knows what the future holds, we would only need one tiny intake opening. The nose would be superfluous. I cannot predict the future status for teeth, and make no formal declaration concerning them. Since all food would be completely utilized, for growth and energy operating function, we could give up our liquid and solid left over evacuation openings. Quite neat, less offensive, far more convenient. Of course this would result in clothing design changes. However, if the loss of these orifices, and baby product feeding lactation stations, would be accompanied by loss of the attendant lusciously curved surrounding anatomy, that adorns such sites on certain members of our female species, I suffer regret.

I can even imagine a possible advanced means of asexual reproduction, asexual means without sex, so unique it could reproduce any object, inanimate or alive, within reasonable size, as another real self. Teeth if those were still used and wanted, a single cigar or a box full, a cup with coffee inside, a flower, even boys and girls with or without teeth, of any age or size. This is not the reproduction of man or woman delivered as child to grow, though that would also be possible. It is a way of really reproducing anything, living or unalive, as a single duplicate, or in greater number if desired, as it exists at the time of reproduction procedure. The method could also make real teeth, of enamel and dentin with nerve inside, of any sizes, shapes, and shades, for dental use.

This reproduction technique tries the imagination within the realm of far out fantasy, yet it is imaginable, seeming potentially possible, using present systems of technology. This is accomplished by a machine yet to be made, which uses television picture and projection techniques, and an atomic conversion unit not yet in existence. This atomic conversion equipment, just as nuclear energy is made from certain substances today, would convert any material, all of which consists of nuclear particles like electrons, protons and neutrons to energy, and energy to electrons, protons and neutrons as desired.

Television is created by viewing an object with a television camera. The image, static or moving, is delivered in a conventional manner to inside the camera on a small tube screen. Within that apparatus, a beam of rapid emitting electrons moves across the screen, many millions in a second, along a top horizontal line. When it reaches the end of the line, the tiny

TEETH TEETH TEETH

sensing beam drops immediately below, to travel another line. It then moves next lower for another line, lower again for another, and for another under that until the bottom of the camera's range. It then jumps to the top, rapidly starting the same fast, thorough, along the lines sequence towards the bottom. This is the sensing of the constant appearing image. Each dotted sense called an element or picture element, varies in intensity from bright white through darkening shades of gray or black, or with a color T.V. camera to elements of respective colors. The television camera broadcasting attachment, continually as all these elements are sensed, converts each to radio waves of varying intensity, broadcast through air or space. They are received by television receivers, most of which are in homes or apartments.

The television receiver converts the radio waves back to electrons, and within its larger receiving tube, emits shooting them at the inside phosphorescent surface of the home television screen. These electrons, each delivering their varied charges for white, grays, black or color at the same speed, along similar lines as picked up by the camera, moving along dropping to lower lines in the same manner, activate light of varying effect on the home receiver phosphorescent screen, creating the images seen.

The future reproduction machine camera scans its object more thoroughly. It uses an X-ray like beam able also to focus exact distances. Its beam begins, adjusted, just before the object to be reproduced. Its sensing elements start emitting, moving above along horizontal lines. Each next element is a distance ahead of its predecessor, the same size as atomic particles, and senses the objects atom particle identity, electron, proton, neutron, at each of their locations. When the line is completed, the beam drops below, a distance again equal to atomic particle size, and scans along sensing another line. It then drops to another, and another below that, all the way to bottom, focused the same distance from the camera before the object. When the entire front face plane is completely scanned, the camera sensing range increases, to move inside the object, to a third dimension of depth, a distance behind exactly equal to atomic particle size. Again at the top it begins its sequence of line sensing. It drops down another line, along the new focused distance, and another and another to the bottom. It then focuses still further back inside, another atom particle distance. This is repeated, at rapid rate, until the entire object is sensed throughout its thickness.

All these atomic particle identities, electron, proton, neutron, and each of their specific locations are delivered constantly, emitted as messages to the asexual reproduction equipment. The atomic conversion unit uses its energy source to deliver instantaneously synchronized, at all respective

TEETH TEETH TEETH

exact locations of sensed places along lines, below each other, and behind each other, through the same atomic distances located, all the needed atom particles, electrons, protons and neutrons to reproduce making a new object thing itself. They could be teeth.

A phase of medicine closer to present practical possibility, we are only now approaching, with which little progress has yet been made, is knowledge of the intimate physical-chemical nature of tissue degeneration. We know relatively nothing of these things at all. Let's not kid ourselves. Even most exacting brain surgery, kidney and heart transplants, precise plastic heart valve and pump installations, clever as they are, are only mechanical correctives. They are merely more intense application of procedures similar to the placement of silver fillings in teeth, or fine dental porcelain bridges. All this is only careful body patching. However such patching, like even the reweaving of a valuable pair of torn or worn trousers, has extended this little we have of our lives. The once 35 year expectancy has gone to 65. The average will soon be 95. Increasing knowledge about to come, will extend life to 155 and then 255. And proportionately along each of these ages, man will be alertly vibrant, more virile than today. Old age is not the number of years elapsed through life. Real living is the fervor of enthusiasm that accompanies youthful living. Old age is a mental attitude enforced upon the one who feels it, by the aging changing of bodies tissues, as they approach their changes towards death. The intimate chemical, physical, biological, atomic knowledge of defects causes that age us will help eradicate those causes one by one. Bodies aging now within sixty five years will have their functional use perpetuated for increasing periods and man may reach on to live forever.

Physicians and dentists who had the M.D. and D.D.S. degree will be almost forgotten like witch doctors of old. The new professional doctors of human welfare will have degrees like D.P.F.P. and D.I.H., Doctor for the Planning of Future Perfection and Doctor of Infinite Happiness. There may be a small remnant of professionals, D.E.R., Doctors of Emergency Repair, for those that never seem to avoid accidents. I can imagine the things described but cannot envision the new society to be.

TEETH TEETH TEETH

At The Denis

Madam: I have a hallowed tooth that suffer me grately.

Sir: Sly down in that legchair Madam and open your gorble wide—your mouse is all but toothless.

Madam: Alad! I have but eight tooth remaining (eight tooth left).

Sir: Then you have lost eighty three.

Madam: Impossyble.

Sir: Everydobby knows there are foor decisives two canyons and ten grundies, which make thirsty two in all.

Madam: But I have done everything to save my tooth.

Sir: Perhumps! but to no avague.

Madam: Ah! why did I not insult you sooner?

Sir: To late, it must be now or neville.

Madam: You will pull it out for me then?

Sir: No, madman, I will excrete it.

Madam: But that is very painfull.

Sir: Let me see it—Crack! there it be madarce.

Madam: But sir I wished to keep (was anxious to keep) that tooth.

Sir: It was all black and moody, and the others are too.

Madam: Mercy—I will have none to eat with soon.

Sir: A free Nasty Heath set is good, and you will look thirty years jungle.

Madam: (Aside) Thirty years jungle; (Aloud) Sir I am no catholic, pull out all my stumps.

Sir: O.K. Gummy.

By John Lennon, one of The Beatles four. From "In His Own Write". Copyright ©1964 by John Lennon. Reprinted by permission of Simon & Schuster Inc.

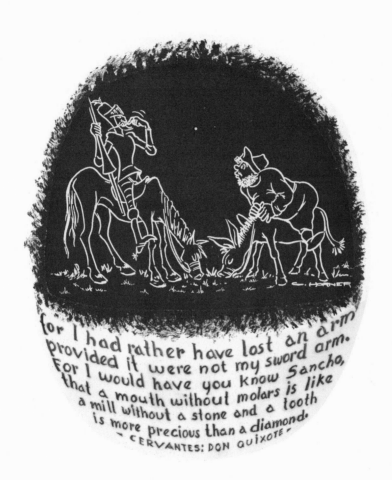

for I had rather have lost an arm
provided it were not my sword arm.
For I would have you know Sancho,
that a mouth without molars is like
a mill without a stone and a tooth
is more precious than a diamond.
– CERVANTES: DON QUIXOTE –

BIBLIOGRAPHY

Dental information in popular literature is limited. Most references given are professional texts unavailable in the average book store or library. They may be found with additional material, in medical dental book stores and libraries. Since all fields of dentistry interrelate, references for individual chapters may also serve others. Some basic science books related to all dentistry are also listed.

1 THE HISTORY OF DENTISTRY
Outline of History *H. G. Wells* McMillan Co., N. Y. 1921
A History of Dentistry *Vincenzo Guerini* Lea & Febiger, Phil. 1909
History of Dentistry & Dentistry in America
B. W. Weinberger C. V. Mosby Co., St. Louis 1948
Story of Dentistry *M. D. K. Bremner* Dental Items of Interest Pub. Co., Bklyn. N. Y. 1959
Piere Fauchard, Surgeon Dentist *B. W. Weinberger* Lancet Press, Minneapolis Minn. 1941
The Folklore of Teeth *L. Kanner* McMillan Co., N. Y. 1933
Dentistry in Ancient India *K. M. Choksey* Popular Book Depot, Bombay India 1953

3 PSYCHOLOGICAL DENTISTRY
Theory and Practice of Psychiatry *W. S. Sadler* C. V. Mosby Co., St. Louis 1936
Psychosomatics & Suggestion Therapy in Dentistry *J. Stolzenberg* Philosophical Lib., N. Y. 1950
Dynamics of Psychosomatic Dentistry *J. Landa* Dental Items of Interest Pub. Co., Bklyn. N. Y. 1953

5 EXAM   6 DIAGNOSIS & TREATMENT PLAN
Dental Radiology *W. W. Wainwright* McGraw-Hill Blakiston Div., N. Y. 1965
Dental Roentgenology *L. M. Ennis, H. M. Berry, S. E. Phillips* Lea & Febiger, Phil. 1967
Oral Diagnosis & Treatment *S. C. Miller* McGraw-Hill Blakiston Div., N. Y. 1957
Dynamics of Oral Diagnosis *E. Cheraskin, L. L. Langley* Year Book Pub. Co., Chicago 1956

7 ANESTHESIA
Practical Anesthesia for Dental & Oral Surgery *H. M. Seldin* Lea & Febiger, Phil. 1967
Conduct. Infiltr. & General Anesth. in Dentistry *M. Nevin* Dental Items of Int. Pub. Co., Bklyn. N. Y. 1959
Clinic. & Exper. Hypnosis in Medicine Dentistry & Psychology *W. S. Kroger* Lippincott, Phil. 1963

8 THE INDIVIDUAL TOOTH
Restorative Dentistry *J. J. Tocchini* McGraw-Hill Blakiston Div., N. Y. 1967
Inlays and Abutments *S. R. Schwartz* Dental Items of Interest Pub. Co., Bklyn. N. Y. 1953

9 PERIDONTIA
Peridontia *Goldman* C. V. Mosby Co., St. Louis 1953
Clinical Peridontology *Glickman* W. B. Saunders Co., Phil. 1959

10 ENDODONTIA
Endodontics *J. Ingle* Lea & Febiger, Phil. 1965
Clinical Endodontics *R. F. Sommer, F. D. Ostrander, M. C. Crowley* W. B. Saunders Co., Phil. 1966

11 ORAL SURGERY
Oral Surgery Vol. 1 & 2 1952; Oral Surgery 1963;
Kurt H. Thoma C. V. Mosby Co., St. Louis
Oral Surgery *S. V. Mead* C. V. Mosby Co., St. Louis 1954

12 PEDODONTIA
Oral Histology and Embryology *B. Orban* C. V. Mosby Co., St. Louis 1949
Baby and Child Care *B. Spock* Cardinal Ed. Pocket Books, N. Y. 1964
Dentistry for Children *J. C. Brauer* The Blakiston Co., N. Y. 1964
Clinical Pedodontics *S. B. Finn* W. B. Saunders Co., Phil. 1957

13 ORTHODONTIA
Textbook of Orthodontia *R. H. W. Strang, A. M. Thompson* Lea & Febiger, Phil. 1958
Technique & Treatment with Light-Wire Appliances *J. R. Jarabak* C. V. Mosby Co., St. Louis 1963

15 FIXED PROSTHODONTICS
Theory & Practice of Crown & Bridge Prosthodontics *S. G. Tyman* C. V. Mosby Co., St. Louis 1965
Modern Practice in Crown & Bridge Prosthodontics *J. F. Johnston* W. B. Saunders Co., Phil. 1965
Implant Dentures *A. Gershkoff & N. Goldberg* J. B. Lippincott Co., Phil. 1957

16 PARTIAL REMOVABLE DENTURES
Essentials of Removable Partial Denture Prosthesis *O. Applegate* W. B. Saunders Co., Phil. 1965
Partial Dentures *L. G. Terkla, W. R. Laney* C. V. Mosby Co., St. Louis 1963

17 FULL REMOVABLE DENTURES
Complete Dentures *M. G. Swenson* C. V. Mosby Co., St. Louis 1959
Denture Prosthesis, Complete Dentures *R. J. Nagle, V. A. Sears* C. V. Mosby Co., St. Louis 1962

18 NUTRITION
Modern Nutrition in Health & Disease *M. G. Wohl, R. S. Goodhard* Lea & Febiger, Phil. 1960
Nutrition in Clinical Dentistry *A. Nizel* W. B. Saunders Co., Phil. 1960
Fluoride Protection of Bone & Teeth *R. F. Sognnaes* Science Nov. 19, 1965 V150, 989-993
Nutrition & Physical Degeneration *W. A. Price* Amer. Acad. of Applied Nutrition, Los Angeles 1950

20 DENTISTRY IN SPORTS
The Encyclopedia of Sports *F. G. Menke* A. S. Barnes & Co., N. Y. 1963
The Heavyweight Championship *N. Fleischer* G. P. Putnams & Sons, N. Y. 1949

21 TEETH BENEATH WATER   22 ANIMAL TEETH
General Zoology *T. I. Storer* McGraw-Hill Book Co., New York 1951
Dental Anatomy, Human & Comparative *C. S. Tomes* P. Blakistons Sons & Co., Phil. 1914
Dental Anatomy, Human & Comparative *Headridge & Gibson* E. & S. Livingston, Edinburgh Britain, 1928
Fishes of North & Middle America *Jordan & Everman* Washington Print. Off., Smithsonian Inst. 1896
Saw of the Sawfish *C. M. Breder Jr.* Copeia 1952 No. 2 90-91 Amer. Mus. of Nat. History, N. Y.
Whales Dolphins Porpoises *K. S. Norris* Univ. Calif. Press, L. A., Berkeley 1966
Dinosaurs *E. Colbert* E. P. Dutton Co., N. Y. 1967
Chimpanzees *R. M. Yerkes* Yale Univ. Press, New Haven, Conn. 1948

BASIC SCIENCE
Microbiology *Kelley & Hite* Appleton-Century-Crofts, New York 1949
Pharmacology and Dental Therapeutics *E. C. Dobbs & H. Prinz* C. V. Mosby Co., St. Louis 1951
Anatomy of the Human Body *H. Gray* Lea & Febiger, Phil. 1951
Oral Pathology *Kurt H. Thoma* C. V. Mosby Co., St. Louis 1954
The Science of Dental Materials *E. W. Skinner, R. W. Philips* W. B. Saunders Co., Phil. 1967

Illustrations are *Bold Italic Numbers*

Illustrations are ***Bold Italic Numbers***

Illustrations are *Bold Italic Numbers*

It is Hoped

This Book,
Explaining Mans Own Dental Parts to Him
Removes Fears, Making Teeth More Treatable

Food they chew more Eatable
Faces lip framed mouths More Beautiful
Pleasures they provide more Enjoyable

That Disease Be Resisted
though should it invade, Pain be Brief
and Being Understood, more Tolerable

That sufferers Seek Relief to Find
Most Dental Disease is Curable

And defects of the Mouth
are often, Perfectly Restorable.

Sydney Garfield

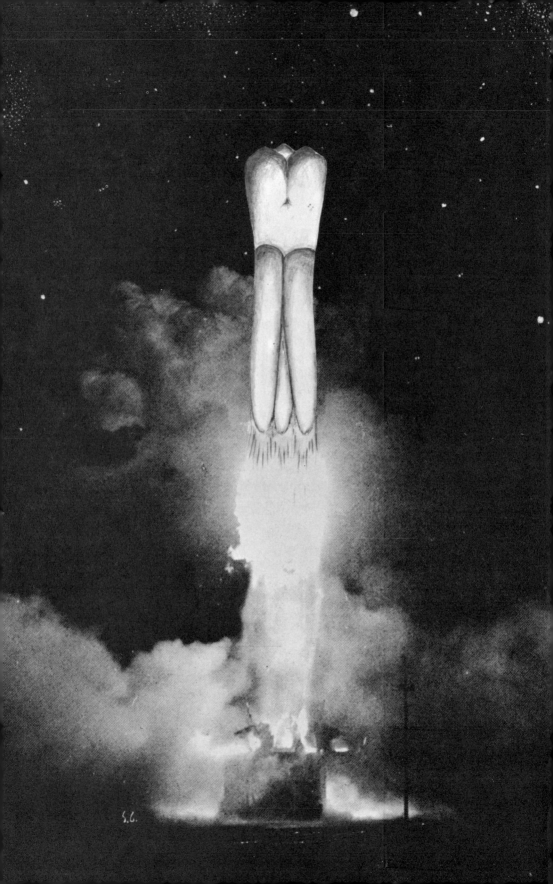